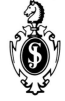

Pancreatic Disease
Progress and Prospects

Edited by
C. D. Johnson and C. W. Imrie

With 65 Figures

Springer-Verlag
London Berlin Heidelberg New York
Paris Tokyo Hong Kong
Barcelona Budapest

C. D. Johnson MChir, FRCS
Senior Lecturer and Honorary Consultant Surgeon, Faculty of
Medicine, University Surgical Unit, Southampton General
Hospital, Tremona Road, Southampton SO1 6HU, UK

C. W. Imrie, ChB, FRCS
Consultant Surgeon, Surgical Unit, Royal Infirmary, Glasgow
G4 OSF, UK

ISBN 3-540-19688-9 Springer-Verlag   Berlin   Heidelberg   New York
ISBN 0-387-19688-9 Springer-Verlag   New York   Berlin   Heidelberg

Cover Illustration: Ch. 3, Fig. 5. Insertion of a metallic Stent (Wallstent,
Schneider).

British Library Cataloguing in Publication Data
Johnson, C. D. (Colin David)
Pancreatic disease
I. Title   II. Imrie, C. W. (Clement William), 1943–
616.37
ISBN 3-540-19688-9

Library of Congress Cataloging-in-Publication Data
Pancreatic disease: progress and prospects / [edited by] C. D. Johnson and C. W.
Imrie
    p.   cm.
Includes index.
ISBN 3-540-19688-9. – ISBN 0-387-19688-9
1. Pancreas–Diseases.   I. Johnson, C. D. (Colin David). 1952–
[DNLM: 1. P Pancreatic Diseases.   WI 800 P1893]
RC857.P33   1991   616.3'7–dc20
DNLM/DLC   91–4880
for Library of Congress   CIP

Typeset by Photo·graphics, Honiton, Devon
Printed by Henry Ling Ltd, The Dorset Press, Dorchester
2128/3830-543210 Printed on acid-free paper

Preface

This book has been produced in association with a meeting, also entitled "Pancreatic Disease – Progress and Prospects", arranged in Southampton in September 1991. It is written by speakers at the meeting, but it is not a standard conference proceedings.

Contributors were asked to provide their manuscripts well in advance so that publication could coincide with the meeting. The book stands in its own right as a contribution to the expanding literature on pancreatic disease. We as editors have tried to highlight areas of particular interest. It is not designed to cover all areas of pancreatic disease in exhaustive detail, but rather to stimulate the reader with up-to-date reviews in areas where progress has been made.

Our contributors have not failed us in our desire to produce a concise and informative book. We are grateful to them for the care with which they prepared their manuscripts, and for meeting the deadlines which enabled a very tight production schedule to proceed. The publishers have also made a significant contribution to this book and have turned out an impressive volume, with illustrations of the highest quality.

Finally however this book must go to our readers. We hope there will be many who will find a stimulus from these pages. All those with an interest in pancreatic disease should find something worthwhile. Topics in surgery, medical gastroenterology, radiology, oncology, paediatrics and endocrine disorders have been addressed in the hope that our readers will include not only established specialists but also those who are developing an interest in the pancreas in their training and in their preparation for professional examinations.

London, May 1991

C. D. Johnson
C. W. Imrie

Contents

Contributors

M. C. Aldridge, MS, FRCS (Edin), FRES, FLS
Senior Registrar in Surgery, Ashford Hospital, Ashford, Middlesex

E. Astudillo, MD
Associate Professor of Surgery, Department of Surgery, Hospital Clinic, Villarroel, 170-08036 Barcelona, Spain

J. P. Bernard, MD
Chef de Clinique, Unité de Recherches de Physiologie et Pathologie Digestives, INSERM U315, 46 Bd de la Gaye, 13258 Marseille Cedex 09, France

W. D. B. Clements, BSc, FRCS
Research Fellow, Department of Surgery, The Queens University of Belfast, Institute of Clinical Science, Grosvenor Road, Belfast BT12 6BJ

M. J. Cooper, MS, FRCS
Consultant Surgeon, Royal Devon and Exeter Hospital (Wonford), Barrack Road, Exeter EX2 5DW

J. C. Dagorn, MD
Directeur, Unité de Recherches de Physiologie et Pathologie Digestives, INSERM U315, 46 Bd de la Gaye, 13258 Marseille Cedex 09, France

M. Davenport, FRCS (Glas & Eng)
Lecturer in Surgery, Department of Hepatobiliary Surgery, Kings College Hospital, Denmark Hill, London SE5 9RS

T. Diamond, BSc, FRCSI
Senior Surgical Registrar, Department of Surgery, The Queen's University of Belfast, Institute of Clinical Sciences, Grosvenor Road, Belfast BT12 6BJ

R. Dinwiddie, FRCP
Consultant Paediatrician, The Hospital for Sick Children, Great
Ormond Street, London WC1N 3JH

L. Fernandez-Cruz, MD
Head, General and Gastrointestinal Surgery, Hospital Clinic, 1
Provincial de Barcelona, Villarroel, 170-08036 Barcelona, Spain

S. Genell, MD
Department of Surgery, University of Lund, Malmö General
Hospital, S-21401 Malmö, Sweden

J. Gillespie, PhD
Research Assistant, Academic Surgical Unit, St Mary's Hospital,
Praed Street, London W2 1NY

D. Giorgi, MD
Cherchuer, Unité de Recherches de Physiologie et Pathologie
Digestives, INSERM U315, 46 Bd de la Gaye, 13258 Marseille
Cedex 09, France

C. N. Hacking, BSc, MRCP, FRCR
Consultant Radiologist, Department of Radiology, Southampton
General Hospital, Southampton SO9 4XY

A. R. W. Hatfield, MD, FRCP
Consultant Gastroenterologist, The Middlesex Hospital, Mortimer
Street, London W1N 8AA

D. I. Heath, MS, FRCS
Surgical Registrar, Law Hospital, Carluke, Lanarkshire ML8 5ER

E. R. Howard, MS, FRCS
Consultant Surgeon, King's College Hospital, Denmark Hill, London
SE5 9RS

C.W. Imrie, MS, FRCS
Consultant Surgeon, Royal Infirmary, Glasgow G4 0SF

B. Isgar, FRCS
Research Registrar, Department of Surgery, Dudley Road Hospital,
Birmingham B18 7QH

C. D. Johnson, MChir, FRCS
Senior Lecturer and Honorary Consultant Surgeon, University
Surgical Unit, Southampton General Hospital, Southampton
SO9 4XY

Miss D. Kelly, FRCSI, MCh
Surgical Registrar, Department of Surgery, St James's Hospital,
James's Street, Dublin 8, Ireland

R. Laugier, MD
Professor of Medicine, Clinique de Maladies de l'Appareil Digestif,
Hopital Sainte-Marguerite, BP29, 13277 Marseille Cedex 09, France

M. Lopez-Boado, PhD, MD
Trauma Surgeon, Hospital Clinic, Villarroel, 170-08036 Barcelona,
Spain

C. N. Mallinson, FRCP
134 Harley Street, London W1N 1AH

D. C. McCrory, FRCSI
Research Fellow, Department of Surgery, The Queen's University
of Belfast, Institute of Clinical Science, Grosvenor Road, Belfast
B12 6BJ

G. McEntee, FRCSI
Senior Registrar in Surgery, Department of Surgery, Royal College
of Surgeons in Ireland, St Stephen's Green, Dublin 2, Ireland

J. Neoptolemos, MA, MD, FRCS
Reader in Surgery, Department of Surgery, Dudley Road Hospital,
Birmingham B18 7QH

K. Ohlsson, MD
Professor of Surgical Pathophysiology, Department of Surgical
Pathophysiology, University of Lund, Malmö General Hospital,
S21401 Malmö, Sweden

J. Pain, MD, FRCS
Senior Registrar in Surgery, The Brook Hospital, Shooters Hill,
London SE18

G. J. Poston, MS, FRCS
Consultant Surgeon, Royal Liverpool Hospital, Prescot Street,
Liverpool L7 8XP

B. J. Rowlands, MD, FRCS, FACS
Professor of Surgery, Queens University of Belfast, Institute of
Clinical Science, Grosvenor Road, Belfast BT12 6BJ

A. Saenz, MD
Trauma Surgeon, Department of Surgery, Hospital Clinic, Villarroel,
170-08036 Barcelona, Spain

Miss H. Sanfey, MCh, FRCSI
Visiting Fellow, Hospital Clinic/Provincial de Barcelona, Villarroel,
170-08036 Barcelona, Spain

H. Sarles, MD
Professeur de Medicine, Clinique de Maladies de l'Appareil Digestif,
Hopital Sainte-Marguerite, 13277 Marseille Cedex 09, France

M. Sarner, MB, FRCP
Consultant Physician, University College Hospital, Gower Street,
London WC1E 6AU

M. G. Shearer, MS, FRCS
Surgical Registrar, Royal Infirmary, Glasgow G4 0SF

P. Watanapa, BSc, MD
Surgical Research Fellow, Department of Surgery, RPMS and Staff
Surgeon, Siriraj Hospital, Mahidol University, Bangkok, Thailand

R. C. N. Williamson, MA, MD, MChir, FRCS
Director of Surgery, Royal Postgraduate Medical School, Hammersmith Hospital, Du Cane Road, London W12 0HS

C. Wilson, MS, FRCS
Surgical Registrar, Division of General Surgery, Stobhill General
Hospital, Glasgow G21 3UW

Section A

Obstructive Jaundice

Chapter 1

Pathophysiology of Obstructive Jaundice

J. Pain

Specific problems may result from obstructive jaundice complicating pancreatic disease, and this is reflected in a higher mortality when surgery is performed in the presence of jaundice. This was recognised by Whipple in 1935 who recommended an initial cholecystogastrostomy to relieve jaundice prior to a pancreatic resection. The main consequences of obstructive jaundice, the underlying pathophysiological factors and possible therapies are shown in Table 1.

Sepsis

In addition to cholangitis and septicaemia, patients with obstructive jaundice have an increased incidence of intraperitoneal, wound, urinary and pulmonary

Table 1. Complications of obstructive jaundice

Complications	Pathophysiology	Prophylaxis/Therapy
Sepsis	Biliary stasis	Biliary drainage
	?Foreign body in bile duct	
	Impaired immunological	Antibiotics
	functions	Biliary drainage
Renal failure	Alterations in fluid	Hydration
	compartments	
	Endotoxaemia	Antiendotoxaemic therapy
Coagulation defects	Decreased vitamin absorption	Vitamin K
	Impaired hepatic function	Fresh frozen plasma
Gastroduodenal bleeding	Coagulation defects	Antiulcer drugs
	?Endotoxaemia	
	?Circulating bile acids	
Impaired wound healing	Malnutrition, malignancy	Mass closure techniques
	?Endotoxaemia	
Pruritus	?Bile acids	Relief of jaundice
	?Opiate receptor stimulation	

infections. Although the biliary tract is a major source of infection, an underlying immunosuppression is also a significant factor in the development of these complications.

Source of infection

Infected bile is a potential source of sepsis and organisms can be cultured from 75%–100% of bile samples when there is calculous obstruction, but the positive culture rate is much lower when the obstruction is due to other causes. Biliary sepsis may result from retrograde contamination from the gastrointestinal tract, but there is evidence to suggest an increased permeability that allows bacteria to pass from the serum into the bile (Ohshio et al. 1988). Deitch et al. (1990) have recently shown that obstructive jaundice may promote bacterial translocation from the gut, and it may be that this route is more important than hitherto realised (Alexander et al. 1990). Endotoxaemia, which is common in obstructive jaundice, can also increase bacterial translocation (Deitch 1988).

Immunosuppression

Immunosuppression may result from malnutrition or malignancy but there is evidence that obstructive jaundice itself leads to impaired cell-mediated immunity with evidence of lymphocyte dysfunction (Keane et al. 1986; Roughneen et al. 1986a, b, 1987) and anergy (Cainzos et al. 1988). Factors implicated in this include impaired interleukin production (Haga et al. 1989) and suppression due to endotoxins (Greve et al. 1990b).

There is impaired hepatic reticuloendothelial (RE) clearance of bacteria (Scott-Conner et al. 1986) and microaggregated albumin (Pain et al. 1987) associated with obstructive jaundice. Kupffer cells, situated in the hepatic sinusoids, are part of the RE system and are normally responsible for the removal of the majority of endotoxin from the portal blood (Pain and Bailey 1987). In obstructive jaundice there is an increased absorption of enteric endotoxin into the portal blood and the Kupffer cell dysfunction allows a spillover of the endotoxin into the systemic circulation.

The mechanism for the RE dysfunction remains obscure. The dysfunction correlates with the presence of cholangitis and plasma bilirubin level but not with transaminase level, or the presence of malignancy. There is no reduction in hepatic sinusoidal blood flow, opsonin levels (fibronectin, immunoglobulin or complement) or serum opsonic activity (Pain 1987). Although the RE dysfunction relates poorly to total plasma bile acid levels there is evidence to suggest that circulating bile acids may affect RE function. Specific surface proteins on macrophages are involved in the recognition of fibronectin-opsonised particles (Rourke et al. 1984) and several modifications of cell membranes and cellular function have been attributed to the detergent properties of bile salts (Keane et al. 1984). Recently van Bossuyt et al. (1990) found that raised bile acid levels reduce the ability of cultured Kupffer cells to bind endotoxin.

Treatment and Prophylaxis

Cholangitis that fails to respond to intravenous antibiotics should be treated by urgent duct drainage. Although second generation cephalosporins are frequently used for elective biliary surgery (Cahill and Pain 1988a), they provide inadequate cover when used alone in jaundiced patients since they have limited activity against *Streptococcus faecalis* and most anaerobes. Prophylactic antibiotics in the form of a single intravenous dose should be given prior to surgery or other form of biliary duct instrumentation.

The depressed RE function in jaundiced animals can be reversed by the administration of an immune stimulator (Pain et al. 1987). In the future such immunomodulation may have a therapeutic role to play in man, but at present the only practical method of reversing the immunosuppression is to relieve the jaundice (Roughneen et al. 1986a; Pain and Bailey 1989).

Renal Failure

Incidence

The overall incidence of postoperative renal failure reported in the last ten years in 1460 patients from 14 studies was 10%, of whom 59% died (Table 2). In non-jaundiced patients undergoing biliary tract surgery, deaths due to postoperative renal failure occur in less than 0.1%.

Pathophysiology

There are two important precipitating factors in the development of renal failure in obstructive jaundice – septicaemia and surgery. The renal lesion

Table 2. Incidence of renal failure

Reference	Date	Number of patients	Renal failure (%)	Renal failure mortality (%)
Ozawa et al.	1979	103	17	72
Pitt et al.	1981	155	18	32
Koyama et al.	1981	220	6	43
Wittenstein et al.	1981	170	9	100
Blamey et al.	1983	89	12	73
Dixon et al.	1983	373	3	62
Ingoldby et al.	1984	27	15	?
Keighley et al.	1984	118	6	71
Al-Fallouji and Collins	1985	50	4	100
Bouillet et al	1985	176	6	50
Pain and Bailey	1986	24	17	50
Gubern et al.	1988	31	10	100
Total		1460	10	59

associated with obstructive jaundice is degeneration of the renal tubular epithelium. The proximal convoluted tubules are principally involved, with changes ranging from swelling and vacuolation of epithelial cells to gross tubular or even cortical necrosis. These changes are compatible with renal tubular ischaemia, which results from a reduction and redistribution of intrarenal blood flow and a consequent fall in glomerular filtration rate. A significant decrease in cortical blood flow has been demonstrated in jaundiced animals (Bomzon and Kew 1983) and the consequent increases in medullary flow and hypertonicity lead to the lack of urinary concentrating ability in jaundice (Massry and Klein 1978). Both the adrenergic nervous system and the renin–angiotensin system appear to be implicated in the pathophysiology, and the increased sympathetic tone and raised levels of circulating catecholamines which occur during abdominal surgery may further decrease renal cortical blood flow. These changes in renal blood flow, together with fibrin deposition in the renal vasculature (Fletcher et al. 1982), result in increased vascular resistance, tubular ischaemia, and tubular or even cortical necrosis – changes characteristic of obstructive jaundice.

Aetiology

A number of different factors have been implicated in the aetiology of these renal vascular changes and altered tubular function (Fig. 1).

Fluid Compartments

In 1960 Williams et al. observed that fatal acute postoperative renal failure in their series of jaundiced patients had always been preceded by a period of hypotension, and they noted that postoperative mortality fell from 13% to 7% if patients were routinely transfused before surgery. Hypotension secondary to hypovolaemia is more common in animals if bile ligation has been performed (Williams et al. 1960; Hishida et al. 1980). Two possible explanations for this response include a reduction in peripheral vascular resistance and an underlying hypovolaemia.

Although there is evidence for a reduction in peripheral resistance with a normal or high cardiac output (Bomzon et al. 1985) there has been contradictory evidence for hypovolaemia in obstructive jaundice. However, Martinez-Rodenas et al (1989) have investigated the changes in body water compartments in rabbits after bile duct ligation. They demonstrated a fall in total body water principally due to a reduction in extracellular water, although plasma volume fell only after prolonged jaundice. It therefore seems that relative hypovolaemia may be a crucial factor in the development of renal dysfunction.

Bilirubin and Bile Salts

Dawson (1965a) found that postoperative renal failure occurred in only 1% of patients when the bilirubin level was below 340 μmol/l, but occurred in 19% when the bilirubin was above this level. Bilirubin uncouples mitochondrial oxidative phosphorylation, potentiates renal ischaemia and may alter renal

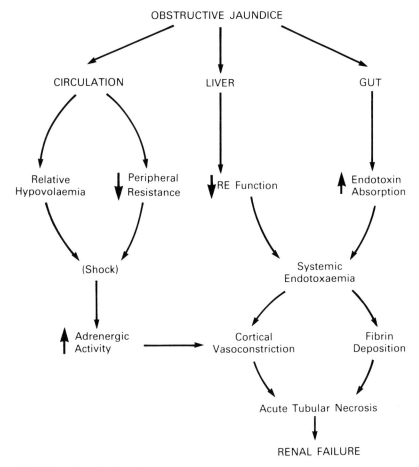

Fig. 1. Principal mechanisms leading to renal failure.

function. However the exposure of the kidney to bile *per se* does not result in acute tubular necrosis (Wait and Kahng 1989). All patients with extrahepatic biliary obstruction have hyperbilirubinaemia, but only some develop renal insufficiency.

Bile salts are retained in obstructive jaundice, but the occurrence of similar patterns of renal failure in fulminant hepatic failure in which bile salts are not retained significantly suggests that they are not of primary aetiological importance. This is supported by animal studies, which show no alteration of renal blood flow or GFR after bile salt infusion (Bomzon et al. 1979).

Endotoxin

Endotoxins are lipopolysaccharides (LPS) derived from the cell walls of Gram-negative bacteria. Structurally there are three distinct segments – a hydrophilic polysaccharide chain, a central acidic core and a hydrophobic lipid A moiety. It is this lipid A moiety, common to all endotoxins, that is the active part of the LPS. Man is exquisitely sensitive to endotoxins and their presence within the systemic blood evokes a wide range of biological responses that affect almost all organ systems. Many of the changes seen during endotoxaemia result from interaction of macrophages with the release of effector substances such as interleukins, tumour necrosis factor and prostaglandins.

Under normal circumstances the kidney is rich in plasminogen activator which protects it from fibrin deposition by fibrinolysis, but this is depressed in obstructive jaundice (Colucci et al. 1988) and there is elevation of acute phase proteins α-1 antitrypsin and α-2 macroglobulin, both of which promote fibrin deposition. The increased fibrinogen turnover in obstructive jaundice is associated with other manifestations of disseminated intravascular coagulation (DIC), and microthrombi in the renal microvascular circulation may contribute to the increased renal vascular resistance and oliguria. Thrombosis of peritubular capillaries combined with peritubular fibrin deposition results in tubular ischaemia and necrosis (Fletcher et al. 1982). These consequences of intravascular coagulation and fibrin deposition on the kidney are identical to those seen in the Sanarelli–Schwartzmann reaction which results from endotoxin exposure.

Endotoxins are also powerful renal vasoconstrictors, and appear to mediate their effects in endotoxaemia through the efferent autonomic renal nerves, and by sympathetic stimulation of renin secretion (Henrich et al. 1982). Endotoxins, direct renal nerve stimulation, and noradrenaline all increase prostaglandin synthesis and release which cause renal vasoactive changes.

Measurement of Endotoxin.   The investigation of the role of endotoxaemia in obstructive jaundice has been hampered by difficulties in quantitating endotoxin levels. The earlier tests relied on gelation of limulus lysate in the presence of endotoxin, and were not quantitative. More recently quantitative assays have been developed using a chromogenic peptide as a substrate for the endotoxin-sensitive limulus enzyme. Although very accurate and sensitive measurements (< 1 pg/ml endotoxin) can be made in non-biological fluids, the measurement of endotoxin in plasma samples is made difficult by the potential for contamination during the collection of samples and the presence of inhibiting and activating proteins within the plasma that interfere with the assay. Various methods of treating plasma samples to remove these proteins are available, but standardisation of "normal" levels and comparisons between the results of different workers are difficult (Pain and Bailey 1987).

Sources of Endotoxin.   Endotoxaemia may arise from a focus of sepsis or the obstructed biliary tree especially during any form of instrumentation (Lumsden et al. 1989) but the main source is the intestinal tract which harbours a vast reservoir of Gram-negative bacteria. Minute amounts of endotoxin can be detected in the portal blood of non-jaundiced subjects, but higher levels are present in obstructive jaundice (Pain and Bailey 1987). Endotoxins are absorbed from the colon as well as from the small intestine (Kiss et al. 1983; Pain and Bailey 1987). Therefore, consideration should be given to the colon as a source of endotoxins when therapeutic methods are designed to prevent endotoxaemia.

Systemic endotoxaemia frequently occurs during or after surgery (Cahill and Pain 1988b). There is RE dysfunction in obstructive jaundice and it is probable that the additional RE depression which occurs during anaesthesia increases the tendency for endotoxin to "spillover" into the systemic circulation. This may be compounded by increased endotoxin absorption resulting from intestinal handling and instrumentation of the biliary tree.

Treatment

Fluids

In view of the evidence of relative hypovolaemia in obstructive jaundice, adequate hydration is probably the simplest and possibly the most effective method of protecting renal function especially for patients undergoing surgery. In a recent study (Pain et al. 1991) in which all patients were fully hydrated prior to surgery, only one of 33 control patients developed transient renal failure and only 34% of patients developed postoperative renal dysfunction, a much lower incidence than previous studies by the same authors (Bailey 1976; Cahill 1983; Pain and Bailey 1986) in which patients did not have routine preoperative hydration.

Mannitol

There are theoretical reasons to support the use of mannitol. As an osmotic diuretic it causes volume expansion, diuresis and natriuresis. Mannitol maintains urine output at low perfusion pressures, and prevents endothelial cell swelling and tubular obstruction by cellular debris (Burke et al. 1983).

Dawson (1964) demonstrated that renal damage in rats with obstructive jaundice could be prevented by a mannitol diuresis. A subsequent study in man (Dawson 1965b) showed that perioperative mannitol given to patients with obstructive jaundice virtually prevented any fall of the creatinine clearance after surgery, whereas in a control group there was a mean fall in excess of 50%. However, in neither the animal study nor the patient study was the control group given a saline infusion of equal volume or equal ability to expand the intravascular space. Furthermore, the patient study was not randomised, and patient age and preoperative creatinine clearance were not balanced between the groups. Mannitol is widely used in the UK (Cahill and Pain 1988a), but a recent randomised study from Spain (Gubern et al. 1988) concluded that mannitol administration did not improve the postoperative renal function of jaundiced patients, nor did it prove beneficial in preventing renal failure. If mannitol is used it is most important to ensure adequate patient hydration to prevent hypovolaemia after the diuresis.

Antiendotoxaemic Therapy

Lactulose. Lactulose, a synthetic disaccharide, is used in the treatment of constipation and for the prevention of hepatic encephalopathy. Lactulose reduces endotoxaemia in parenchymal liver disease, decreases mortality in rats with obstructive jaundice (Pain and Bailey 1986; Greve et al. 1990c) and in a non-randomised study of patients with obstructive jaundice preoperative oral lactulose reduced both portal and systemic endotoxaemia and protected against postoperative renal failure (Pain and Bailey 1986). A subsequent randomised study has confirmed this beneficial role (Pain et al. 1991). The mechanism of action is unknown. It has a direct antiendotoxic action in vitro and in animals but this is more modest than that of bile salts (Pain and Bailey 1986, 1988). It may reduce the availability of colonic endotoxin for absorption by its laxative effect and by an alteration of colonic bacterial flora. If lactulose is absorbed from the intestine of jaundiced patients it may exert a systemic action, since it reduces tumour necrosis factor (TNF) release by macrophages in response to endotoxin (Greve et al. 1990a).

Bile Salts.   Bile salts are detergents and have a direct antiendotoxic action in vitro, causing inactivation of the endotoxin molecule (Shands and Chun 1980). The enhanced absorption of enteric endotoxin in obstructive jaundice is associated with the absence of bile salts from the gut lumen. The clinical effects of endotoxaemia cannot be induced in healthy animals by the oral administration of endotoxin even if doses 500–3000 times the minimal lethal parenteral dose are given (Bertok 1977). The increased absorption of orally administered endotoxin in obstructive jaundice can be prevented if the endotoxin is incubated with a bile salt prior to its oral administration (Filkins 1971), if oral bile salts are administered (Bailey 1976), or if internal biliary drainage is performed (Gouma et al. 1986). Sodium deoxycholate also inhibits TNF production through a direct effect on the response of monocytes to endotoxin (Greve et al. 1989).

In patients with obstructive jaundice, oral sodium deoxycholate prevents both portal and systemic endotoxaemia and protects postoperative renal function (Cahill 1983). However, chenodeoxycholic acid is less effective in these roles (Cahill et al. 1987) and ursodeoxycholic acid has no clinical benefit (Thompson et al. 1986). This suggests that different bile salts have different antiendotoxic activities. These activities have recently been compared in vitro and in vivo and were found to relate to their known detergent activities (Pain and Bailey 1988). Deoxycholic acid and its conjugates were the most effective antiendotoxaemic agents in vitro and in vivo whereas ursodeoxycholic acid was the least effective.

Lactulose or sodium deoxycholate?   The question of which antiendotoxaemic agent to use remains open. Both lactulose and sodium deoxycholate were effective in protecting renal function in a recent randomised study (Pain et al. 1991). Lactulose is widely available and safe, but in the doses used (30 ml six hourly for three days before surgery) may cause diarrhoea which requires reduction of the dose. Sodium deoxycholate (500 mg eight hourly for two days before surgery) is not commercially available as a drug and has to be made up in the hospital pharmacy. Clinical experience of its use is limited, but no serious side effects have been observed.

Other Methods

The cyclic polypeptide antibiotics Polymixin B and colistin interact with endotoxin, with a consequent loss of most of its toxic properties. Polymixin B prevents endotoxaemia in rats with obstructive jaundice (Ingoldby 1980), but in man it has proved disappointing in the prevention of endotoxaemia in cirrhosis and obstructive jaundice (Ingoldby et al. 1984). This agent must be used with caution because of its nephrotoxic properties.

Bowel preparation to reduce the endotoxin releasing Gram-negative bacteria should decrease the endotoxin available for absorption, but was ineffective in practice (Hunt et al. 1982). Oral antibiotics may be actually detrimental, as destruction of Gram-negative organisms may increase the free endotoxin available for absorption (Goto and Nakamura 1980). Mechanical preparation by whole bowel irrigation decreases bacterial numbers, and has been shown to prevent endotoxaemia in patients with inflammatory bowel disease (Wellman et al. 1984). This technique might also decrease endotoxin absorption in obstructive jaundice, but orally administered bile salts or lactulose are effective and less unpleasant for the patient.

Immunotherapy

Passive or active immunisation against endotoxin may, in the future, form the basis of an effective therapy against endotoxaemia. All three parts of the LPS molecule exhibit immunogenic properties. The large number of different O antigens of Gram-negative bacteria precludes them as a source of antibody production for therapeutic use. However, lipid A from virtually all enterobacteria share common determinants and are serologically cross-reactive. McCabe et al. (1972) found that death from septicaemia is reduced among patients with high titres of antibody to the LPS core (R antigen). Freeze-dried human plasma concentrates rich in anti-LPS IgG, and human antiserum to LPS core have both been shown to lower mortality in septicaemic patients (Ziegler et al. 1982; Lachman et al. 1984).

Another approach to abrogate the effects of endotoxaemia that may become applicable is to direct therapy against the TNF produced in response to the endotoxaemia. Antibodies to TNF (Tracey et al. 1986) or to recombinant human TNF (Sheppard et al. 1989) reduce mortality in animals even when administered after the onset of endotoxaemia.

Preoperative Biliary Drainage

The role of preoperative biliary drainage is discussed in Chapter 2.

Coagulation Disorders

In 1936 Hawkin and Brinkhouse demonstrated that dogs with bile fistulae had a haemorrhagic diathesis associated with decreased levels of prothrombin. The preoperative administration of vitamin K to jaundiced patients has dramatically lowered coagulation problems, but bleeding may still be a problem especially in the presence of portal hypertension. This can be compounded by DIC and thrombocytopenia secondary to endotoxaemia (Takeda et al. 1977).

Gastrointestinal Haemorrhage

Gastrointestinal haemorrhage may complicate obstructive jaundice and several mechanisms have been implicated in the pathogenesis of gastric erosions and ulceration. These include hyperacidity, reduced gastric mucus, increased H^+ back diffusion, reduced gastric mucosal blood flow and alteration of energy metabolism (Mizumoto et al. 1986). How these mechanisms are mediated in obstructive jaundice is unknown but possible mediators are endotoxaemia and serum bile acids.

Endotoxin increases gastric secretion in animals. Patients with obstructive jaundice who have postoperative bleeding from peptic ulceration have raised levels of circulating endotoxins (Nakagawa et al. 1986). Alteration of bowel microflora by the administration of oral antibiotics to stressed animals prevents ulceration yet this protection is lost if endotoxin is also administered (Rosoff and Goldman 1968). The action of endotoxins appears to be mediated via increased parasympathetic tone since protection is afforded by atropine (Rosoff and Goldman 1968). In cirrhosis and following portacaval shunting, conditions also associated with endotoxaemia, increased gastric acid output, haemorrhagic gastritis and peptic ulceration occur (Clemente et al. 1977). Endotoxaemia also reduces blood flow to the body of the stomach leading to the formation of erosions (Richardson et al. 1973), and histological examination of such lesions shows microvascular fibrinous thrombi occluding mucosal vessels close to the erosions (Margaretten and McKay 1971). This may result from DIC induced by endotoxin.

Intragastric bile acids can break the gastric mucosal barrier by inhibiting gastric cellular microsomal and mitochondrial function (Harmon et al. 1978). The increased circulating levels of plasma bile acids present in obstructive jaundice may have similar effects. Continuous intravenous bile acid infusion in rats, although reducing gastric acid output, also reduces mucus content and increases susceptibility to stress-induced ulceration (Mizumoto et al. 1986).

Series in the beginning of the 1980s reported that 5%–14% of jaundiced patients developed postoperative gastrointestinal haemorrhage (Table 3). Whether this incidence has been reduced with the widespread adoption of prophylaxis against haemorrhage has yet to be shown.

Impaired Wound Healing

Obstructive jaundice leads to delayed wound healing in animals (Bayer and Ellis 1976). In man there is an increased incidence of both wound dehiscence and incisional herniae following surgery for obstructive jaundice. Before 1980 the incidence of abdominal wound dehiscence after surgery for obstructive jaundice was about 15% (Ellis and Heddle 1977; Irvin et al. 1978) but this has since fallen to 0–6% (Wittenstein et al. 1981; Blamey et al. 1983; Armstrong et al. 1984b; Taube and Ellis 1987; Grande et al. 1990). This reduction is almost certainly due to improved wound closure materials and techniques.

Table 3. Studies from early 1980s reporting the high incidence of postoperative gastrointestinal haemorrhage in patients with obstructive jaundice

Reference	Date	Patients	Postoperative haemorrhage
Pitt et al.	1981	155	6%
Wittenstein et al.	1981	133	7%
Blamey et al.	1983	89	11%
Armstrong et al.	1984a	120	14%
Dixon et al.	1984	409	7%
McPherson et al.	1984	58	5%

In obstructive jaundice there are reduced fibroblast migration and reduced levels of prolyl hydroxylase (Grande et al. 1990), which reflect the rate of collagen synthesis. It is likely that these changes are not due to the obstructive jaundice per se but are related to the presence of malnutrition or malignancy. Armstrong et al. (1984b) showed that decreased wound healing was unrelated to bilirubin level, but was consequent upon poor nutritional status, malignancy and postoperative sepsis. Recently, Grande et al. (1990) have shown that the reduced skin prolyl hydroxylase levels present in obstructive jaundice are unrelated to bilirubin or albumin levels, but whereas the levels rapidly return to normal after surgery for benign biliary obstruction they remain depressed if there is an underlying malignancy.

An association between wound healing and endotoxaemia has been suggested by Askew et al. (1984) who showed improved wound healing in jaundiced rats following treatment with oral bile salts. With the widespread adoption of mass wound closure techniques, wound dehiscence is likely to become rare.

Pruritus

Pruritus is usually the most distressing symptom for patients with obstructive jaundice. It is believed to be the result of the interaction of skin nerve endings with one or more substances retained in obstructive jaundice. Although bile acids have been implicated, the evidence is conflicting. Experimental administration of bile acids may produce pruritus, but the levels of bile acids in the skin do not correlate with the degree of pruritus, and relief of pruritus may occur without a fall in serum bile acid levels (Bartholomew et al. 1982). Resins such as cholestyramine, which bind bile acids in the intestine can reduce pruritus, but its beneficial action may not simply be due to the binding of bile acids. Cholestyramine binds many other substances and has been reported to reduce pruritus in patients with uraemia and polycythaemia which are not associated with bile acid retention. A theoretical contraindication to the use of cholestyramine in patients with obstructive jaundice is its effect to reduce intestinal bile acid levels and thereby increase endotoxin absorption.

Recently it has been suggested that the pruritus is not due to a local interaction within the skin, but of central neurogenic origin involving the opiate receptor system (Jones and Bergasa 1990). Pruritus is a recognised side effect of morphine. Patients with chronic liver disease have evidence of increased stimulation of opiate receptors by agonist ligands and administration of opiate receptor antagonists can relieve the pruritus (Jones and Bergasa 1990).

References

Al-Fallouji MAR, Collins REC (1985) Surgical relief of obstructive jaundice in a district general hospital. J R Soc Med 78:211–216

Alexander JW, Boyce ST, Babcock GF et al. (1990) The process of microbial translocation. Ann Surg 212:496–512.

Armstrong CP, Dixon JM, Taylor TV, Davies GC (1984a) Surgical experience of deeply jaundiced patients with bile duct obstruction. Br J Surg 71:234–238

Armstrong CP, Dixon JM, Duffy SW, Elton RA, Davies GC (1984b) Wound healing in obstructive jaundice. Br J Surg 71:267–270

Askew AR, Bates GJ, Balderson G (1984) Jaundice and the effect of sodium taurocholate taken orally upon abdominal wound healing. Surg Gynecol Obstet 159:207–209

Bailey ME (1976) Endotoxin, bile salts and renal function in obstructive jaundice. Br J Surg 63:774–778

Bartholomew TC, Summerfield JA, Billing BH, Lawson AM, Setchell KDR (1982) Bile acid profiles in human serum and skin interstitial fluid and their relationship to pruritus studied by gas chromatography–mass spectrometry. Clin Sci 63:65–73

Bayer I, Ellis H (1976) Jaundice and wound healing: an experimental study. Br J Surg 63:392–396

Bertok L (1977) Physico-chemical defense of vertebrate organisms: the role of bile acids in defense against bacterial endotoxins. Perspect Biol Med 21:70–76

Blamey SL, Fearon KCH, Gilmour WH, Osborne DH, Carter DC (1983) Prediction of risk in biliary surgery. Br J Surg 70:535–538

Bomzon L, Kew MC (1983) Renal blood flow in experimental obstructive jaundice. In: Epstein M (ed) The kidney in liver disease. Elsevier Biomedical, New York, pp 313–326

Bomzon L, Mendelsohn D, Wilton PB, Kew MC (1979) Bile salts, obstructive jaundice and renal blood flow. Isr J Med Sci 15:169–171

Bomzon L, Gali D, Better OS et al. (1985) Reversible suppression of the vascular contractile response in rats with obstructive jaundice. J Lab Clin Med 105:568–572

Bouillot J-L, Ledorner G, Alexandre J-H (1985) Facteurs de risque de chirurgie des icteres obstructifs. Etude retrospective apropos de 176 patients. Gastroenterol Clin Biol 9:238–243

Burke TJ, Arnold PE, Schrier RW (1983) Prevention of ischemic acute renal failure with impermeant solutes. Am J Physiol 244:F646–649

Cahill CJ (1983) Prevention of post-operative renal failure in patients with obstructive jaundice – the role of bile salts. Br J Surg 70:590–595

Cahill CJ, Pain JA (1988a) Current practice in biliary surgery. Br J Surg 75:1169–1172

Cahill CJ, Pain JA (1988b) Obstructive jaundice: renal failure and other endotoxin-related complications. Surg Ann 20:17–37

Cahill CJ, Pain JA, Bailey ME (1987) Bile salts, endotoxin and renal function in obstructive jaundice. Surg Gynecol Obstet 165:519–522

Cainzos M, Potel J, Puente JL (1988) Anergy in jaundiced patients. Br J Surg 75:147–149

Clemente C, Bosch J, Rodes J, Arroyo V, Mas A, Margall S (1977) Functional renal failure and haemorrhagic gastritis associated with endotoxaemia in cirrhosis. Gut 18:556–560

Colucci M, Altomare DF, Chetta G, Triggiani R, Cavallo LG, Semeraro N (1988) Impaired fibrinolysis in obstructive jaundice – evidence from clinical and experimental studies. Thromb Haemost 60:25–29

Dawson JL (1964) Jaundice and anoxic renal damage: protective effect of mannitol. Br Med J 1:810–811

Dawson JL (1965a) The incidence of postoperative renal failure in obstructive jaundice. Br J Surg 52:663–665.

Dawson JL (1965b) Post-operative renal function in obstructive jaundice: effect of a mannitol diuresis. Br Med J 1:82–86

Deitch A, Sittig K, Li M, Berg R, Specian RD (1990) Obstructive jaundice promotes bacterial translocation from the gut. Am J Surg 159:79–84

Deitch EA (1988) The immunocompromised host. Surg Clin North Am 68:181–190

Dixon JM, Armstrong CP, Duffy SW, Davies GC (1983) Factors affecting morbidity and mortality after surgery for obstructive jaundice: a review of 373 patients. Gut 24:845–852

Dixon JM, Armstrong CP, Duffy SW, Elton RA, Davies GC (1984) Upper gastrointestinal bleeding. A significant complication after surgery for relief of obstructive jaundice. Ann Surg 199:271–275

Ellis H, Heddle R (1977) Does the peritoneum need to be closed at laparotomy? Br J Surg 64:733–736

Filkins JP (1971) Decreased shock lethality in rats with surfactant treated endotoxin. Proc Soc Exp Biol Med 136:466–468

Fletcher MS, Westwick J, Kakkar VV (1982) Endotoxin, prostaglandins and renal fibrin deposition in obstructive jaundice. Br J Surg 69:625–629

Goto H, Nakamura S (1980) Liberation of endotoxin from *Escherichia coli* by addition of antibiotics. Jpn J Exp Med 50:35–43

Gouma DJ, Coelho JCU, Fisher JD, Schlegel JF, Li YF, Moody FG (1986) Endotoxaemia after relief of biliary obstruction by internal and external drainage in rats. Am J Surg 151:476–479

Grande L, Garcia-Valdecasa JC, Fuster J, Visa J, Pera C (1990) Obstructive jaundice and wound healing. Br J Surg 77:440–442

Greve JW, Gouma DJ, Buurman WA (1989) Bile acids inhibit endotoxin-induced release of tumour necrosis factor by monocytes: an in vitro study. Hepatology 10:454–458

Greve JW, Gouma DJ, van Leuwen PAM, Buurman WA (1990a) Lactulose inhibits endotoxin induced tumour necrosis factor production by monocytes. An in vitro study. Gut 31:198–203

Greve JW, Gouma DJ, Soeters PB, Buurman WA (1990b) Suppression of cellular immunity in obstructive jaundice is caused by endotoxins. A study with germ-free rats. Gastroenterology 98:478–485

Greve JW, Maessen JG, Tiebosch T, Buurman WA, Gouma DJ (1990c) Prevention of postoperative complications in jaundiced rats. Internal biliary drainage versus oral lactulose. Ann Surg 212:221–227

Gubern JM, Sancho JJ, Simo J, Sitges-Serra A (1988) A randomized trial on the effect of mannitol on postoperative renal function in patients with obstructive jaundice. Surgery 103:39–44

Haga Y, Sakamoto K, Egami H et al. (1989) Changes in production of interleukin-1 and interleukin-2 associated with obstructive jaundice and biliary drainage in patients with gastrointestinal cancer. Surgery 106:842–848

Harmon JW, Doong T, Gadacz TR (1978) Bile acids are not equally damaging to the gastric mucosa. Surgery 84:79–86

Hawkin WB, Brinkhouse KM (1936) Prothrombin deficiency: the cause of bleeding in bile fistula dogs. J Exp Med 63:795–801

Henrich WL, Hamasaki Y, Said SI, Campbell WB, Cronin RE (1982) Dissociation of systemic and renal effects in endotoxaemia. J Clin Invest 69:691–699

Hishida H, Honda N, Sudo N, Nagase M (1980) Mechanisms of altered renal perfusion in the early stages of obstructive jaundice. Kidney Int 17:223–230

Hunt DR, Allison MEM, Prentice CRM, Blumgart LH (1982) Endotoxaemia, disturbance of coagulation and obstructive jaundice. Am J Surg 144:325–329

Ingoldby CJ (1980) The value of polymixin B in endotoxaemia due to experimental obstructive jaundice and mesenteric ischaemia. Br J Surg 67:565–567

Ingoldby CJ, McPherson GAD, Blumgart LH (1984) Endotoxemia in human obstructive jaundice. Effect of Polymixin B. Am J Surg 147:766–771

Irvin TT, Vassilakis JS, Chattopadhyay DK, Greaney MG (1978) Abdominal wound healing in jaundiced patients. Br J Surg 65:521–522

Jones EA, Bergasa NV (1990) The pruritus of cholestasis: from bile acids to opiate agonists. Hepatology 11:884–887

Keane RM, Gadaccz TR, Munster AM, Birmingham W, Winchurch RA (1984) Impairment of human lymphocytic function by bile salts. Surgery 95:439–443

Keane RM, Collins PB, Johnson AH, Hayes DB (1986) Delayed homograft rejection following common bile duct ligation: in vivo evidence that obstructive jaundice is immunosuppressive. Ir J Med Sci 155:143–146

Keighley MR, Razay G, Fitzgerald MG (1984) Influence of diabetes on mortality and morbidity following operations for obstructive jaundice. Ann R Coll Surg Engl 66:49–51

Kiss A, Ferenci P, Graninger W, Pamperl H, Potzi R, Meryn S (1983) Endotoxaemia following colonoscopy. Endoscopy 15:24–26

Koyama K, Takagi Y, Ito K, Sato T (1981) Experimental and clinical studies on the effect of biliary drainage in obstructive jaundice. Am J Surg 142:293–299

Lachman E, Pitsoe SB, Gaffin SL (1984) Anti-lipopolysaccharide immunotherapy in management of septic shock of obstetric and gynaecological origin. Lancet i:981–983

Lumsden AB, Henderson JM, Alspaugh J (1989) Endotoxemia during percutaneous manipulation of the obstructed biliary tree. Am J Surg 158:21–24

Margaretten W, McKay DG (1971) Thrombotic ulcerations of the gastrointestinal tract. Arch Intern Med 127:250–253

Martinez-Rodenas F, Oms LM, Carulla X et al. (1989) Measurement of body water compartments after ligation of the common bile duct in rabbits. Br J Surg 76:461–464

Massry SG, Klein K (1978) Effects of bile duct ligation on renal function. In: Epstein M (ed) The kidney and liver disease. Elsevier, New York, pp 155–165

McCabe WR, Kreger BE, Johns M (1972) Type-specific and cross-reactive antibodies in Gram-negative bacteremia. N Engl J Med 287:261–267

McPherson GAD, Benjamin IS, Hodgson HJF, Bowley NB, Allison DJ, Blumgart LH (1984) Pre-operative percutaneous transhepatic biliary drainage: the results of a controlled trial. Br J Surg 71:371–375

Mizumoto S, Harada K, Takano S, Misumi A, Akagi M (1986) Mechanisms of acute gastric mucosal lesion accompanying obstructive jaundice – role of bile acids in plasma. Gastroenterol Jpn 21:6–16

Nakagawa K, Matsubara S, Ouchi K, Owada Y, Yajima Y (1986) Endotoxemia after abdominal surgery. Tohuku J Exp Med 150:273–280

Ohshio G, Manabe T, Tobe T, Yoshioka H, Hamashima Y (1988) Circulating immune complex, endotoxin and biliary infection in patients with biliary obstruction. Am J Surg 155:343–347

Ozawa K, Yamada T, Tanaka J, Ukikusa M, Tobe T (1979) The mechanism of suppression of renal function in patients and rabbits with jaundice. Surg Gynecol Obstet 149:54–60

Pain JA (1987) Reticuloendothelial function in obstructive jaundice. Br J Surg 74:1091–1094

Pain JA, Bailey ME (1986) Experimental and clinical study of lactulose in obstructive jaundice. Br J Surg 73:775–778

Pain JA, Bailey ME (1987) Measurement of operative endotoxin plasma levels in jaundiced and non-jaundiced patients. Eur Surg Res 19:207–216

Pain JA, Bailey ME (1988) Prevention of endotoxaemia in obstructive jaundice – a comparative study of bile salts. HPB Surgery 1:21–27

Pain JA, Bailey ME (1989) Effects of surgery on reticuloendothelial function in jaundiced patients. Surg Res Commun 5:239–244

Pain JA, Collier DStJ, Ritson A (1987) Reticuloendothelial system phagocytic function in obstructive jaundice and its modification by a muramyl dipeptide analogue. Eur Surg Res 19:16–22

Pain JA, Cahill CJ, Gilbert JM, Johnson CD, Trapnell JE, Bailey ME (1991) Prevention of postoperative renal dysfunction in obstructive jaundice – a multicentre study of bile salts and lactulose. Br J Surg 78: 467–469

Pitt HA, Cameron JL, Postier RG, Gadacz TR (1981) Factors affecting mortality in biliary tract surgery. Am J Surg 141:66–72

Richardson RS, Norton LW, Sales JEL, Eisenmann B (1973) Gastric blood flow in endotoxin-induced stress ulcer. Arch Surg 106:191–195

Rosoff CB, Goldman H (1968) Effect of intestinal bacterial flora on acute gastric ulceration. Gastroenterology 55:212–222

Roughneen PT, Gouma DJ, Kulkarni AD, Fanslow WF, Rowlands BJ (1986a) Impaired specific cell mediated immunity in experimental biliary obstruction and its reversibility by internal biliary obstruction. J Surg Res 41:113–125

Roughneen PT, Kulkarni AD, Gouma DJ, Fanslow WC (1986b) Suppression of host-versus-graft response in experimental biliary obstruction. Transplantation 42:687–689

Roughneen PT, Drath DB, Kulkarni AD, Rowlands BJ (1987) Impaired nonspecific cellular immunity in experimental cholestasis. Ann Surg 206:578–582

Rourke FJ, Blumestock FA, Kaplan JE (1984) Effect of fibronectin fragments on macrophage phagocytosis of gelatinized particles. J Immunol 1342:1931–1936

Scott-Conner CEH, Bernstein JM, Scher KS, Mack ME (1986) The effect of biliary obstruction on a gram-negative bacteremic challenge: a preliminary report. Surgery 6:679–682

Shands JW, Chun PW (1980) The dispersion of gram-negative lipopolysaccharide by deoxycholate. J Biol Chem 255:1221–1226

Sheppard BC, Fraker DL, Norton JA (1989) Prevention and treatment of endotoxin and sepsis lethality with recombinant human tumor necrosis factor. Surgery 106:156–162

Takeda S, Takaki A, Ohsato K (1977) Occurrence of disseminated intravascular coagulation (DIC) in obstructive jaundice and its relation to biliary tract infection. Jpn J Surg 7:82–89

Taube M, Ellis H (1987) Mass closure of abdominal wounds following major laparotomy in jaundiced patients. Ann R Coll Surg Engl 69:276–278

Thompson JN, Cohen J, Blenkharn JI, McConnell JS, Barr J, Blumgart LH (1986) A randomized clinical trial of oral ursodeoxycholic acid in obstructive jaundice. Br J Surg 73:634–636

Tracey KJ, Beutler B, Lowry SF et al. (1986) Shock and tissue injury induced by recombinant human cachetin. Science 234:470–474

van Bossuyt H, Desmaretz C, Gaeta GB, Wisse E (1990) The role of bile acids in the development of endotoxaemia during obstructive jaundice in the rat. J Hepatol 10:274–279

Wait RB, Kahng KU (1989) Renal failure complicating obstructive jaundice. Am J Surg 157:256–263

Wellman W, Fink PC, Schmidt FW (1984) Whole-gut irrigation as anti-endotoxinaemic therapy in inflammatory bowel disease. Hepatogastroenterology 31:91–93

Whipple AO, Parsons WB, Mullins CR (1935) Treatment of carcinoma of the ampulla of Vater. Ann Surg 102:763–779

Williams RD, Elliot DW, Zollinger RM (1960) The effect of hypotension in obstructive jaundice. Arch Surg 81:334–340

Wittenstein BH, Giacchino JL, Pickleman JR et al. (1981) Obstructive jaundice: the necessity for improved management. Am Surg 47:116–120

Ziegler EJ, McCutchen A, Fierer J et al. (1982) Treatment of gram-negative bacteremia and shock with human antiserum to a mutant *Escherichia coli*. N Engl J Med 307:1225–1230

Chapter 2

Effects of Biliary Drainage in Obstructive Jaundice

B. J. Rowlands, T. Diamond, D. C. McCrory and W. D. B. Clements

Introduction

Obstructive jaundice is often a clinical manifestation of diseases of the extrahepatic biliary system and pancreas. Surgical procedures in these patients are associated with significant mortality and morbidity due mainly to the development of postoperative complications such as sepsis, bleeding disorders and renal failure (Armstrong et al. 1984; Pain et al. 1985). Therapeutic endoscopic and radiological procedures carry similar risks although their frequency is less well documented. Clinical and experimental studies have identified several aetiological factors including hypotension, impaired nutritional status, impaired immune function, hepatic dysfunction and the presence of toxic substances (bilirubin, bile salts) in the circulation. Wardle and Wright (1970) reported an association between renal insufficiency and endotoxaemia in obstructive jaundice and since that time there has been increasing recognition of the role of circulating endotoxins in the development of many of the complications of obstructive jaundice (Wilkinson et al. 1976; Hunt 1980). This has led to the investigation of factors that result in the development of endotoxaemia, including the absence of intraluminal bile salts and impairment of immunological function. These in turn initiated studies on therapeutic measures to reduce endotoxaemia, such as oral replacement of bile salts, percutaneous and endoscopic decompression of the biliary tract, stimulation of immune function and the use of antibiotics and antiendotoxin agents (Diamond and Rowlands 1991). This chapter will concentrate on the critical evaluation of the effects of biliary drainage in obstructive jaundice in animal and clinical studies, and their implications for current therapeutic strategies.

Risk Factors in Biliary Surgery

Several risk factors associated with surgery in obstructive jaundice have been identified. This enables the patients who are at high risk of complications to be closely monitored and supported and for some to be offered and to benefit from an alternative form of therapy (e.g. percutaneous or endoscopic biliary drainage). A high serum bilirubin level in jaundiced patients undergoing pancreatic resection is recognised as a predictor of a high mortality rate and is associated with an increased frequency of renal insufficiency, septic complications and postoperative haemorrhage (Braasch and Gray 1977).

Hunt (1980) reported that a high serum bilirubin (> 300 μmol/l), low glomerular filtration rate (< 50 ml/min), the presence in plasma of fibrinogen degradation products and of endotoxaemia were associated with an increased mortality. Pitt et al. (1981) analysed 15 clinical and laboratory parameters in 155 consecutive jaundiced patients undergoing bile duct surgery in an attempt to define a subpopulation at greatest risk. They found eight parameters which correlated with morbidity and mortality (malignancy, age > 60 years, haematocrit $< 30\%$, white cell count $> 10\ 000/\text{mm}^3$, albumin < 30 g/dl, bilirubin > 170 μmol/1, alkaline phosphatase > 100 IU and creatinine > 115 μmol/1). In a retrospective study of 373 patients undergoing surgery for relief of biliary obstruction Dixon et al. (1983), using multivariate analysis, demonstrated only three factors which correlated with morbidity and mortality (haematocrit $<30\%$, bilirubin > 200 μmol/l and malignancy). In a prospective study of patients with benign biliary obstruction, only serum bilirubin correlated with mortality (Armstrong et al. 1984) whereas in a retrospective study of a similar group of patients three factors (creatinine, albumin and bilirubin) correlated with mortality (Blamey et al. 1983). In all these studies serum bilirubin, reflecting the severity of the jaundice, serum creatinine, serum albumin and the haematocrit seem to be the most significant factors determining outcome. These observations led to the suggestion that relief of obstructive jaundice by surgical, radiological or endoscopic techniques, thereby lowering serum bilirubin, might lead to improvement in renal, liver synthetic and haematological abnormalities and consequent improved mortality and morbidity.

Clinical Aspects of Biliary Drainage

Decompression of the biliary tract to reduce serum bilirubin prior to definitive surgery for carcinoma of the ampulla of Vater was first recommended by Whipple et al. (1935). A two-state procedure was used consisting of surgical drainage of the biliary tract (cholecyst-gastrostomy) followed 3–4 weeks later by resection of the tumour. Although the effect of biliary decompression was favourable, intra-abdominal adhesions made the second operation more complex and mortality was not significantly improved. The introduction of the Chiba needle for percutaneous liver puncture and of ultrasonography and

endoscopic retrograde cholangiopancreatography (ERCP) provided new diagnostic and therapeutic options in the management of patients with obstructive
jaundice. External biliary drainage was used to provide decompression of the
biliary tract as a first stage in the preparation of jaundiced patients for operation
(Nakayama et al. 1978). It was postulated that this would improve liver function
and reduce toxic effects and complications when a definitive operation was
carried out 2–3 weeks later (Blumgart 1978).

Several early reports showed improvement in operative morbidity and
mortality following preoperative external biliary drainage (Nakayama et al.
1978; Gouma et al. 1983; Gundry et al. 1984). These early reports were not
based on prospective, randomised, controlled, clinical trials and the initial
enthusiasm for this technique was tempered by the conclusive demonstration
of several studies that preoperative external biliary drainage does not improve
operative morbidity and mortality in jaundiced patients (Hatfield et al. 1982;
McPherson et al. 1984; Pitt et al. 1985). Hatfield et al. (1982) and McPherson
et al. (1984) highlighted the significant incidence of local complications such
as cannula sepsis, bleeding and biliary leakage associated with external drainage
and Pitt et al. (1985) highlighted the significant increase in hospital cost. These
reservations regarding local complications have been emphasised by others
(Sirinek and Levine 1989). In addition, although hyperbilirubinaemia returns
rapidly towards normal, there is little impact on impaired renal, haematological,
and immunological function and hepatic synthetic function takes several weeks
to recover fully. In a review of all reports on preoperative external biliary
drainage from 1974 to 1984, Gouma and Moody (1984) concluded that the
hazards of the technique outweighed any possible advantages. Preoperative
external biliary decompression has been abandoned by most surgeons.

The failure of external biliary drainage to improve outcome led to an interest
in the efficacy of preoperative internal biliary drainage but clinical experience
with this technique is limited. Theoretically, internal drainage may produce
better results by preventing external loss of fluid and electrolytes and avoidance
of the disruption of the enterohepatic bile salt circulation. In a randomised
trial of patients undergoing surgical resection for carcinoma of the head of the
pancreas, endoscopic internal biliary drainage significantly reduced the incidence
of biliary infection, bacteraemia and intraoperative bleeding when compared
with external drainage (Lygidakis et al. 1987). Trede and Schwall (1988)
reported that preoperative endoscopic internal biliary drainage decreased
postoperative complications in patients with pancreatic carcinoma. Smith et al.
(1985) demonstrated improved renal function and fewer surgical complications
in patients who had a percutaneous stent to allow internal biliary drainage
compared to a control group who had immediate surgery. In a randomised
comparison of endoscopic versus percutaneous stent insertion for palliative
therapy, Speer et al. (1987) demonstrated a higher success rate for relief of
jaundice and a lower 30-day mortality for the endoscopic method. The higher
mortality after percutaneous drainage was due to complications associated with
liver puncture. Endoscopic stenting to provide internal biliary drainage has
also been shown to be as effective and probably superior to operative bypass
in the palliation of malignant biliary obstruction in patients who have a poor
prognosis (Bornman et al. 1986; Anderson et al. 1989).

Experimental Aspects of Biliary Drainage

The recognition that circulating endotoxins play an important role in the development of complications in obstructive jaundice may explain why preoperative biliary drainage failed to improve outcome despite the theoretical advantage of biliary decompression and reversal of hyperbilirubinaemia (Diamond and Rowlands 1991). In addition to local septic and haemorrhagic complications and biliary leakage it is possible that failure to restore bile flow into the gut lumen could be a reason for the poor results with external drainage. Gouma et al. (1986) showed that following relief of biliary obstruction in rats by internal drainage, endotoxaemia was reduced but following external drainage, endotoxaemia was unaffected. In addition, using a surgical stress model of caecal ligation and puncture, they showed that mortality in jaundiced rats was reduced following internal drainage, but following external drainage, mortality was unaffected (Gouma et al. 1987). They concluded that these differences between internal and external drainage were due to the return of bile to the gut which occurs with internal drainage but not with external drainage.

The Origin and Development of Endotoxaemia

This has been reviewed extensively in Chapter 1. Briefly, it is postulated that in obstructive jaundice there are two major contributing factors in the development of endotoxaemia. First, the absence of bile salts in the gut results in a much greater pool of endotoxin in the large bowel, for absorption into the portal circulation (Kocsar et al. 1969; Bailey 1976). Second, impairment of hepatic Kupffer cell phagocytic function in obstructive jaundice allows spillover of endotoxin into the systemic circulation with subsequent development of systemic complications (Bradfield 1974; Holman and Rikkers 1982; Pain 1987). Other factors such as the production of antiendotoxin secretory IgA from the liver (Rank and Wilson 1983), changes in mucosal permeability and blood flow (Papa et al. 1983) and the passage of bacteria and bacterial toxins from the gut lumen to the portal circulation (Deitch et al. 1990) may all be influenced by obstructive jaundice to the detriment of the host. Systemic endotoxaemia activates mediators of the inflammatory response, initiating an inflammatory cascade that leads ultimately to impairment of organ function. The study of some of these phenomena in obstructive jaundice has been carried out using a variety of animal models.

Bile Duct Ligation (BDL)

The rat bile duct ligation model is well established for the study of many aspects of obstructive jaundice including endotoxaemia, renal function, wound healing, and immunological function (Bailey 1976; Bayer and Ellis 1976; Holman and Rikkers 1982; Pain and Bailey 1986). The bile duct should be doubly ligated and divided between the ligatures to reduce the possibility of spontaneous recanalisation (Lee 1972). Other animal models for biliary obstruction are available. Bile duct ligation in dogs has been used to investigate the effect of biliary obstruction on hepatic reticuloendothelial function (Cardoso et al. 1982). Changes in reticuloendothelial and lymphocytic immune function have been studied in the rabbit subject to biliary obstruction followed by internal drainage, via a cholecystjejunostomy (Vane et al. 1988). Larger animals have a gallbladder (unlike the rat) and a reversal procedure such as cholecystjejunostomy is technically easy to perform but no convenient model for external biliary drainage in these animals is routinely available.

Mice have been used to study bacterial translocation in obstructive jaundice and convenient techniques for the harvest and quantitative culture of the spleen and mesenteric lymph nodes are available (Deitch et al. 1990). Unfortunately, with this model, simple techniques for internal and external biliary drainage are not available.

The rat is the most widely used experimental animal for studies in obstructive jaundice as larger numbers can be used, they are relatively inexpensive, and internal and external drainage procedures have been described. However, rats are highly resistant to the pathophysiological effects of endotoxaemia. Zwiefach (1961) reported relative LD_{75} for circulatory collapse following endotoxin challenge in various animals: cat 1; rabbit 2.5; dog 8; guinea pig 20 and rat 300. Thus, in order to overcome this high resistance to endotoxaemia and to allow widespread use of the rat for studies on the development and effects of endotoxaemia in various circumstances, including obstructive jaundice, a technique involving the administration of lead acetate has been developed to produce sensitivity to endotoxin (Filkins 1970).

Internal Drainage: choledochoduodenostomy

This rat model was first described by Ryan et al. (1977) and is used to study reversal of biliary obstruction by internal drainage and return of bile to the gastrointestinal tract. The operation involves a laparotomy at a given time (e.g. 2 or 3 weeks) following bile duct ligation and anastomosis of the dilated proximal common bile duct to the duodenum. The anastomosis is splinted by a Teflon tube. The procedure is reported to be well tolerated with negligible mortality and rats have survived and appeared healthy for up to 12 weeks (Ryan et al. 1977).

The procedure has several disadvantages. The reversal operation is carried out on a dilated, thin walled, friable bile duct making insertion of a purse string difficult and biliary leakage may occur. The bile duct may also require mobilisation which can cause significant bleeding, or inadvertent puncture of the biliary tree may occur. Diamond et al. (1991) have overcome these problems by a modification of the procedure. At the initial bile duct ligation a silastic cannula is introduced into the bile duct. This is held in place with silk ties passed around the duct. The lower end of the cannula is then kinked and ligated to allow biliary obstruction to occur. The reversal operation is then simply a matter of dividing the ligature and introducing the cannula into the duodenum through a purse-string suture.

External Drainage

Biliary Fistula

This model involves cannulation of the rat common bile duct and exteriorisation of the cannula via a subcutaneous tunnel to the skin surface. The cannula may be connected to the cage via a swivel joint so that free movement of the rat is possible and bile may be drained and collected continuously (Balabaud et al. 1981). The model mimics percutaneous external biliary drainage in humans, where biliary obstruction is relieved, but bile is not returned to the gastrointestinal tract. It has been used to study the effect of absence of gastrointestinal bile flow on the development of endotoxaemia (Kocsar et al. 1969) and in studies to compare reversal of endotoxaemia by internal and external biliary drainage (Gouma et al. 1986, 1987). This rat biliary fistula model has several disadvantages, including dislodgement of the cannula, biliary leakage, twisting and kinking of the cannula and chewing of the cannula by the rat. A more serious problem is that of infection of the cannula and the biliary system, which could provide an external source of infection and endotoxin in the biliary system. This may account for the poor results of external drainage in the prevention of endotoxaemia and renders studies on its origin difficult to interpret.

Choledochovesical Fistula

Burke et al. (1977) described a choledochovesical fistula (CDVF). The common bile duct is drained into the urinary bladder via a silastic cannula. This was further modified by Diamond and Rowlands (1990). At the initial procedure a silastic cannula is inserted into the bile duct and held in place with silk ligatures. The lower end is introduced into the urinary bladder through a purse-string suture. The middle portion of the cannula is then kinked and ligated to produce biliary obstruction. At the reversal operation the ligature is divided, to allow bile flow from the biliary tree to the urinary bladder and hence the exterior. When these cannulas were cultured no bacteria were grown, which confirms that this is a sterile model for external biliary drainage.

With all biliary obstruction models there is a choloresis after relief of obstruction (Accatino et al. 1979). Internal drainage returns the bile to the small bowel and enterohepatic circulation, but with external drainage the bile is lost to the exterior and must be replaced by daily subcutaneous injections of saline for the first 4–5 days after the reversal procedure (Gouma et al. 1987).

Other Drainage Models

To study the effects of the absence of bile from the small intestine without prior biliary obstruction, Bergesen et al. (1985) developed a choledochocolic fistula, diverting bile from the bile duct to the colon. Ascending cholangitis occurred with this model, so it appears that the CDVF is a better model to study absence of bile without intercurrent infection. The direct toxic effects of bile salts in the systemic circulation have been studied by Byers and Friedman (1952) who constructed a choledochocaval shunt by anastomosing the common bile duct to the inferior vena cava. This is a technically difficult procedure with a high mortality and is used infrequently.

Results from Animal Experiments

Many aspects of obstructive jaundice have been studied using animal models but caution is advised in the interpretation of the results and their clinical applications. BDL has been used to show that in cholestasis there is depressed wound healing (Arnaud et al. 1981), portal hypertension and liver structural damage (Johnston and Lee 1976; Franco et al. 1979) significant portal and systemic endotoxaemia (Gouma et al. 1986; Diamond and Rowlands 1989), decreased bacterial trapping (Katz et al. 1984), increased sensitivity to septic challenge (Tanaka et al. 1985), decreased reticuloendothelial cell function (Holman and Rikkers 1982), depressed T cell responses (Roughneen et al. 1986), depressed non-specific cell-mediated immunity (Roughneen et al. 1987), decreased bacterial clearance (Cardoso et al. 1982) and increased bacterial translocation (Deitch et al. 1990). Deitch et al. (1990) found increased bacterial translocation and ileal structural damage in bile duct-ligated mice. They postulated that ileal damage due to a lack of bile salts may cause breakdown of the intestinal mucosal barrier and allow bacterial translocation, but they did not administer bile salts to bile duct-ligated mice to see if these changes could be reversed. Earlier work by Deitch et al. (1987), demonstrated ileal structural damage after administration of endotoxin to normal mice and it could be argued that endotoxin released from infected bile in bile duct-ligated mice might cause ileal damage and bacterial translocation. Using the choledochocolic fistula model, Bergesen et al. (1987) did not detect any ileal damage in the absence of bile. However, when the duodenal papilla was transplanted to the mid small intestine, Altmann (1971) showed an increase in villous growth. Furthermore, by selectively transplanting only pancreatic secretions, greater villous enlargement was seen than with purely biliary secretions. This area would repay further investigation, for example, with the CDVF to study ileal structure in the absence of bile, without prior biliary obstruction, and by treating BDL animals with bile salts to see if ileal structural damage and bacterial translocation can be prevented.

The results following reversal of cholestasis have also been conflicting. After internal drainage rats with BDL survived a septic insult better than those reversed by external drainage (Gouma et al. 1987). A higher level of endotoxin was found in externally drained animals (Gouma et al. 1986) but bacteria may have ascended the exteriorised cannula and produced endotoxins in the bile. Using the CDVF model, Diamond, et al. (1990) showed that internal and external drainage were equally effective in reversing endotoxaemia. The mortality after septic challenge was similar in both reversal groups. This may be due to the sterile nature of the CDVF as a form of biliary drainage, which prevents ascending biliary infection and endotoxaemia. T cell suppression in obstructive jaundice is reversed by biliary decompression (Roughneen et al. 1986). Thompson et al. (1990) showed that T cell dysfunction returns to normal more quickly with internal biliary drainage. Greve et al. (1990) demonstrated that T cell function was depressed in bile duct-ligated rats with normal gut flora, but not in bile duct-ligated germ-free rats. This would imply that endotoxin released from the normal bacterial flora produced the immune suppression.

Conclusions

Animal models of biliary obstruction and drainage have increased our knowledge of the basic pathophysiology of obstructive jaundice and its complications. Several important features – biliary obstruction, lack of intraluminal bile salts and altered gastrointestinal structure and function – appear to be important in the development of endotoxaemia. When hepatic dysfunction allows the "spillover" of endotoxin into the systemic circulation, complications occur. Relief of biliary obstruction, preferably into the gastrointestinal tract, may produce some improvement in the clinical condition but is unlikely to improve substantially the mortality and morbidity unless the internal drainage is combined with other therapeutic strategies that combat the effects of endotoxin. Further clinical studies are obviously needed to test the efficacy of such a regimen.

References

Accatino L, Contreras A, Fernandez S, Quintana C (1979) The effect of complete biliary obstruction on bile flow and bile acid excretion: post-cholestatic choloresis in the rat. J. Lab Clin Med 93:706–717

Altmann GG (1971) Influence of bile and pancreatic secretions on the size of intestinal villi in the rat. Am J Anat 132:167–168

Anderson JR, Sorenson SM, Kruse A, Rokkjaer M, Matzen P (1989) Randomized trial of endoscopic endoprosthesis versus operative bypass in malignant obstructive jaundice. Gut 30:1132–1135

Armstrong CP, Dixon JM, Taylor TV, Davies GC (1984) Surgical experience of deeply jaundiced patients with bile duct obstruction. Br J Surg 71:234–238

Arnaud JP, Humbert WH, Eloy MR, Adloff M (1981) Effect of obstructive jaundice on wound healing. Am J Surg 141:593–596

Bailey ME (1976) Endotoxin, bile salts and renal function in obstructive jaundice. Br J Surg 66:392–397

Balabaud C, Saric J, Gonzalez P, Delphy C (1981) Bile collection in free moving rats. Lab Anim Sci 31:273–275

Bayer I, Ellis H (1976) Jaundice and wound healing: an experimental study. Br J Surg 63:392–396

Bergesen O, Schjonsby H, Schjerven L (1985) Effect of bile on vitamin B12 absorption in rats. Scand J Gastroenterol 20:589–594

Bergesen O, Schjonsby H, Andersen KJ, Schjerven L (1987) Intestinal epithelial function and villous surface area in rats with bile fistulae. Scand J Gastroenterol 22:731–736.

Blamey SL, Fearon KCH, Gilmour WH, Osbourne DH, Carter DC (1983) Prediction of risk in biliary surgery. Br J Surg 70:535–538.

Blumgart LH (1978) Biliary tract obstruction: new appoaches to old problems. Am J Surg 135:19–31

Bornman PC, Harries-Jones EP, Tobias R, Van Stiegmann G, Terblanche J (1986) Prospective controlled trial of transhepatic biliary endoprosthesis versus bypass surgery for incurable carcinoma of the head of pancreas. Lancet i:69–71

Braasch JW, Gray BN (1977) Considerations that lower pancreatoduodenectomy mortality. Am J Surg 133:480–484

Bradfield JWB (1974) Control of spillover: the importance of Kupffer cell function in clinical medicine. Lancet ii:883–886

Burke V, Stone DE, Beaman J (1977) Effects of biliary diversion on intestinal microflora in the rat. J Med Microbiol 10:241–244

Byers SO, Friedman M (1952) Observations concerning the production and excretion of cholesterol in mammals. J Exp Med 95:12–24

Cardoso V, Pimenta A, Correia da Fonesca J, Rodrigues JS, Machado MJ (1982) The effect of cholestasis on hepatic clearance of bacteria. World J Surg 6:330–334

Deitch EA, Bery R, Specian R (1987) Endotoxin promotes translocation of bacteria from the gut. Arch Surg 122:185–190

Deitch EA, Sittig K, Li M, Berg R, Specian RD (1990) Obstructive jaundice promotes bacterial translocation from the gut. Am J Surg 159:79–84

Diamond T, Rowlands BJ (1989) Endotoxaemia in obstructive jaundice: the role of gastrointestinal bile flow. Surg Res Comm 5:11–16

Diamond T, Rowlands BJ (1990) Choledochovesical fistula: a model for sterile 'external' biliary drainage. Surg Res Comm 8:131–138

Diamond T, Rowlands BJ (1991) Endotoxaemia in obstructive jaundice. HPB Surgery (in press)

Diamond T, Dolan S, Thompson RLE, Rowlands BJ (1990) Development and reversal of endotoxaemia and endotoxin related death in obstructive jaundice. Surgery 108:370–375

Diamond T, Dolan S, Rowlands BJ (1991) An improved technique for choledochoduodenostomy in the rat with obstructive jaundice. Lab Animal Sci (in press)

Dixon JM, Armstrong CP, Duffy SW, Davies GC (1983) Factors affecting morbidity and mortality after surgery for obstructive jaundice: a review of 373 patients. Gut 24:845–852

Filkins JP (1970) Bioassay of endotoxin inactivation in the lead-sensitised rat. Proc Soc Exp Biol Med 134:610–612

Franco D, Gigou M, Szekely AM, Bismuth N (1979) Portal hypertension after bile duct obstruction. Arch Surg 114:1064–1067

Gouma DJ, Moody FG (1984) Preoperative percutaneous biliary drainage: use or abuse. Surg Gastroenterol 3:74–80

Gouma DJ, Wesdorp RIC, Oostenbroek RJ, Soeters PB, Greep JM (1983) Percutaneous transhepatic drainage and insertion of an endoprosthesis for obstructive jaundice. Am J Surg 145:763–767

Gouma DJ, Coelho JCU, Fisher JD, Schlegel JF, Li YF, Moody FG (1986) Endotoxaemia after the relief of biliary obstruction by internal and external biliary drainage in rats. Am J Surg 151:476–479

Gouma DJ, Coelho JCU, Schlegel JF, Li YF, Moody FG (1987) The effect of preoperative internal and external biliary drainage on mortality in jaundiced rats. Arch Surg 122:731–734

Greve JW, Gouma DJ, Soeters PB, Buurman WA (1990) Suppression of cellular immunity in obstructive jaundice is caused by endotoxins: a study with germ free rats. Gastroenterology 98:478–485

Gundry SR, Strodel WE, Knol JA, Eckhauser FE, Thompson NW (1984) Efficacy of preoperative biliary tract decompression in patients with obstructive jaundice. Arch Surg 119:703–708

Hatfield ARW, Terblanche J, Fattar S et al. (1982) Preoperative external biliary drainage in obstructive jaundice: a prospective controlled clinical trial. Lancet ii:896–899

Holman JM, Rikkers LF (1982) Biliary obstruction and host defence failure. J Surg Res 32:208–213

Hunt DR (1980) The identification of risk factors and their application to the management of obstructive jaundice. Aust NZ J Surg 50:476–480

Johnstone JMS, Lee EG (1976) A quantitative assessment of the structural changes in the rat's liver following obstruction of the common bile duct. Br J Exp Pathol 57:85–94

Katz S, Grosfeld JC, Gross K, Plager DA, Ross D, Rosenthal RS, Hull M, Weber TR (1984) Impaired bacterial clearance and trapping in obstructive jaundice. Ann Surg 199:14–20

Kocsar LT, Bertok L, Varteresz V (1969) Effect of bile acids on intestinal absorption of endotoxin in rats. J. Bacteriol 100:220–223

Lee E (1972) The effect of obstructive jaundice on the migration of reticuloendothelial cells and fibroblasts into early experimental granulomata. Br J Surg 59:875–877

Lygidakis NJ, Van der Heyde MN, Lubbers MJ (1987) Evaluation of preoperative biliary drainage in the surgical management of pancreatic head carcinoma. Acta Chir Scand 153:665–668

McPherson GAD, Benjamin IS, Hodgson HJF, Bowley NB, Allison DJ, Blumgart LH (1984) Preoperative percutaneous transhepatic biliary drainage: the results of a controlled trial. Br J Surg 71:371–375

Nakayama T, Ikeda A, Okuda K (1978) Percutaneous transhepatic drainage of the biliary tract. Technique and results in 104 cases. Gastroenterology 74:554–559

Pain JA (1987) Reticuloendothelial function in obstructive jaundice. Br J Surg 74:1091–1094

Pain JA, Bailey ME (1986) Experimental and clinical study of lactulose in obstructive jaundice. Br J Surg 73:775–778

Pain JA, Cahill CJ, Bailey ME (1985) Perioperative complications in obstructive jaundice: therapeutic considerations. Br J Surg 72: 942–945

Papa M, Halperin Z, Rubenstein E, Orenstein A, Gafin S, Adar R (1983) The effect of ischaemia on the dog's colon on transmural migration of bacteria and endotoxin. J. Surg Res 35:264–269

Pitt HA, Cameron JL, Postier RG, Gadacz TR (1981) Factors affecting mortality in biliary tract surgery. Am J Surg 141:66–72

Pitt HA, Gomes AS, Lois JF, Mann LL, Deutsch LS, Longmire WP (1985) Does preoperative percutaneous biliary drainage reduce operative risk or increase hospital cost? Ann Surg 201:545–553

Rank J, Wilson ID (1983) Changes in IgA following varying degrees of biliary obstruction in the rat. Hepatology 3:241–247

Roughneen PT, Gouma DJ, Kulkarni AD, Fanslow WF, Rowlands BJ (1986) Impaired specific cell mediated immunity in experimental biliary obstruction and its reversibility by internal biliary drainage. J Surg Res 41:113–125

Roughneen PT, Drath DB, Kulkarni AD, Rowlands BJ (1987) Impaired nonspecific cellular immunity in experimental cholestasis. Ann Surg 206:578–582

Ryan CJ, Than T, Blumgart LH (1977) Choledochoduodenostomy in the rat with obstructive jaundice. J Surg Res 23:321–331

Sirenek, KR, Levine BA (1989) Percutaneous transhepatic cholangiography and biliary decompression. Arch Surg 124:885–888

Smith RC, Pooley M, George CRP, Faithful GR (1985) Preoperative percutaneous transhepatic internal drainage in obstructive jaundice: a randomized controlled trial examining renal function. Surgery 96:641–647

Speer AG, Russell RCG, Hatfield ARW et al. (1987) Randomised trial of endoscopic versus percutaneous stent insertion in malignant obstructive jaundice. Lancet ii:57–62

Tanaka N, Christensen P, Ryder S, Klofver-Stahl B, Bengmark S (1985) Biliary obstruction and susceptibility to biliary sepsis in rats. Res Exp Med (Berl) 185:115–119

Thompson RLE, Hoper M, Diamond T, Rowlands BJ (1990) Development and reversibility of T lymphocyte dysfunction in experimental obstructive jaundice. Br J Surg 77:1229–1232

Trede M, Schwall G (1988) The complications of pancreatectomy. Ann Surg 207:39–41

Vane DW, Redlich P, Weber T, Leapman S, Siddiqui AR, Grosfield JL (1988) Impaired immune function in obstructive jaundice. J Surg Res 45:287–293

Wardle EN, Wright NA (1970) Endotoxin and acute renal failure associated with obstructive jaundice. Br Med J 4:472–474

Whipple AO, Parsons WB, Mullins CR (1935) Treatment of carcinoma of the Ampulla of Vater. Ann Surg 102:763–779

Wilkinson SP, Moodie H, Stamatakis JD, Kakkar VV, Williams R (1976) Endotoxaemia and renal failure in cirrhosis and obstructive jaundice. Br Med J 2:1415–1418

Zwiefach BW (1961) Aspects of comparative physiology of laboratory animals relative to the problem of experimental shock. Fed Proc 20:18–29

Chapter 3

Percutaneous Techniques for the Relief of Jaundice

C. N. Hacking

Introduction

Obstructive jaundice is a common clinical problem for which a variety of percutaneous techniques is available for both diagnosis and treatment. Percutaneous transhepatic cholangiography (PTC) superseded intravenous cholangiography and although endoscopic retrograde cholangiopancreatography (ERCP), where available, is the investigation of choice, PTC is still valuable where ERCP fails or as a prelude to transhepatic interventional procedures.

The surgical management of malignant biliary obstruction is difficult. Localised bile duct carcinoma, ampullary carcinomas and some early or localised pancreatic tumours may be cured by radical surgery. In the majority of cases the nature of the tumour, its extent and the age and general medical condition of the patient prevent any such surgical cure and palliation of the distressing jaundice and pruritus is all that can be offered. Surgical bypass operations successfully relieve these symptoms, but are invasive and carry a mortality of between 5% and 33% depending on the patient's clinical status (Pitt et al. 1981; Blumgart et al. 1984).

Over the past 20 years non-operative techniques have been developed to achieve palliation without surgery with lower morbidity, mortality and a shorter hospital stay. These techniques include percutaneous biliary drainage (PBD), percutaneous transhepatic stent insertion (PSI) and endoscopic retrograde stent insertion (ESI).

Percutaneous Transhepatic Cholangiography (PTC): Percutaneous Biliary Drainage (PBD)

Diagnostic PTC, first introduced in the early 1960s, was rarely used for therapeutic purposes, but by the end of the decade temporary external biliary drainage (EBD) was achieved via a teflon tube with satisfactory relief of jaundice (Kaude et al. 1969) and this quickly gained a place in the management of patients prior to surgery and for long-term palliation in patients thought unsuitable for surgery.

The indications for EBD are summarised in Table 1. Permanent EBD is rarely used now with internal/external biliary drainage (I/EBD) favoured in the USA and internal stents used more commonly in Europe and Japan. It is, however, often an interim stage of a more complicated percutaneous transhepatic procedure.

The technique now employed for PTC and EBD is to opacify the ducts with a fine needle (22–23 gauge) inserted via an intercostal approach in the midaxillary line for right duct punctures and an anterior subcostal approach close to the xiphisternum for left duct punctures. Following intravenous sedation with Diazemuls (diazepam) and pethidine a local anaesthetic (lignocaine 1%) is injected into the skin, subcutaneous tissues and liver capsule.

Through a small incision, the skinny needle is advanced quickly during suspended mid inspiration to a point midway between the gas in the duodenal cap and the dome of the diaphragm. This corresponds to a point just cephalad to the porta hepatis at the level of T10–T12. Under direct X-ray control, the needle is withdrawn slowly whilst simultaneously injecting small puffs of dilute contrast medium.

Rapid flow of contrast towards the midline indicates hepatic vein puncture and rapid peripheral flow indicates puncture of a portal vein radical. Slow, progressive filling occurs after puncture of the bile ducts or gallbladder, but lymphatic puncture and particularly puncture of the extravascular portal tract can be misleading if not recognised quickly. If no bile ducts are encountered the needle is withdrawn to within about 1 cm of the liver surface, re-angled slightly and re-advanced. This is repeated until successful puncture is obtained.

When a bile duct has been successfully punctured dilute contrast is gently injected taking care not to increase the intrabiliary pressure too greatly. This is particularly important in cholangitis, as reflux of bile into the bloodstream will lead to bacteraemia. If bile duct puncture is not achieved despite repeated attempts percutaneous transhepatic gallbladder puncture is permissible.

Gallbladder puncture is most easily performed under ultrasound control, but can be achieved blind by angling the fine needle anteriorly and inferiorly from the original intercostal puncture site. Bile is aspirated and replaced first with

Table 1. Indications for EBD

Failed ERCP
Cholangitis
Palliation of unpassable obstructions
Prior to internal/external biliary drainage
Prior to percutaneous stent insertion
Prior to combined stent insertion
Prior to combined sphincterotomy
Gallstone extraction
Postsurgical or traumatic biliary leak
Dilatation of primary and anastomotic strictures

---

saline until the bile is almost clear and then with contrast. Good filling of the intrahepatic ducts can be achieved with the patient tipped head down, provided that the cystic duct is not occluded by tumour or calculus.

Following satisfactory opacification a suitable intrahepatic duct is chosen to give the optimal path down to the obstructing lesion. The duct chosen should not be too close to the hilum, particularly with proximal disease, but should be of a sufficient diameter to accommodate the final catheter without too much dilatation. Unless the duct punctured initially is suitable, a further 22 gauge needle, which will allow the passage of a fine guide wire (0.018 in platinum tip) is used to puncture this selected duct under direct screening. Dilatation over this wire with larger catheters enables placement of larger guide wires. Alternatively an 18 gauge sheathed needle can be used for this second duct puncture to allow the passage of a larger guide wire without further dilatation.

Over a stiff 0.035 in wire a series of dilators is passed and then a drainage catheter, usually 6–9F with multiple side holes, is placed in a secure part of the biliary tree above the obstructing lesion. This is secured to the skin and drains into an external catheter bag (Fig. 1). Once catheter access to the ducts has been achieved the initial fine needle can be removed.

When initial duct opacification has occurred via the gallbladder, and if it still proves impossible to cannulate and intrahepatic duct, satisfactory drainage

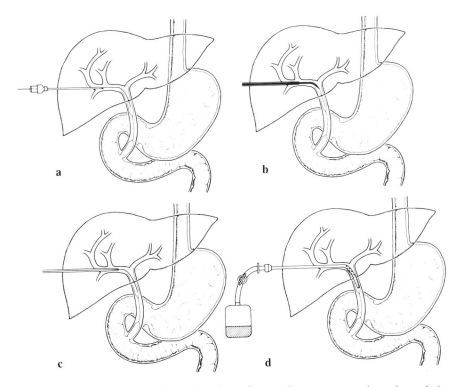

Fig. 1. External biliary drain. Conversion from fine needle puncture to large bore drain. **a** Insertion of 0.018 in stiff wire through 22G needle. **b** A 3.3/5.5F coaxial catheter is passed over the wire. **c** 3.3F catheter and 0.018 in wire are removed and the 0.035 in wire is inserted. **d** An 8.3F drainage catheter is inserted following tract dilatation.

can be established using a cholecystostomy catheter introduced over a wire and using serial dilators (Elyaderani and Gabriele 1979; Pearse et al. 1984).

Internal/External Biliary Drainage (I/EBD)

Conversion of an existing EBD to internal drainage was first described in 1974 (Molnar and Stockum). This requires manipulation of a catheter and guide wire combination through the obstructing lesion. This can be performed during initial duct puncture in over half of cases, but where cholangitis is present and where there is gross duct dilatation it is preferable to perform I/EBD in two sessions separated by at least 24–48 h. An angled biliary manipulation catheter (Cook) and a variety of guide wires are used and the stricture is dilated with catheters or a balloon to accept the final 8–12F drainage catheter. The tip of this catheter is placed in the duodenum and its side holes are positioned both above and below the stricture (Fig. 2). This catheter allows early external drainage, but when any bleeding has subsided and injected contrast flows freely through the catheter, the external tap can be closed to allow bile to drain antegradely into the duodenum.

The principal advantages of this technique are that fluid and electrolyte losses do not occur, percutaneous access to the ducts is maintained and change

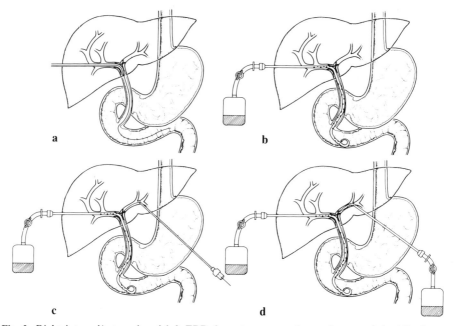

Fig. 2. Right internal/external and left EBD for a tumour at the confluence of the bile duct. **a** 0.035 in wire and 6.5F biliary manipulation catheter are passed through the tumour. **b** Following dilatation an 8.3F I/EBD catheter is placed across the tumour with its tip in the duodenum. Side holes are placed above and below the tumour. **c** Left duct puncture. **d** Left EBD and right I/EBD in place.

of catheter is a simple procedure which can be performed easily on a day case basis. The patient or his relatives quickly learn to manage the catheter at home and to flush them with sterile saline three or more times a week. The catheter is changed routinely every 2–3 months and the patient is instructed that if signs of obstruction occur they are to recommence external drainage and contact the hospital.

The disadvantages are that many patients do not like the constant reminder of their underlying malignancy, the catheters provide a route for infection, pericatheter leakage is not uncommon and skin irritation and infection can occur.

Palliation of symptoms and relief of jaundice is usual if over one-third of the liver is drained. Hilar lesions or intrahepatic tumour may require separate right and left drains (Fig. 2), but more than two drains should be avoided as the potential benefit of complete drainage is outweighed by the inconvenience and increased risk of infection.

Complications of PBD are summarised in Table 2. They can be divided into early and late. Sepsis and haemorrhage are the most frequent early problems, but these can be reduced by careful attention to technique and the use of adequate antibiotics (Ferrucci et al. 1980; Carrasco et al. 1984). Recurrent jaundice can be due to catheter blockage or tumour growth with liver metastases or hilar extension leading to further duct occlusion.

Percutaneous Transhepatic Stent Insertion (PSI)

The dissatisfaction of patients with long-term external catheters of both types described above has led to a number of developments allowing full internalisation of drainage by endoprostheses or stents. PSI was first described in 1978 (Pereiras et al. 1978; Burcharth 1978). It was modified over the next few years and was widely available by the early 1980s. In 1980 the first description of endoscopic stent insertion (ESI) appeared in the literature (Soehendra and Reynders-Frederix 1980). These two techniques developed in parallel and were used as alternatives according to local skills and expertise.

Following successful bile duct puncture the obstructing lesion is negotiated as described above either as a one- or two-stage procedure and a period of

Table 2. Complications of PBD

Early	Late
Cholangitis	Jaundice
Septicaemia	Cholangitis
Biliary peritonitis	Septicaemia
Haemorrhage	Hydroelectrolyte loss
Catheter dislodgement	Pericatheter leakage
Biliary-pleural fistula	Tumour seeding

I/EBD allowed. After at least 48 h this catheter is removed over a stiff 0.035 in or 0.038 in guide wire. The track and malignant stricture are then carefully dilated up to 10–12F with serial dilators. An angioplasty balloon catheter can be used if the structure is particularly resistant.

A variety of transhepatic stent designs is available, but with the exception of the newer metallic stents all are introduced over the stiff guide wire and positioned with a pusher tube. Some designs have a suture attached to their proximal end to allow more accurate positioning and retrieval. The position and length of the stricture are carefully assessed with the wire. A stent is then chosen and when this is satisfactorily placed the pusher tube is withdrawn (Fig. 3).

Temporary EBD is re-established by partially withdrawing the guide wire through the stent and introducing a catheter over this wire to lie alongside the endoprosthesis or in an adjoining duct. Haemobilia after track and stricture dilatation is common and this period of EBD allows the haemobilia to settle before internal drainage is finally established. A cholangiogram after a further 24–48 h is performed and if stent position and patency are satisfactory then the external catheter is removed. Antibiotics are given for a further 48 h or longer if sepsis is suspected.

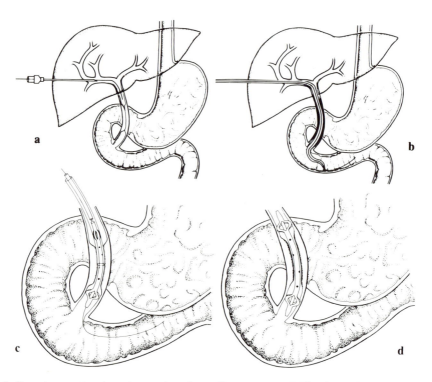

Fig. 3. Percutaneous transhepatic stent insertion. **a** Duct puncture. **b** The obstruction is negotiated with the guide wire. **c** A 12F Miller double mushroom stent (Cook) is introduced through a sheath and pushed into position. **d** The stent in position with one mushroom end above and below the tumour within the bile duct.

Results and Complications of PSI

Technical success for both PSI (Coons and Carey 1983; Burcharth 1984; Dick et al. 1987) and endoscopic stent insertion (ESI) (Huibregtse and Tytgat 1982; Speer et al. 1987) are similar (70%–100%), with good palliation and relief of jaundice. Hilar and intrahepatic obstructions are easier to stent percutaneously (75%–95% vs 65%–85%) as the shorter catheter and guide wires allow more precise control and the percutaneous route allows a more accurate selection of the most appropriate segments to drain. Technical difficulties encountered endoscopically include duodenal diverticula and previous upper gastrointestinal (GI) surgery, whereas percutaneous access and subsequent cannulation is only really contraindicated in uncorrectable coagulopathies.

The complications of PSI are the same as those described for PBD, but the larger bore stents (12–14F) cause more pain during insertion and have a significantly greater early morbidity and perhaps a higher 30-day mortality compared with ESI. The longer time required for the procedure and the increased radiation doses to the operator have also been cited as reasons for abandoning PSI as a first-line treatment in management of these patients (Mendez et al. 1984).

There are only two randomised prospective studies to date which compare complication rates after PSI or conventional bypass surgery (Bornman et al. 1986) and PSI or ESI (Speer et al. 1987). Fifty patients with localised but unresectable carcinoma of the head of the pancreas were randomised for surgical bypass or PSI. Technical success was achieved in 84% for PSI and 76% for surgery. Procedural complication rates were 28% and 32% respectively and the 30-day mortality rate was 8% and 20%. The median survivals were 19 and 15 weeks. None of these observed differences reached statistical significance. In the second study 75 patients with hilar or low strictures were randomised for either PSI or ESI. None were considered suitable for surgery. Technical success was 61% and 81% for PSI and ESI respectively. The procedural morbidity was 67% and 19% and the 30-day mortality 33% and 15%. Other non-randomised studies have shown lower complication rates for PSI, but it is now generally felt that the first treatment should be endoscopic stent insertion when the expertise is available. PSI should be considered if this proves impossible.

Combined Endoscopic and Percutaneous Stent Insertion (CSI)

We have developed a combination of endoscopic and percutaneous techniques in order to increase the technical success of ESI. This has been termed the rendezvous procedure or combined stent insertion (CSI) (Robertson et al. 1987).

This technique of percutaneous assistance for the endoscopist was first used in the treatment of common duct stones to allow sphincterotomy to be performed on patients in whom initial endoscopic biliary cannulation was unsuccessful (Mason and Cotton 1981; Shorvon et al. 1985).

Following failed ERCP access to a suitable bile duct is obtained by the techniques described under PBD. If a catheter and guide wire can be manipulated through the obstruction a one-stage procedure is performed, but if this is not possible, or there is cholangitis, or an endoscopist is unavailable, a two-stage procedure is planned.

The bile duct is drained externally for a short period with a 6F catheter whether or not the catheter has been passed through into the duodenum. If the EBD catheter remains above the obstruction after the first stage then the initial task of the interventional radiologist at the second stage is to manipulate a wire and catheter through into the duodenum. The wire is used to calculate the exact length of the stricture and its distance above the ampulla. A 450 cm guide wire is then placed through a biliary manipulation catheter (Cook) into the duodenum.

The patient is then turned into a prone–oblique position, sedated further if necessary and a large channel side viewing duodenoscope is passed to visualise the ampulla. The catheter and guide wire show the position of the ampulla even if it is deep inside a diverticulum.

A Dormia basket is passed through the endoscope to collect the tip of the long wire. This task is simplified if the radiologist can see the endoscopic view, either through a side arm or on a video monitor. He withdraws the manipulation catheter until only its deflected tip lies outside the ampulla and then withdraws the wire until it protrudes a few millimetres beyond the catheter tip. The endoscopist lines up the Dormia basket close to the ampulla and the radiologist advances the wire whilst turning the catheter if necessary.

The wire is grasped and then withdrawn up the endoscope until it emerges through the top of the operating channel. It is important for both operators to ensure that the passage of this wire is carefully controlled.

At this point the long wire is held by the radiologist, it passes through the skin, liver, biliary tree, ampulla and endoscope and its other end is controlled by the endoscopist's assistants. A 7F guiding catheter is passed over the endoscopist's end of the wire and fed down the endoscope with the bridge locked. When it reaches the bridge this is unlocked and with the biliary manipulation catheter withdrawn above the stricture and the wire held taut by the radiologist the guiding catheter is passed through the ampulla, up the common bile duct and through the obstructing tumour (Fig. 4).

The endoscopist then passes a 10–11F stent over the guiding catheter and down through the endoscope with the aid of a pusher tube. Once again this is performed with the bridge locked to prevent looping of the guiding catheter and wire in the duodenum. The bridge is unlocked and the stent is pushed up the bile duct to the level of the tumour. The radiologist keeps the wire taut as the endoscopist pushes the stent through the tumour. If resistance is met then careful withdrawal of the percutaneous wire pulls the guiding catheter and stent up through the lesion as the endoscopist pushes. In our hands this combination of pushing and pulling has enabled all lesions to be intubated.

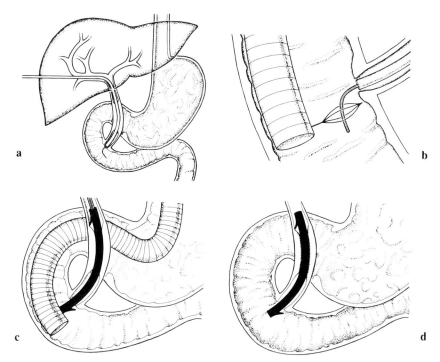

Fig. 4. Combined endoscopic and percutaneous stent insertion. **a** The catheter and wire are negotiated through the tumour into the duodenum. **b** 450 cm long guide wire is grasped by a Dormia basket and is then pulled up through the endoscope. **c** The stent is pushed out of the endoscope and pushed/pulled into position. **d** Final position of the stent.

Results and Complications of CSI

No controlled studies have yet been published comparing CSI with PSI, but it seems that the overall success rate of endoscopic stenting can be increased from about 70%–80% to almost 100% by the addition of the combined technique (Robertson et al. 1987). Morbidity and 30-day mortality are not significantly different from PSI, but patient discomfort is reduced, as CSI requires percutaneous insertion of only a 5 or 6F catheter as opposed to a 12–14F dilator, and the length of time the radiologist spends with his or her hands close to the X-ray beam is reduced (Hall et al. 1989). For these reasons in many institutions CSI has replaced PSI in the majority of cases following failed ESI.

A further advantage of CSI over PSI is that if recurrent jaundice occurs with or without cholangitis, stent change can usually be performed endoscopically with only occasional need for a further combined procedure. Conversely replacement of a percutaneously placed stent can be difficult particularly if the distal end of the stent is left in the common duct above the ampulla and therefore out of reach of the endoscopist. This position is chosen intentionally to try to maintain competence of the ampulla and prevent reflux of bacteria and food particles up the stent. Several authors have described ways of performing stent changes by puncturing the proximal end of the transhepatic stent with a fine needle. An 0.018 in wire can be threaded through this needle and then dilating catheters passed over this wire until a 0.035 in wire can be accepted. This wire can then be used to re-bore the lumen of the stent, but if stent change is still necessary a balloon catheter can be fed along the wire and into the lumen of the stent. The balloon is then partially inflated and the stent can be either pushed through into the duodenum or removed through a percutaneous sheath (Harries-Jones et al. 1982; Adam 1987).

Choices Available for Palliative Treatment

Satisfactory palliation of symptoms and relief of jaundice can be achieved with all the non-operative methods described above. Patients prefer an internal stent for long-term drainage. EBD can be used for short-term drainage prior to stent insertion or for the emergency treatment of cholangitis. ESI is the safest technique for internal drainage and should be attempted first. After failure of this technique, CSI will usually achieve success. Surgical bypass can therefore be reserved for patients with impending duodenal obstruction who need duodenal bypass as well as a biliary drainage procedure. Surgical bypass is also appropriate for those younger, fitter patients with tumours thought to be resectable on all imaging criteria, but who at operation are found to have irresectable tumours.

Factors Controlling Stent Function

All currently available stents suffer from a number of problems. Many will become clogged with biliary sludge after a few months, and tumour overgrowth or stent migration can occur. The many different types of stents available testify to the various ways that these problems have been tackled.

Stent clogging occurs following the deposition of bacteria and sludge on the inside of the stent (Speer et al. 1986). Crystals form and the ensuing concretions increase until luminal patency is lost. Different stent materials have varying resistance to encrustation. Polyurethane is better than polyethylene which in turn is better than teflon.

Antibiotics have been incorporated into catheter materials (Trooskin et al. 1985). This should in theory prolong stent patency. Biomechanical methods which attempt to mimic the normal cellular membrane as closely as possible (and so reduce bacterial adherence) show early promise (Dooley, personal communication).

Stent diameter also plays an important part in patency and so ever larger stents have been used. The limitations of endoscopic channel size and the dangers of over dilatation of the transhepatic tract have led to the intro-duction of expandable metal stents with internal diameter of 1 cm. (Gilliams et al. 1990). Two types show excellent promise. Placement of the Wallstent

(Schneider) is achieved by withdrawing a plastic membrane which holds the stent in its compressed form. As the membrane is pulled back the self-expanding stent springs open, shortening as it does so, and dilates the stricture (Fig. 5). The stent in its compressed form can be delivered on a 7F catheter, which avoids the need for excessive tract dilatation. Before its final release the stent can be withdrawn into a satisfactory position. The stent will expand slowly over a two-week period, but in tough strictures balloon inflation inside the stent has been advocated to achieve a larger internal diameter more quickly. The second stent, the Gianturco Z-stent (Cook), in its present form is not so suitable for malignant strictures, due to tumour growth directly into the lumen, but is perhaps the stent of choice for benign strictures (Dick, personal communication).

Initial experience with the Wallstent suggested that the duration of stent patency was not significantly longer than for conventional stents (Gilliams et al. 1990), but many of the occlusions were due to the earliest available stents being too short. This led to suboptimal stent placement and tumour overgrowth. Another series with a choice of stent lengths has been more encouraging with only three stents blocking in 41 patients. All these occlusions were from tumour overgrowth and none as yet from bile encrustation (Adam et al. 1991).

There are two problems with this technique. Tumour in-growth through the fine wire mesh of the Wallstent has been reported, and the present cost of

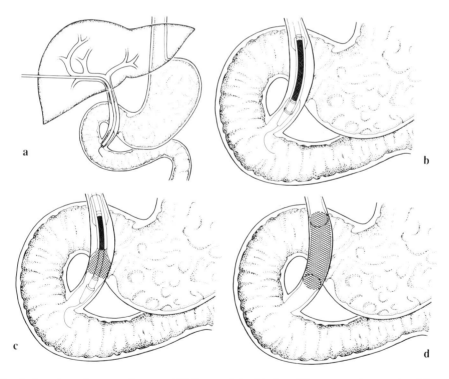

Fig. 5. Insertion of a metallic stent (Wallstent, Schneider). **a** The tumour is negotiated by a catheter/wire combination. **b** Stent introducer system is placed across the stricture. **c** Withdrawal of the membrane releases the self-expanding metallic mesh stent. **d** Stent in position.

these stents has prevented their introduction into common usage.

It is likely that they will gain in popularity for the treatment of hilar cholangiocarcinomas, where there is a relatively long life expectancy, and the need for left and right duct drainage often occurs. The endoscopist is least successful in this group. The Wallstent can now be inserted endoscopically, but this approach is likely to be reserved for patients with a better prognosis and more distal disease.

The problem of stent migration has been addressed by a variety of different designs with varying degrees of success. The metallic stents have not been reported to migrate; in fact it is very difficult to remove them at all, even surgically.

Benign Biliary Strictures

Table 3 shows the causes of the most common causes of biliary stricture. The post surgical strictures are the most amenable to balloon dilatation. Duct injury at cholecystectomy is the commonest cause; following surgical repair of this up to 90% will restricture within seven years.

Balloon dilatation of these strictures compares favourably with surgery and after multiple reconstructive operations may be the only available approach if further anastomotic strictures occur. Patency rates of 67% at three years for all strictures and 76% for iatrogenic strictures have been reported (Mueller et al. 1986).

Limited technical success has been met in dilating strictures in sclerosing cholangitis (Skolkin et al. 1989), but this can adversely affect subsequent liver transplantation and so should be avoided if possible.

Access to the ducts for dilatation of benign strictures can be achieved via right or left hepatic duct punctures as described above. Where recurrent strictures at a biliary-enteric anastomosis occur, success has been reported with direct percutaneous puncture of a subcutaneously positioned jejunal loop. This is fixed in the right side of the abdomen and marked with a ring of metal clips. A fine needle is used to puncture the loop under radiographic control and if an injection of contrast proves this to be in the desired loop, a wire is introduced and the track dilated to accept a biliary manipulation catheter which is then used for retrograde cannulation of the anastomosis.

With a stiff wire through the stricture from either above or below a low

Table 3. Types of biliary stricture

Malignant	
Benign	Iatrogenic or post-traumatic
	Anastomotic
	Sclerosing cholangitis
	Stone-related
	Pancreatitis

profile balloon catheter is inserted, placed across the stricture and inflated. A high pressure balloon (Olbert biliary balloon – Meadox) is essential as pressures of 12–15 atmospheres are often needed to dilate these fibrotic strictures. The balloon is held inflated for 1–2 min or until the stricture is seen to dilate. Biliary access is maintained with an external drain and a further cholangiogram is performed at 24–48 h. This may show further stricturing, which necessitates further dilatations. Only when the cholangiogram shows a satisfactory result should the drainage catheter be removed. Dilating these fibrotic strictures can be extremely painful and since many of the patients will be anxious and have had several operations in the past it is advisable to perform the procedure under general anaesthetic or heavy sedation/analgesia.

Gallstones

Obstructive jaundice secondary to gallstones is now most commonly managed endoscopically with sphincterotomy and retrograde stone removal. Where ERCP is not available or where for technical or anatomical reasons endoscopic removal proves impossible there are a number of percutaneous techniques which should be considered (Table 4).

Extraction Through T-Tube Track

Retained stones after cholecystectomy, although often dealt with endoscopically, can equally easily be removed through a mature T-tube track; this approach has a lower morbidity (Burhenne 1980). The T-tube is removed over a guide wire and a sheath is inserted into the CBD. A second safety wire is placed in the ducts and a steerable catheter inserted (10–12F). A three- or four-wire basket can then be passed through this steerable catheter to collect any stones and deliver them into the duodenum. Large stones can be crushed with mechanical, electromagnetic or ultrasonic contact lithotripsy and balloon sphincteroplasty can be performed if necessary.

Table 4. Percutaneous gallstone removal

Extraction through T-tube track
Transhepatic extraction
Intrahepatic
Extrahepatic
Balloon sphincteroplasty
Balloon stricturoplasty
Biliary lavage
Contact lithotripsy
Dissolution therapy
Combined percutaneous and endoscopic extraction

Transhepatic Stone Extraction

Stones in intrahepatic or extrahepatic bile ducts can be managed percutaneously by using many of the techniques described above (Clouse and Falchuk 1983; Haskin and Teplik 1985).

Percutaneous cholangiography or cholecystography is performed to outline the ductal anatomy and position of any stones and their relationship to co-existing benign or malignant strictures. A suitable duct is chosen, punctured and catheterised in the way described. A period of EBD for 2–3 days is advisable as infection is present in up to 90% of patients. The drain is removed over a wire, a sheath is inserted and a second safety wire is placed in the duct. A basket is then fed through an open-ended 8F catheter, the stones are flushed down into the distal CBD, collected and deposited in the duodenum.

Strictures are dilated with high-pressure biliary dilatation balloons (Olbert). Biliary lavage may be necessary to clear large numbers of small stones and sludge. Giant stones can be dealt with by mechanical, contact or if available, extracorporeal shock wave lithotripsy. Balloon sphincteroplasty with balloons up to 15 mm in diameter can be used safely (Berkman et al. 1988) and resistant stones, particularly if high in cholesterol, can be reduced in size with a 5–7 day infusion of mono-octanoin (3–5 ml/h) and then dealt with using the techniques just described (Haskin et al. 1984).

Combined Percutaneous and Endoscopic Extraction

Technical and anatomical reasons for failure to cannulate the ampulla endoscopically can be overcome by using percutaneous assistance (Mason and Cotton 1981; Shorvon et al. 1985). The technique is as described for combined stent insertions and once again its advantage is the use of smaller gauge transhepatic catheters.

References

Adam A (1987) Use of the modified introduction set for transhepatic removal of obstructed Carey–Coons biliary endoprosthesis. Clin Radiol 38:171–174

Adam A, Chetty N, Roddie M et al. (1991) Self-expandible stainless steel endoprostheses for treatment of malignant bile duct obstruction. AJR 156:321–325

Berkman WA, Bishop AF, Palagallo GL et al. (1988) Transhepatic balloon dilatation of the distal common bile duct and ampulla of Vater for removal of calculi. Radiology 167:453–455

Blumgart LH, Hadjis N, Benjamin IS et al. (1984) Surgical approaches to cholangiocarcinoma at confluence of hepatic ducts. Lancet i:66–70

Bornman C, Tobias R, Harries-Jones EP et al. (1986) Prospective controlled trial of transhepatic biliary endoprosthesis versus bypass surgery for incurable carcinoma of the pancreas. Lancet i:69–71

Burcharth F (1978) A new endoprosthesis for non-operative intubation of the biliary tree in malignant obstructive jaundice. Surg Gynecol Obstet 146:76–78

Burcharth F (1984) Results of the percutaneous implantation of endoprosthesis. In: Classen M, Geenan J, Kawai K (eds) Non-surgical biliary drainage. Springer-Verlag, Berlin, pp 47–55

Burhenne HJ (1980) Percutaneous extraction of retained biliary tract stones: 661 patients. AJR 134:888–898

Carrasco CH, Zornoza J, Bechtel WJ (1984) Malignant biliary obstruction: complications of percutaneous biliary drainage. Radiology 152:343–346

Clouse ME, Falchuk KR (1983) Percutaneous transhepatic removal of common duct stones. Gastroenterology 85:815–819

Coons HG, Carey PH (1983) Large-bore, long biliary endoprostheses (biliary stents) for improved drainage. Radiology 148:89–94

Dick R, Platts A, Gilford J et al. (1987) The Carey–Coons percutaneous biliary endoprosthesis: a three-centre experience in 87 patients. Clin Radiol 38:175–178

Elyaderani M, Gabriele OF (1979) Percutaneous cholecystostomy and cholangiography in patients with obstructive jaundice. Radiology 130:601–602

Ferrucci JT, Mueller PR, Harbin WP (1980) Percutaneous transhepatic biliary drainage. Radiology 135:1–13

Gilliams A, Dick R, Dooley JS et al. (1990) Self-expandible stainless steel braided endoprosthesis for biliary strictures. Radiology 174:137–140

Hall RI, Denyer ME, Chapman AH (1989) Palliation of obstructive jaundice with a biliary endoprosthesis. Comparison of insertion by the percutaneous–transhepatic and combined percutaneous–endoscopic routes. Clin Radiol 40:186–189

Harries-Jones EP, Fataar S, Tuft RJ (1982) Repositioning of biliary endoprosthesis with Gruntzig balloon catheters AJR 138:771–772

Haskin PH, Teplik SK (1985) Percutaneous management of biliary stones. Semin Intervent Radiol 2:81–96

Haskin PH, Teplik SK, Gambescia et al. (1984) Percutaneous transhepatic removal of a common duct stone after monooctanoin. Radiology 151:247–248

Huibregtse K, Tytgat GN (1982) Palliative treatment of obstructive jaundice by transpapillary introduction of large bore bile duct endoprosthesis. Gut 23:371–375

Kaude JV, Weidenmier CH, Agee OF (1969) Decompression of bile ducts with the percutaneous transhepatic technic. Radiology 93:69–71

Mason RR, Cotton PB (1981) Combined duodenoscopic and transpapillary approach to stenosis of the Papilla of Vater. Br J Radiol 54:678

Mendez G, Russell E, Le Page JR et al. (1984) Abandonment of endoprosthetic drainage technique in malignant biliary obstruction. AJR 143:617–622

Molnar W, Stockum AE (1974) Relief of obstructive jaundice through percutaneous transhepatic catheter – a new therapeutic method. AJR 122:356–367

Mueller PR, van Sonnenberg E, Ferrucci JT Jr et al. (1986) Biliary stricture dilatation: multicenter review of clinical management in 73 patients. Radiology 160:17–22

Pearse DM, Hawkins IF Jr, Shaver R et al. (1984) Percutaneous cholecystostomy in acute cholecystitis and common duct obstruction. Radiology 152:365–367

Pereiras RV, Rheingold OJ, Hutson D et al. (1978) Relief of malignant obstructive jaundice by percutaneous insertion of a permanent prosthesis in the biliary tree. Ann Intern Med 89:589–593

Pitt HA, Cameron JL, Postier RG et al. (1981) Factors affecting mortality in biliary tract surgery Am J Surg 141:66–71

Robertson DAF, Hacking CN, Birch S et al. (1987) Experience with a combined percutaneous and endoscopic approach to stent insertion in malignant obstructive jaundice. Lancet ii:1449–1452

Shorvon PJ, Cotton PB, Mason RR (1985) Percutaneous transhepatic assistance for duodenoscopic sphincterotomy. Gut 26:1373–1376

Skolkin MD, Alspaugh JP, Casarella WJ et al. (1989) Sclerosing cholangitis: palliation with percutaneous cholangioplasty. Radiology 170:199–206

Soehendra N, Reynders-Frederix V (1980) Palliative bile duct drainage; a new endoscopic method of introducing a transpapilliary stent. Endoscopy 12:8–11

Speer AG, Farrington H, Costerton JW et al. (1986) Bacteria, biofilms and biliary sludge. (Abstract) Gut 27:A601

Speer G, Russell RCG, Hatfield ARW et al. (1987) Randomised trial of endoscopic versus percutaneous stent insertion in malignant obstructive jaundice. Lancet ii:57–62

Trooskin SZ, Donetz AP, Harvey RA et al. (1985) Prevention of catheter sepsis by antibiotic bonding. Surgery 97:547–551

Adenocarcinoma of the Pancreas

Chapter 4

The Molecular Biology of Pancreatic Adenocarcinoma

Judith Gillespie and G. J. Poston

Carcinoma of the exocrine pancreas is now the fifth leading cause of death from malignant disease in Western society (Carter 1990) yet there has been little improvement in the outcome of treatment for pancreatic cancer since the beginning of this century. What improvement there has been is largely due to the use of radical surgery with low mortality in specialist centres of excellence (Trede and Schwall 1988). As a conseqeunce, the diagnosis of carcinoma of the pancreas still remains a virtual death sentence for the vast majority of patients, the overall five-year survival rate being less than 2%. Unfortunately, most epidemiological studies show an increasing incidence of the disease, particularly among the elderly, in whom it appears to have trebled over the last 50 years (Carter 1990). Although the aetiological environmental factors which have been associated with pancreatic cancer have been well documented (Poston and Williamson 1990) and include smoking, high fat/protein diet, coffee, alcohol and exposure to industrial carcinogens, none has been shown to be directly causative.

This chapter explores the molecular biology of pancreatic cancer, and examines some of the potential avenues of treatment which may arise from this knowledge in order to develop new treatment strategies for this otherwise awful disease.

Endocrine Regulation of Pancreatic Cancer

The idea that cancers which arise from hormone target organs might maintain their hormone responsiveness has evolved into the classification of cancers as hormone dependent or independent and has led to the development of treatment regimens aimed at arresting tumour growth by either hormone deprivation or administration of antagonistic agents of these hormones, including other hormones whose actions oppose those hormones which promote tumour growth. The concept of growth factor and hormone regulation of cancer has been extensively and recently reviewed by Goustin et al. (1986). Townsend et al. (1988) have specifically reviewed the role of growth factors in intestinal neoplasms.

Direct Effects of Hormones on Pancreatic Carcinogenesis

Chronic elevation of plasma cholecystokinin (CCK) in rats by long-term feeding with raw soya flour (for more than four months) will cause hyperplastic foci of pancreatic acinar cells (McGuinness et al. 1987). If the diet is continued for up to 36 weeks, some of these hyperplastic foci will progress to pancreatic cancer, even without the addition of carcinogens (McGuinness et al. 1987). The link between CCK and carcinogenesis, however, is not straightforward since Pour et al. (1988) have shown in the hamster model of pancreatic ductal carcinogenesis that exogenous CCK, given simultaneously with or shortly before the carcinogen BOP, inhibited cancer induction. On the other hand, Satake et al. (1986) found that weekly administration of caerulein enhanced the carcinogenic effect of BMP. Similarly, Howatson and Carter found that both CCK (1985) and secretin (1987) enhanced BOP pancreatic carcinogenesis in hamsters. It may be that the studies which failed to show any effect used insufficient dosages of caerulein to achieve the necessary hyperplastic response. The inhibitory studies may relate to the observation that caerulein also inhibits the growth in nude mice of a human cholangiocarcinoma, known to possess CCK receptors (Hugh et al. 1987). Epidermal growth factor (EGF) promotes BOP pancreatic carcinogenesis in hamsters (Chester et al. 1986) and both the somatostatin analogue RC-160 and luteinising hormone-releasing hormone (LH-RH) reduce BOP pancreatic carcinogenesis and prolong survival in hamsters (Zalatnai and Schally 1989).

Hormone Regulation of Established Tumours

CCK and Secretin

There are good data to show that CCK will promote the growth of established pancreatic cancers in the same way that CCK stimulates normal pancreatic growth. Townsend et al. (1981) reported that the combination of caerulein and secretin (but neither agent alone) produced significant stimulation of growth in a transplantable hamster pancreatic ductal cancer (H2T). Receptors for both hormones have been found in a human pancreatic cancer cell line (Estival et al. 1981). Asperlicin, a competitive non-peptide CCK antagonist, significantly inhibits the growth in nude mice of a human pancreatic adenocarcinoma (SKI) that possesses CCK receptors (Alexander et al. 1987), probably by inhibiting the effect of endogenous CCK. A similar effect is seen in rats with azaserine-induced pancreatic cancer in which tumour growth promoted by exogenous CCK is reduced by the CCK antagonist CR-1409 (Douglas et al. 1989). Upp et al. (1987) reported that the presence of CCK receptors on a human pancreatic cancer (SKI) will predict the response of this cancer to caerulein treatment. Caerulein produced a significant growth response in SKI in vivo. Growth of a tumour without CCK receptors was not affected by caerulein treatment. Furthermore, caerulein treatment enhanced the presence of high affinity binding receptors for CCK in the SKI tumour.

Bombesin

Bombesin, a member of the gastrin releasing peptide (GRP) family of peptide hormones normally promotes pancreatic growth (Stock-Damge et al. 1987) and will promote the growth of azaserine-induced rat acinar tumours (Douglas et al. 1989). However, chronic treatment with bombesin will inhibit the growth of human ductal pancreatic cancers when grown as xenografts in nude mice, while at the same time it stimulates the growth of the normal nude mouse pancreas (Alexander et al. 1988).

VIP

Vasoactive intestinal peptide (VIP) receptors exist on both normal and neoplastic (Yao et al. 1987) pancreatic tissue. Binding of VIP to these receptors promotes intracellular cAMP accumulation which may be a regulatory factor in cell division and growth (Fernandez-Moreno et al. 1985). Poston et al. (1988) have shown that chronic treatment with VIP inhibits the growth of hamster pancreatic cancer in vivo, but not human pancreatic cancer. This effect may be related to the presence of two VIP receptor types (one with molecular weight 66 kDa, and the other with mol.wt 90 kDa) on the hamster pancreatic cancer cells whereas only one type of VIP receptor (mol. wt, 66 kDa) was detectable on the human cancer cell lines (Yao et al. 1987).

Somatostatin

Somatostatin inhibits the growth of a number of malignant tumours and tumour cell lines and its effect on pancreatic carcinogenesis has been described earlier. The oncological application of somatostatin and its analogues has been extensively reviewed by Schally (1988).

In 1984 Redding and Schally described the inhibition of both rat and hamster pancreatic cancer by administration of somatostatin. Subsequently Upp et al. (1988) reported that the somatostatin analogue SMS 201-995 inhibits the growth of human pancreatic cancer in nude mice. Recent reports suggest that this response may be potentiated by the oestrogen antagonist tamoxifen (Poston et al. 1990). In vitro, somatostatin reverses the growth-potentiating effect of EGF on MIA PACA-2 human pancreatic cancer cells (Liebow et al. 1989) and H2T hamster ductal pancreatic cancer cells (unpublished data), which may be through promotion of tyrosine phosphatase activity interacting with the EGF receptor (Liebow et al. 1990).

Not only does somatostatin treatment prolong tumour doubling time but it may result in programmed cell death (apoptosis) in carcinogen-induced pancreatic cancer in hamsters; in some cases completely preventing the development of carcinogen-induced tumours (Szende et al. 1989, 1990). In addition to causing tumour regression long-term treatment of hamster ductal pancreatic cancers with somatostatin analogue RC-160 also down-regulated insulin like growth factor 1 (IGF-1) receptor expression. IGF-1 has been demonstrated to be trophic to human pancreatic cancer cell lines in vitro (Ohmura et al. 1990). Although evidence exists from studies in vitro for a directly mediated response (Fekete et al. 1989), somatostatin may also affect tumour growth in vivo by inhibiting other hormones such as CCK which may promote tumour growth. We have recently demonstrated somatostatin analogue inhibition of EGF and growth of pancreatic cancer stimulated by transforming growth factor alpha in a hamster model (unpublished data).

Membrane receptors for somatostatin have been demonstrated on a number of experimental models of hamster pancreatic cancer (Fekete et al. 1989 and unpublished data) in addition to a number of human pancreatic cancers (Fekete et al. 1989 and Dr Pomila Singh, Galveston, TX, personal communication).

Epidermal Growth Factor and Transforming Growth Factors

Epidermal growth factor (EGF) promotes pancreatic carcinogenesis in hamsters (Chester et al. 1986) and promotes the growth of human pancreatic cancer cells in vitro (Liebow et al. 1989).

Normally, stimulation of the EGF receptor down-regulates EGF receptor expression, so reducing the number of available EGF receptors (Korc and Magun 1985). This occurs by phosphorylation of membrane proteins (Hierowski et al. 1985). The pancreas is one of the richest sources in the body of mRNA for prepro-EGF (Rall et al. 1985), which suggests the possibility of autocrine growth stimulation of pancreatic cancer by EGF production. The EGF receptor is the cellular homologue of the avian erythroblastosis virus erb-B proto-oncogene (Downward et al. 1984). The genes for pancreatic neuropeptide Y (NPY) and erb B overlap on human chromosome 7 (Takeuchi et al. 1986). Korc et al. (1986) have shown that human pancreatic cancer cells overexpress the gene for EGF receptor with concomitant changes on chromosome 7. These increases in expression of EGF receptor may be as great as 100-fold (Chen et al. 1990).

Normal fibroblasts must attach to a surface to grow in vitro. However, if exposed to substances which reversibly transform them, these same fibroblasts can grow in suspension; such factors have been termed transforming growth factors (TGF). Two groups of TGF have been identified: TGF-alpha is a 5.6 kDa polypeptide structurally related to EGF with which it exhibits a 35% homology, with six cysteine residues in the same relative positions, and it can bind to and stimulate the EGF receptor (Korc 1989). TGF-beta constitutes a separate distinct polypeptide family of about 25 kDa in size with no sequence homology with TGF-alpha (Roberts et al. 1983). TGF-betas do not bind to the EGF recptor but stimulate a separate unique receptor to induce c-sis oncogene mRNA expression which in turn induces a mitogenic response through production of platelet-derived growth factor (PDGF) (Leof et al. 1986). However, in contrast to their effect on mesenchymal cells, TGF-betas are the most potent growth inhibitory peptide known for a number of epithelial cells (Moses et al. 1985). Both TGF-alpha and -beta are produced by breast (Lippmann et al. 1986) and colon cancers (Coffey et al. 1986).

Several cultured human pancreatic cancer cell lines produce TGF-alpha in addition to EGF. TGF-alpha is 10–100 times more potent that EGF in stimulating anchorage-independent growth of these cell lines (Ohmura et al. 1990). TGF-alpha binds to pancreatic EGF receptors where it is degraded following receptor stimulation (Korc 1989). In addition, Derynck's group have demonstrated in NRK fibroblasts that transmembrane TGF-alpha precursors can activate adjacent EGF/TGF-alpha receptors in the cell membrane and so stimulate anchorage-dependent cell growth (Brachmann et al. 1989). However, the binding of TGF-alpha to the EGF receptor does not down-regulate the expression of the EGF receptor, which normally occurs with EGF stimulation (Korc and Magun 1985; Korc 1989) and so binding of TGF-alpha may result in an uncontrolled autocrine growth effect. This effect is reversed in cell cultures on soft agar containing anti-TGF-alpha monoclonal antibody. On the other hand, some pancreatic cancer cells have been shown to produce TGF-beta which in turn inhibits their own growth (Korc 1989). These findings suggest that TGF-alpha participates in the regulation of pancreatic cancer cell proliferation and point to the possible existence of a TGF-alpha/EGF receptor autocrine cycle whose function may be modulated by TGF-beta (Smith et al. 1987). We have recently demonstrated that exogenous administration of TGF-alpha stimulates the growth of hamster pancreatic cancer in vivo (unpublished data).

In a seminal paper, Beauchamp et al. (1990) have been able to dissect out the interrelationship of TGF-alpha, TGF-beta 1 and 3, basic fibroblast growth factor (b-FGF), and c-sis (PDGF-beta) in human pancreatic cancer cell lines. Both MIA PACA 2 and PANC 1 expressed mRNA for all these factors by Northern blot analysis. However, only PANC 1 expressed TGF-beta 2 transcripts. TGF-beta activity was detectable in medium conditioned by either cell line, but TGF-alpha-like activity was not detected in medium from either cell line by radioreceptor assay. Both TGF-alpha and EGF caused a concentration-dependent stimulation of soft agar colony growth of MIA PACA-2 cells on soft agar, but only TGF-alpha promoted the growth of PAN 1 in the same system. Similarly, b-FGF caused a concentration-dependent stimulation of MIA PACA 2 but not PANC 1 and PDGF had no effect on the growth of either cell line. Although both cell lines exhibited high affinity, saturable TGF-beta binding sites, and TGF-beta 1 was capable of autoinduction of TGF-beta 1 mRNA expression in PANC 1 cells, TGF-beta had no stimulatory or inhibitory effect on soft agar colony growth of either cell line. They concluded that the ability of pancreatic cancer cells to respond to positive growth regulatory factors, coupled with the loss of responsiveness to negative growth factors may be important in determining the pathogenicity of these tumours in vivo.

Pancreatic secretory trypsin inhibitor (PSTI) is a peptide of 56 amino acid residues which is present in pancreatic acinar cells and is secreted into pancreatic juice where it is believed to protect the pancreas against prematurely activated proteases (Freeman et al. 1990). PSTI has some sequence homology with EGF and their corresponding genes share nearly 50% homology (Hunt et al. 1974). PSTI has been detected in some pancreatic cancers (Ogata 1988). Freeman et al. (1990) have recently reported that PSTI promotes the growth of the rat acinar pancreatic cancer cell line AR4-2J in vitro but this response does not appear to be mediated via the EGF receptor.

Steroids and LH-RH

Analogues and antagonists of leuteinising hormone-releasing hormone (LH-RH) have been shown to inhibit the growth, and in some case to cause tumour regression with apoptosis, of carcinogen-induced ductal pancreatic cancers in hamsters (Schally et al. 1984). Membrane receptors for LH-RH have been demonstrated on both experimental hamster pancreatic cancers and human pancreatic cancers (Fekete et al. 1989).

There has been recent interest in the use of steroid hormones and their antagonists in the therapy of pancreatic cancer (Andren-Sandberg 1986). Certainly, oestrogen receptors can be demonstrated on normal (Tesone et al. 1979) and neoplastic (Greenway et al. 1981) pancreatic tissue in both man and carcinogen-induced rat acinar tumours. Androgen receptors are found on both normal pancreas and pancreatic cancers (Corbishley et al. 1986) and both glucocorticoids and sex steroid hormones play a regulatory role in normal exocrine pancreatic secretion and growth (Gullo et al. 1982).

In the laboratory it is much more difficult to induce pancreatic cancers with azaserine in female rats than it is in male rats, but this can be overcome with prior oophorectomy and tamoxifen treatment (Lhoste et al. 1986). Similarly, oestrogen therapy and castration inhibit the early stages of acinar pancreatic carcinogenesis following azaserine treatment in male rats (Sumi et al. 1989). There is good evidence that 4-hydroxytamoxifen inhibits the growth of human pancreatic cancer cells through specific antioestrogen binding sites, although these effects bear little relationship to oestrogen receptor content (Benz et al. 1986).

Plasma levels of circulating androgens are decreased in patients, particularly men, with pancreatic cancer (Greenway et al. 1983) and this has led some to claim that low levels of testosterone may be an endocrine marker for the disease (Tulassy et al. 1988). It is true that studies on rat pancreatic cancer (Hayashi and Katayama 1981) and human pancreatic cancer in nude mice (Greenway et al. 1983) and tissue culture (Benz et al. 1986) show a trophic effect of androgens on the growth of the tumour cells. This may be one reason for the higher incidence of the disease in males. However, in male hamsters, castration promotes the growth of transplantable ductal cancers, although this effect may be mediated by increased release of endogenous gastrin (Lawrence et al. 1988). Testosterone may act either directly on the cancer cells or it may be converted by aromatase into oestrogen or by 5α-reductase to the more potent 5α-dihydrotestosterone, after internalisation into the pancreatic cancer cells (Iqbal et al. 1983).

Glucocorticoids stimulate the growth of human pancreatic cancer cells and rat AR42J acinar cancer cells in vitro and also promote the synthesis of amylase mRNA, production of secretory organelles and enzyme secretion by these cells in tissue culture (Logsdon et al. 1985).

Other Peptides

High affinity receptors for human tumour necrosis factor-alpha (TNF-alpha) and interferon-gamma have been detected on a number of human pancreatic cancer cell lines (Raitano et al. 1990). Although a dose-dependent inhibitory effect of TNF-alpha could be demonstrated, which correlated with the presence and number of cytokine receptors, no such relationship could be demonstrated for interferon-gamma. However, incubation of one of the cell lines, COLO 357, with both labelled TNF and interferon led to internalisation of both agents. It was concluded, on the basis of these observations, that any response to cytokines by pancreatic cancer cell lines was governed by post-receptor events rather than by differences in receptor number or affinity.

Intracellular Mechanisms

The function of regulatory peptides and steroids is to transmit information. However, a specific receptor must exist for each peptide to initiate its own specific response. Molecules of similar structure, such as CCK and gastrin or EGF and TGF-alpha may act on unique receptors, related receptors or the same receptor, particularly if they may stimulate two or more separate responses from the same cell. For example, CCK will both stimulate acinar secretion of enzymes and also promote acinar cell division. The receptor proteins for peptide hormones exist on the cell membrane whereas those for steroid hormones exist either in the cytosol or within the nucleus (Williams 1987). In the case of CCK the initial site of peptide receptor binding in acinar cells is the basolateral membrane domain. At physiological temperatures (30–37°C) the bound hormone is subsequently internalised and localised within specific intracellular compartments where it may have direct actions (Goldfine and Williams 1983). Similarly insulin, IGF II, EGF and somatostatin are all internalised in the acinar cells following receptor binding, although to varying degrees and extents (Logsdon and Williams 1984; Mossner et al. 1984a). The main problem in interpretation of these data is that whereas Scatchard analysis of binding of radiolabelled agonist to receptor ligand will give the number and binding affinity of membrane receptors in each sample, this technique produces a static picture which does not clarify the events occurring beyond the membrane once internalisation has occurred. On the other hand, autoradiographic studies of radiolabelled agonist bound to receptors either on microscopy or following gel electrophoresis of lysed cells will give information about receptor size and site but not about the kinetics of the initial reaction. Thus most of the data derived so far about number of functional receptors per cell at any given moment are probably inaccurate.

Cell receptor populations are not static, but are constantly increased (up-regulation) or decreased (down-regulation) by alterations in the rate of receptor synthesis and degradation in response to stimulus drive and target cell response. Down-regulation of acinar receptors has been demonstrated in vitro for insulin and acetylcholine (Mossner et al. 1984b); Hootman et al. 1986). Binding characteristics of specific receptors are also affected by the occupancy of totally separate hormone-receptor species. For instance, somatostatin enhances binding of oestradiol to its cytosolic protein in the rat pancreas (Band et al. 1983) and treatment with CCK decreases the binding of EGF, IFG-II and somatostatin to their respective receptors (Sakamoto et al. 1984; Matozaki et al. 1986).

In general, those hormones which stimulate the release of pancreatic enzymes are mediated intracellularly by Ca^{2+} and diacylglycerol (DAG) whereas those hormones which regulate ductal secretion are mediated via cyclic AMP (cAMP) (Williams and Hootman 1986), although this division is not absolute. A third class of hormone regulators which are primarily concerned with metabolism and induction of protein synthesis activate tyrosine kinase (Liebow et al. 1990). Unlike the stimulatory peptides, somatostatin regulates growth by stimulation of tyrosine phosphatase to produce activated tyrosine phosphatase which in turn activates serine kinase and so inhibits cell division and growth (Liebow et al. 1989).

Although oestrogen binding proteins exist in pancreatic cytosol with high binding affinity (Sandberg and Rosenthal 1974), they exhibit different reaction kinetics and are of different molecular size to the high binding affinity oestrogen receptors found in uterine cytosol (Boctor et al. 1983). A separate atypical low affinity oestrogen binding site which requires a peptide cofactor has also been described in the pancreas (Boctor et al. 1981). Pancreatic oestradiol binding proteins are found in both ductal and acinar cells (Boctor et al. 1983) and are known to act in the region of the endoplasmic reticulum.

Second Messengers

As discussed above hormone and growth factor signals generally require the stimulation of a second intracellular chemical messenger (transduction) in order to begin the initiation of a response by the cell. These transduction pathways exhibit autoregulation and directly interact at a number of important modulatory steps (Gorelick 1987). The initial generation of the calcium signal with release of neutral lipids is mediated by the breakdown of phosphatidylinositol (PI) and changes in cyclic nucleotide levels involve the activation of adenylate cyclase.

The breakdown of PI is initiated through the action of a series of phospholipase C and kinases to produce neutral lipids (which activate protein kinase C), inositol triphosphate (IP3) and arachidonic acid (Rasmussen 1986a, b). Subsequent studies have demonstrated the action of some transforming oncogenes on PI turnover (Nishizuka 1984), the effect of phorbol esters on cell transformation (Nishizuka 1986), and the influence of kinase C on both the EGF receptor (Roos et al. 1986) and the transferrin receptor (May et al. 1986). The PI pathway promotes intracellular Ca^{2+} through inositol 1,4, 5-triphosphate (IP3). This soluble product is seen immediately after a hormone–receptor interaction which is subsequently mediated via Ca^{2+} (Rasmussen 1986a,b). Raised intracellular Ca^{2+} activates further enzyme pathways by binding to calmodulin, a calcium binding protein (Gorelick 1987). Increases in the intracellular concentrations of calmodulin have been found in cells undergoing malignant transformation (Means and Dedman 1980). Lastly PI breakdown generates inositol phosphate mediators from arachidonate, probably through the action of phospholipase A2 on phosphatidyl choline or phosphatidylethanolamine (Nishizuka 1984, 1986).

The adenylate cyclase system responds to ligand receptor interaction with the generation of cyclic nucleotides, either promoting of inhibiting cyclase activity (Rasmussen 1986a,b). The G proteins of the cyclase system influence the affinities of receptors for ligand and so may play a role in receptor sensitisation and desensitisation (Sibley and Lefkowitz 1985). Adenylate cyclase has three primary components: G_s, a stimulating subunit; G_i, an inhibiting subunit; and a third, catalytic, subunit (Gilman 1984).

Polyamines

Polyamines (putrescine, spermidine and spermine) are ubiquitous highly charged cations that are required for growth and differentiation in all eukaryotic cells and are particularly important in the regulation of DNA, RNA and protein synthesis (Pegg 1986). Membrane stability and cyclic AMP-independent protein kinases are apparently also influenced by polyamines (Pegg 1986). The mechanisms by which polyamines exert their effects are poorly understood, though their polybasic nature is thought to be an important factor (Scalabrino and Ferioli 1981). High levels of polyamines are found in rapidly dividing cells and a depletion of intracellular polyamines causes a slowing and eventual cessation of cell growth (Janne et al. 1978).

The biosynthesis of polyamines in mammalian systems begins with the decarboxylation of ornithine by the enzyme ornithine decarboxylase (ODC) to form the diamine putrescine. This is the first, and probably rate-limiting step in the polyamine biosynthetic pathway, and ODC activity is greatly elevated during cell division (McCann 1980). Subsequently putrescine is converted by spermidine synthase into spermidine which in turn is converted into spermine by spermine synthase. These last two steps are potentially reversible by polyamine oxidase (Dowling et al. 1985).

During caerulein-stimulated normal pancreatic growth there are increases in content and concentration of all three polyamines within 12–96h after the onset of caerulein administration (Baylin et al. 1978; Morriset and Benrezzak 1984). Total spermidine and spermine content also correlates with the rates of increase in both pancreatic weight and DNA content (Baylin et al. 1978). Because of their antimitogenic potential, numerous pharmacological inhibitors of polyamine biosynthesis have been developed (Scalabrino and Ferioli 1981), most importantly against ODC because of its key regulatory role (Scalabrino and Ferioli 1982). Treatment with one of these, alpha-difluoromethyl-ornithine, (DFMO), suppresses the increase in pancreatic weight induced by caerulein (Benrezzak and Morriset 1984) and this effect can be reversed by administration of putrescine, the biosynthetic product of ODC (Morriset and Benrezzak 1985). Thus, the stimulation of pancreatic DNA synthesis by caerulein appears to be dependent on polyamine synthesis.

ODC activity is greatly elevated in hamster pancreatic cancer cell lines (Black and Chang 1982) and inhibition of ODC with DFMO inhibits the growth of both human and hamster pancreatic cancers (Marx et al. 1983; Chang et al. 1984). This effect is reversed by administration of exogenous putrescine (Chang et al. 1984), and is potentiated by addition of cyclosporine both in vitro and in vivo (Saydjari et al. 1986).

Nuclear Events

Little is known of what occurs after intracellular second messenger promotion during events which stimulate pancreatic growth. However, more is known about the regulation of pancreatic enzyme production during the same dietary changes which promote pancreatic growth (Schick et al. 1984). It seems reasonable, therefore, to review these pathways since some inference may be drawn from stimulatory events which promote both pancreatic secretion and growth. In the pancreas, the synthesis of functional groups of enzymes is regulated by specific hormones, whether these hormones are administered exogenously or produced endogenously (Kern et al. 1987).

Production of proteins by the cell, whether for use within the cell or for export, commences with transcription of the DNA code of a particular gene by RNA polymerase II. Within the nucleus this primary messenger RNA (mRNA) transcript is processed either by the removal of intron sequences by splicing mechanisms, or by addition of a poly(A) tail to the 3' terminus (Kern et al. 1987). The processed mRNA is now transported to the cytoplasm and binds to the 40S and 60S ribosome subunits before the coding sequence of the mRNA is translated into protein (Darnell 1982). The protein product is then either utilised or packaged for export. Regulation of gene expression as protein product can therefore occur at several points (Fig. 1). The events which regulate gene expression involve the interaction of regulatory proteins with specific nucleotide sequences on DNA (Dynan and Tjian 1985). RNA polymerase II initiates transcription after binding to the promoter (TATA) sequence of the gene, which usually lies 30 nucleotides upstream from the DNA nucleotide at which transcription begins. The RNA polymerase then moves downstream from the promoter site, unwinding the DNA and polymerising a single strand of mRNA. This is further regulated by enhanced gene sequences which lie upstream in the 5' flanking region of genes. Enhanced elements either regulate gene expression in a tissue-specific fashion or in

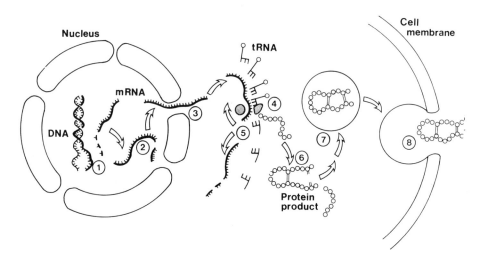

Fig. 1. Pathway of protein synthesis from gene transcription, showing the eight main points of regulation between transcription of the gene from DNA to mRNA to the point of release of protein at the cell membrane. 1, Transcription of DNA to mRNA; 2, Post-transcriptional processing of mRNA; 3, Rate of mRNA transport; 4, Translation of mRNA; 5, Breakdown or recycling of mRNA; 6, Post-translational processing and cleavage of protein product; 7, Storage of protein product; 8, Release or internal use of protein product.

response to individual hormones (Scheele 1986). However, our knowledge of hormone regulation is largely confined to steroid hormones which have receptor proteins that bind directly to DNA (Scheidereit et al. 1983) and so regulate gene expression at the level of transcription.

Little is understood of the regulation of gene expression by peptide hormones and growth factors. Scheele and Kern with their groups have carefully analysed the response to CCK and secretin in the exocrine pancreas (Wicker et al. 1985). They have shown that pronounced changes in individual enzyme biosynthesis were not accompanied by changes in mRNA levels, at least during the first 6h of stimulation, which suggests that these initial changes in gene expression are due to alterations in post-translational processing. This time-related difference in the mechanism of gene expression is probably because exocrine pancreatic product mRNAs have relatively long half-lives of up to 6 h and therefore sudden increases in demand for protein synthesis can be met both at and beyond the translational level, which is the rate-limiting step in protein synthesis. Changes at this level may involve nucleotide signals in the 5'-non-translated region of mRNAs and the interaction of these signals or sequences with either regulatory proteins or regulatory RNA molecules (Kern et al. 1987).

In general, growth factors such as insulin, IGF-1, EGF and platelet-derived growth factor (PDGF) all stimulate phosphorylation of the ribosomal protein S6, but the subsequent effect on promotion or inhibition of cell growth and mitosis is cell type specific (Cochran 1985). In 3T3 fibroblasts, treatment with PDGF stimulates expression of the c-*myc* and c-*fos* oncogenes (Armelin et al. 1984) and similar changes in expression of these oncogenes are seen in many cancer cells.

Little is known about oncogene activity and the role of oncogenes in human pancreatic cancer. As discussed earlier c-*sis* activity (expressed as PDGF-beta) is increased in pancreatic cancer but as yet there is no evidence that PDGF-beta is either a stimulatory or inhibitory growth factor in pancreatic cancer. Increased c-*erb* activity may be the mechanism of overexpression of the EGF/TGF-alpha receptor postulated by Korc (1989). Cooper et al. (1984) have characterised expression of activated *ras*^k gene in human pancreatic cancer cell lines. Activation of this gene appears to be due to an amino acid change on position 12 of the *ras*^k-2 sequence (O'Hara et al. 1986). Oncogenes of the *ras* family encode membrane-bound proteins which possess guanine nucleotide-binding and hydrolytic activities that enable signal transduction across the cell membrane. Single point mutations in *ras* proto-oncogenes activate their oncogenic potential. It has now been shown that mutant c-K-*ras* oncogenes are detectable in over 70% of cytological aspirates from pancreatic malignancies (Shibata et al. 1990), and somatic point mutations at codon 12 in the c-K-*ras* gene exist in the majority of human pancreatic cancers (Almoguera et al. 1988; Smit et al. 1988; Grunewald et al. 1989).

Palmiter and Brinster have created a transgenic model of acinar pancreatic cancer in mice by fusing the SV-40 tumour virus to the elastase 1 gene which is only expressed in the pancreas (Ornitz et al. 1987). These mice develop pancreatic cancer by three months of age and will prove a powerful tool in the dissection of molecular events leading to the induction of pancreatic cancer.

Tumour cells characteristically exhibit an increased rate of glycolysis (Warburg 1956), but little is known of the regulation of this mechanism in pancreatic cancer cells. Schek et al. (1988), using complementary DNA (cDNA) probes have shown that there is an overexpression of mRNA for glyceraldehyde-3-phosphate dehydrogenase, enolase and glucose transporter protein which may play a role in the Warburg effect.

Clinical Potentials of Molecular Biology

Initial studies related to advances in the molecular biology of pancreatic cancer have concentrated on therapeutic strategies related to the presence of sex-steroid hormone receptors on the majority of pancreatic cancers. Relatively high amounts of the active metabolite of tamoxifen, 4-hydroxytamoxifen, have been found in the normal pancreas as long as 24 h after administration to spayed female mice (Wilking et al. 1982). These findings led to early clinical trials in patients with pancreatic cancer, which have claimed some limited success for anti-oestrogens (Theve et al. 1983) and LH-RH antagonists (Gonzalez-Barcena et al. 1986). However, in the only large-scale prospective randomised trial to assess tamoxifen theapy in pancreatic cancer, tamoxifen 30 mg daily gave the same results as no treatment at all (Bakkevold et al. 1990). Of course this study may have used an insufficient dose of tamoxifen, but as oestrogen is not the major trophic drive for the pancreas it is unlikely that oestrogen receptor antagonists will inhibit the growth of pancreatic cancer.

It is more likely that an agent with specific antiproliferative properties would be of some benefit as a biotherapy for pancreatic cancer. For example somatostastin has now been developed into several long-acting cyclic octapeptide analogues, each with differing antisecretory, antimotility and antiproliferative effects. Trials with the Sandoz analogue SMS 201–995 (Sandostatin) have been disappointing (Klijn et al. 1990). This is perhaps not surprising in view of the specific antisecretory potential of this analogue.

Under the auspices of the Cancer Research Campaign and in collaboration with Dr Andrew Schally of Tulane University Medical School, New Orleans, we have now started clinical trials of RC-160, a long-acting somatostatin analogue, for the treatment of pancreatic cancer. We are being extremely cautious in this Phase 1B study because of the potential side effects of somatostatin on other gastrointestino-pancreatic hormones, and particularly on the regulation of serum glucose (Osei and O'Dorisio 1985). We have now recruited 22 patients with histologically confirmed irresectable carcinoma of the pancreas. Patients receive RC-160 500 μg three times a day by self-administered subcutaneous injection. There have been three treatment failures due either to unacceptable symptoms or failure to administer treatment. After 15 months, seven patients are still alive and median survival on treatment is 150 days which compares favourably with historical controls of 90 days (Klijn et al. 1990) and 105 days (Bakkevold et al. 1990). Our next series of studies will compare long-term treatment of varying dosage regimens of RC-160 before we progress to an evaluation of a combination of somatostatin analogues with other hormonal agents such as LH-RH analogues and cytotoxic chemotherapy regimens.

Conclusions

We now have an understanding of the biology of exocrine pancreatic cancer which allows us to predict and test its response to various biological agents using different models of the disease in the laboratory. The molecular biologists continue to dissect all the pathways and mechanisms involved. These extend from the hormone and growth factor receptors on the cell membrane and within the cytosol to the expression of oncogenes which are responsible for pancreatic cancer. It is conceivable that this work will be completed before the end of this century, commensurate with the mapping of the human genome. It now behoves clinicians to grasp this new biology and apply it to clinical pancreatic cancer. We must aim to give this dreadful disease the same prognosis that is now possible with lymphomas and leukaemias, which only 20 years ago carried an equally appalling prognosis.

Acknowledgement. This work is supported by the British Digestive Foundation of which Mr Poston is the Amelie Waring scholar, and by the Cancer Research Campaign (Project Grant PO1).

References

Alexander RW, Upp JR Jr, Singh P et al. (1987) Asperlicin inhibits the growth of a xenografted human pancreatic carcinoma. Gastroenterology 92:1293A (abstract)

Alexander RW, Upp JR Jr, Poston GJ et al. (1988) Bombesin inhibits growth of human pancreatic adenocarcinoma in nude mice. Pancreas 3:297–302

Almoguera C, Shibata D, Forrester K et al. (1988) Most human carcinomas of the exocrine pancreas contain mutant c-K-*ras* genes. Cell 53:549–554

Andren Sandberg A (1986) Estrogens and pancreatic cancer: some recent aspects. Scand J Gastroenterol 21:129–133

Armelin HA, Armelin MCS, Kelly K et al. (1984) Functional role for C-myc in mitogenic response to platelet derived growth factor. Nature 310:655–660

Bakkevold KE, Pettersen A, Arnesjo B, Espehaug B (1990) Tamoxifen therapy in unresectable adenocarcinoma of the pancreas and the papilla of Vater. Br J Surg 77:725–730

Band P, Richardson SB, Boctor AM, Grossman A (1983) Somatostatin enhances binding of [³H]estradiol to a cytosolic protein in rat pancreas. J Biol Chem 258:7284–7287

Baylin SB, Stevens SA, Shakir KMM (1978) Association of diamine oxidase and ornithine decarboxylase with maturing cells in rapidly proliferating epithelium. Biochim Biophys Acta 541:415–419

Beauchamp RD, Lyons RM, Yang EY et al. (1990) Expression of and response to growth regulatory peptides by two human pancreatic carcinoma cell lines. Pancreas 5:369–380

Benrezzak O, Morriset J (1984) Effects of alpha-difluoromethylornithine on pancreatic growth induced by caerulein. Regul Pept 9:143–153

Benz C, Hollander C, Miller B (1986) Endocrine-responsive pancreatic carcinoma: steroid binding and cytotoxicity studies in human tumour cell lines. Cancer Res 46:2276–2281

Black O Jr, Chang BK (1982) Ornithine decarboxylase enzyme activity in human and hamster pancreatic tumour cell lines. Cancer Lett 17:87–93.

Boctor AM, Band P, Grossman A (1981) Requirement for an accessory factor for binding of [³H]estradiol to protein in the cytosol fraction of rat pancreas. Proc Natl Acad Sci USA 78:5648–5651

Boctor AM, Band P, Grossman A (1983) Analysis of binding of [³H]estradiol to the cytosol fraction of rat pancreas: comparison with sites in the cytosol of uterus. Endocrinology 113:453–462

Brachmann R, Lindquist PB, Nagashima M et al. (1989) Transmembrane TGF-a precursors activate EGF/TGF-a receptors. Cell 56:691–700

Carter DC (1990) Cancer of the pancreas. Gut 31:494–496

Chang BKR, Black O Jr, Gutman R (1984) Inhibition of growth of human or hamster pancreatic cancer cell lines by alpha-difluoromethylornithine alone and combined with *cis*-diaminedichloroplatinum (II). Cancer Res 44:5100–5104

Chen YF, Pan G-Z, Hou X et al. (1990) Epidermal growth factor and its receptors in human pancreatic carcinoma. Pancreas 5:278–283

Chester JF, Gaissert MA, Ross JA, Malt RA (1986) Pancreatic cancer in the Syrian hamster induced by *N*-nitroso bis (2-oxopropyl)-amine: carcinogenic effect with epidermal growth factor. Cancer Res 46:2954–2970

Cochran AB (1985) The molecular action of platelet derived growth factor. Adv Cancer Res 45: 183–216

Coffey RJ Jr, Shipley GD, Moses HL (1986) Production of transforming growth factors by human colon cancer lines. Cancer Res 46:1164–1169

Cooper CS, Blair DG, Oskarsson MK et al. (1984) Characterization of human transforming genes for chemically transformed, teratocarcinoma, and pancreatic carcinoma cell lines. Cancer Res 44:1–10

Corbishley TP, Iqbal MJ, Wilkinson ML, Williams R (1986) Androgen receptors in human normal and malignant pancreatic tissue and cell lines. Cancer 57:1922–1995

Darnell IE (1982) Variety in the level of gene control in eukaryotic cells. Nature 297:365–371

Douglas BR, Wortersen RA, Jansen JBM et al. (1989) Influence of cholecystokinin antagonist on the effects of cholecystokinin and bombesin on azaserine induced lesions on rat pancreas. Gastroenterology 96:462–469

Dowling RH, Hosomi M, Stace NM et al. (1985) Hormones and polyamines in intestinal and pancreatic adaptation. Scand J Gastroenterol 20:Suppl 112:84–95

Downward J, Yarden Y, Mayes E et al. (1984) Close similarity of epidermal growth factor receptor and V-erb-B oncogene protein sequences. Nature 307:521–527

Dynan WS, Tjian R (1985) Control of eukaryotic messenger RNA synthesis by sequence specific DNA-binding proteins. Nature 316:774–778

Estival A, Clemente F, Ribet J (1981) Adenocarcinoma of the human exocrine pancreas: presence of secretin and caerulein receptors. Biochem Biophys Res Commun 102:1336–1341

Fekete M, Zalatnai A, Comaru-Schally A-M, Schally AV (1989) Membrane receptors for peptides in experimental and human pancreatic cancers. Pancreas 4:521–528

Fernandez-Moreno MD, Diaz-Juarez JL, Arilla E, Prieto JC (1985) Effect of resection of small intestine in the interaction of vasoactive intestinal peptide with rat colonic epithelial cells. Horm Metab Res 17:289–292

Freeman TC, Curry BJ, Calam J, Woodburn JR (1990) Pancreatic secretory trypsin inhibitor stimulates the growth of rat pancreatic carcinoma cells. Gastroenterology 99:1414–1420

Gilman AG (1984) G proteins and dual control of adenylate cyclase. Cell 36:577–579

Goldfine ID, Williams JA (1983) Receptors for insulin and CCK in the acinar pancreas: relationship to hormone action. Int Rev Cytol 85:1–38

Gonzalez-Barcena D, Rangel-Garcia NE, Perez-Sanchez PL et al. (1986) Response to D-TRP-6-LH-RH in advanced adenocarcinoma of the pancreas. Lancet ii:154

Gorelick FS (1987) Second messenger systems and adaptation. Gut 28:S1:79–84

Goustin AS, Leof EB, Shipley GD, Moses HL (1986) Growth factors and cancer. Cancer Res 46:1015–1029

Greenway B, Iqbal MJ, Johnson PJ, Williams R (1981) Oestrogen receptor proteins in malignant and fetal pancreas. Br Med J 283:751–753

Greenway B, Iqbal MJ, Johnson PJ, Williams R (1983) Low serum testosterone concentration in patients with carcinoma of the pancreas. Br Med J 286:93–95

Grunewald K, Lyons J, Frohlich A et al. (1989) High frequency of K-*ras* codon mutations in pancreatic adenocarcinomas, Int J Cancer 43:1037–1041

Gullo L, Priori P, Laro G (1982) Influence of adrenal cortex on exocrine pancreatic function. Gastroenterology 83:92–96

Hayashi Y, Katayama H (1981) Promoting effect of testosterone propionate on experimental exocrine pancreatic tumours by 4-hydroxy amino quinoline 1-oxide in rats. Toxicol Lett 9:349–354

Hierowski MT, Liebow C, du Sapin K, Schally AV (1985) Stimulation by somatostatin of dephosphorylation of membrane proteins in pancreatic cancer MIA PaCa-2 cell lines. FEBS Lett 179:252–256

Hootman SR, Brown ME, Williams JA, Logsdon CD (1986) Regulation of muscarinic acetyl choline receptors in cultured guinea pig pancreatic acini. Am J Physiol 251:G75–G83

Howatson AG, Carter DC (1985) Pancreatic carcinogenesis enhancement by cholecystokinin in the hamster–nitrosamine model. Br J Cancer 51:107–114

Howatson AG, Carter DC (1987) Pancreatic carcinogenesis: effect of secretin in the hamster–nitrosamine model. J Natl Cancer Inst 78:101–105

Hugh T, Alexander RW, Upp JR et al. (1987) Caerulein inhibits growth of a human cholangiocarcinoma with cholecystokinin receptors. Gastroenterology 92:1801 (abstract)

Hunt LT, Barker WC, Dayhoff MO (1974) Epidermal growth factor: internal duplication and probable relationship to pancreatic trypsin inhibitor. Biochem Biophys Res Commun 60:1020–1028

Iqbal MJ, Greenway B, Wilkinson ML et al. (1983) Sex steroid enzyme, aromatase and 5-alpha-reductase in the pancreas: a comparison of normal adult, foetal and malignant tissue. Clin Sci 65:71–75

Janne J, Poso H, Raina A (1978) Polyamines in rapid growth and cancer. Biochim Biophys Acta 473:241–293

Kern HF, Rausch U. Scheele GA (1987) Regulation of gene expression in pancreatic adaptation to nutritional substrate or hormones. Gut 28:S1:89–94

Klijn JGM, Hoff AM, Planting AST et al. (1990) Treatment of patients with metastatic pancreatic and gastrointestinal tumours with the somatostatin analogue Sandostatin: a phase II study including endocrine effects. Br J Cancer 62:627–630

Korc M (1989) Regulation of pancreatic cancer cell proliferation by an autocrine cycle coupled to the epidermal growth factor receptor. Pancreas 4:262–263 (abstract)

Korc M, Magun BE (1985) Recycling of epidermal growth factor in a human pancreatic carcinoma cell line. Proc Natl Acad Sci USA 82:6172–6175

Korc M, Meltzer P, Trent J (1986) Enhanced expression of epidermal growth factor receptor correlates with alterations of chromosome 7 in human pancreatic cancer. Proc Natl Acad Sci USA 83:5141–5144

Lawrence JP, Poston GJ, Townsend CM et al. (1988) Stimulatory effect of castration on the growth of hamster pancreatic cancer in vivo: mediating role of gastrin. Gastroenterology 94:A253 (abstract)

Leof EB, Proper JA, Goustin AS et al. (1986) Induction of C-*sis* mRNA and activity similar to platelet derived growth factor beta: a proposed model for indirect mitogenesis involving autocrine activity. Proc Natl Acad Sci USA 83:2453–2457

Lhoste EF, Roebuck BD, Longnecker DS (1986) Effect of steroids on the early stage of azaserine-induced pancreatic carcinogenesis in the rat. Dig Dis Sci 31:1139 (abstract)

Liebow C, Reilly C, Serrano M, Schally AV (1989) Somatostatin analogues inhibit growth of pancreatic cancer by stimulating tyrosine phosphatase. Proc Natl Acad Sci USA 86: 2003–2007

Liebow C, Lee MT, Schally AV (1990) Antitumor effects of somatostatin mediated by the stimulation of tyrosine phosphatase. Metabolism 39:163–166

Lippmann ME, Dickson RB, Bates S et al. (1986) Autocrine and paracrine growth regulation of humann breast cancer. Breast Cancer Res Treat 7:59–70

Logsdon CD, Williams JA (1984) Intracellular Ca^{2+} and phorbol esters synergistically inhibit EGF intermediaries in pancreatic acini. Biochem J 223:893–400

Logsdon CD, Mossner J, Williams JA, Goldfine ID (1985) Glucocorticoids increase amylase mRNA levels, secreting organelles, and secretion in pancreatic acinar AR42J cells. J Cell Biol 100:1200–1208

Marx M, Townsend CM Jr, Barranco SC et al. (1983) Treatment of pancreatic cancer by alpha-difluoromethylornithine (DFMO), an inhibitor of polyamine synthesis. Dig Dis Sci 28:941 (abstract)

Matozaki T, Saramoto C, Nagao M, Baba S (1986) Phorbol ester or diacylglycerol modulates somatostatin binding to its receptors on rat pancreatic acinar cell membranes. J Biol Chem 261:1414–1420

May WS, Sayhoun N, Jacobs S et al. (1986) Mechanism of phorbol diester-induced regulation of surface transferrin receptor involves the action of activated protein kinase C and intact cytoskeleton. J Biol Chem 260:9419–9426

McCann PP (1980) Regulation of ornithine decarboxylase in eukaryotic cells. In: Gangas JM (ed) Polyamines in biomedical research. Wiley, New York, pp 109–123

McGuinness EE, Morgan RGH, Wormsley KG (1987) Fate of pancreatic nodules induced by raw soya flour in rats. Gut 28:S1:207–212

Means AR, Dedman JR (1980) Calmodulin – an intracellular calcium receptor. Nature 285:73–77

Morisset J, Benrezzak O (1984) Polyamines and pancreatic growth induced by caerulein. Life Sci 35:2471–2480

Morisset J, Benrezzak O (1985) Reversal of alpha dimethyl fluoroornithine inhibition of caerulein induced pancreatic growth by putrescine. Renal Pept 11:201–208

Moses HL, Tucker RF, Leof EB et al. (1985) Type beta transforming growth factor is a growth stimulant and growth inhibitor. In: Feremisco J et al. (eds) Growth factors and transformation. Cold Spring Harbour, Cold Spring Harbour Laboratory, pp 65–71

Mossner J, Logsdon CD, Petau N et al. (1984a) Effect of intracellular Ca^{2+} in insulin like growth factor II internalisation into pancreatic acini: role of insulin and cholecystokinin. J Biol Chem 259:12350–12356

Mossner J, Logsdon CD, Goldfine ID, Williams JA (1984b) Regulation of pancreatic acinar cell insulin receptors by insulin. Am J Physiol 247:G155–G160

Nishizuka Y (1984) The role of protein kinase C in cell surface signal transduction and tumour promotion. Nature 308:693–698

Nishizuka Y (1986) Studies and perspectives of protein kinase C. Science 233:305–312

Ogata N (1988) Demonstration of pancreatic secretory trypsin inhibitor in serum-free culture medium conditioned by the human pancreatic carcinoma cell line CAPAN-1. J Biol Chem 263:13427–13431

O'Hara BM, Oskarsson M, Tainsky MA, Blair DG (1986) Mechanism of activation of human *ras* gene cloned from a gastric adenocarcinoma and a pancreatic carcinoma cell line. Cancer Res 46:4695–4700

Ohmura E, Okada M, Onada N et al. (1990) Insulin-like growth factor 1 and transforming growth factor alpha as autocrine growth factors in human pancreatic cancer cell growth. Cancer Res 50:103–107

Ornitz DM, Hammer RE, Messing A et al. (1987) Pancreatic regulation induced by SV40 T-antigen expression in acinar cells of transgenic mice. Science 238:188–193

Osei K, O'Dorisio TM (1985) Malignant insulinoma: effects of a somatostatin analogue (compound 201–996) on serum glucose, growth and gastro-entero-pancreatic hormones. Ann Intern Med 103:223–225

Pegg AE (1986) Recent advances in the biochemistry of polyamines in eukaryocytes. Biochem J 234:249–262

Poston GJ, Williamson RCN (1990) Causes, diagnosis and management of exocrine pancreatic cancer. Compr Ther 16:36–42

Poston GJ, Yao CZ, Upp JR Jr et al. (1988) Vasoactive intestinal peptide inhibits the growth of hamster pancreatic cancer but not human pancreatic cancer in vivo. Pancreas 3:439–443

Poston GJ, Townsend CM Jr, Rajaraman S et al. (1990) Effect of somatostatin and tamoxifen on the growth of human pancreatic cancers in nude mice. Pancreas 5:151–157

Pour PM, Hegelson S, Lawson T et al. (1988) Effect of cholecystokinin on pancreatic carcinogenesis in the hamster model. Carcinogenesis 9:597–601

Raitano AB, Scuderi P, Korc M (1990) Binding and biological effects of tumor necrosis factor and gamma interferon in human pancreatic carcinoma cells. Pancreas 5:267–277

Rall LB, Scott J, Bell GJ et al. (1985) Mouse prepro-epidermal growth factor synthesis by kidney and other tissues. Nature 313:228–231

Rasmussen HR (1986a) The calcium messenger system: part 1. N Engl J Med 314:1095–1101

Rasmussen HR (1986b) The calcium messenger system: part 2. N Engl J Med 314:1164–1170

Redding TW, Schally AV (1984) Inhibition of growth of pancreatic carcinomas in animal models by analogues of hypothalamic hormones. Proc Natl Acad Sci USA 81:248–252

Roberts AB, Anzano MA, Meyers CA et al. (1983) Purification and properties of a type B transforming growth factor from bovine kidney. Biochemistry 22:5692–5698

Roos W, Fabbro D, Kung W et al. (1986) Correlation between hormone dependency and the regulation of epidermal growth factor receptor by tumour promoters in human mammary carcinoma lines. Proc Natl Acad Sci USA 83:991–995

Sakamoto C, Goldfine ID, Williams JA (1984) The somatostatin receptor on isolated pancreatic acinar cell plasma membranes J Biol Chem 259:9623–9627

Sandberg AA, Rosenthal HE (1974) Estrogen receptors in the pancreas. J Steroid Biochem 5:969–957

Satake K, Mukai R, Kato Y, Umeyama K (1986) Effect of caerulein on the normal pancreas and an experimental pancreatic carcinoma in the Syrian golden hamster. Pancreas 1:246–253

Saydjari R, Townsend CM Jr, Barranco SC et al. (1986) Effects of cyclosporine A and alpha-difluoromethylornithine on the growth of pancreatic cancer in vitro. JNCI 77:1087–1092

Scalabrino G, Ferioli ME (1981) Polyamines in mammalian tumours, part I. Adv Cancer Res 35:152–268

Scalabrino G, Ferioli ME (1982) Polyamines in mammalian tumours, part II. Adv Cancer Res 36:1–102

Schally AV, Comaro-Schally M, Redding T (1984) Antitumor effects of analogues of hypothalamic hormones in endocrine dependent cancers. Proc Soc Exp Biol Med 175:259–281

Schally AV (1988) Oncological applications of somatostatin analogues. Cancer Res 48:6977–6985

Scheele GA (1986) Regulation of gene expression in the exocrine pancreas. In: Go VLW et al. (eds) The exocrine pancreas: biology, pathology and disease, Raven Press, New York, pp 55–67

Scheidereit C, Greisse S, Westphal HW, Beato M (1983) The glucocorticoid receptor binds to defined nucleotide sequences near the promoter of mouse mammary tumour tissue. Nature 304:749–752

Schek N, Hall BL, Finn OJ (1988) Increased glyceraldehyde-3-phosphate dehydrogenase gene expression in human pancreatic adenocarcinoma. Cancer Res 48:6354–6359

Schick J, Verspohl R, Kern HF, Scheele GA (1984) Two distinct adaptive responses in the synthesis of exocrine pancreatic enzymes to inverse changes in proteins and carbohydrates in the diet. Am J Physiol 247:G611–616

Shibata D, Almoguera C, Forrester K et al. (1990) Detection of c-K-*ras* mutations in fine needle aspirates from human pancreatic adenocarcinomas. Cancer Res 50:1279–1283

Sibley DR, Lefkowitz RJ (1985) Molecular mechanisms of receptor desensitisation using the beta-adrenergic receptor-coupled adenylate cyclase system as a model. Nature 317:124–129

Smit VT, Boot AJ, Smits AA et al. (1988) K-*ras* codon 12 mutations occur very frequently in pancreatic adenocarcinomas. Nucleic Acids Res 16:7773–7782

Smith JJ, Derynck R, Korc M (1987) Production of transforming growth factor alpha in human pancreatic cancer cells: evidence of a superagonist autocrine cycle. Proc Natl Acad Sci USA 84:7567–7570

Stock-Damge C, Lhoste E, Aprahamian M, Pousse A (1987) Effect of chronic bombesin on pancreatic size, composition and secretory function in the rat. Gut 28:S1:1–7

Sumi C, Longnecker D, Roebuck BD, Brinck-Johnson T (1989) Inhibitory effect of estrogen and castration on the early stages of pancreatic carcinogenesis in Fischer rats treated with azaserine. Cancer Res 49:2332–2336

Szende B, Zalatnai A, Schally AV (1989) Programmed cell death (apoptosis) in pancreatic cancer of hamsters after administration of analogs of luteinizing hormone releasing hormone and somatostatin. Proc Natl Acad Sci USA 86:1643–1647

Szende B, Srkalovic G, Schally AV et al. (1990) Inhibitory effects of analogs of luteinizing hormone-releasing hormone and somatostatin on pancreatic cancers in hamsters, events that accompany tumor regression. Cancer 65:2279–2290

Takeuchi T, Gumucio DL, Yamada T et al. (1986) Genes encoding pancreatic polypeptide and neuropeptide Y are on human chromosomes 17 and 7. J Clin Invest 77: 1038–1041

Tesone M, Chazenbalk D, Ballesos G, Charreau EH (1979) Estrogen receptors in rat pancreatic islets. J Steroid Biochem 11:1309–1314

Theve NO, Pousette A, Carlstrom K (1983) Adenocarcinoma of the pancreas – a hormone sensitive tumour. A preliminary report on nolvadex treatment. Clin Oncol 9:193–197

Townsend CH Jr, Franklin RB, Watson LC et al. (1981) Stimulation of pancreatic cancer growth by caerulein and secretin. Surg Forum 32:228–230

Townsend CM Jr, Beauchamp RD, Singh P, Thompson JC (1988) Growth factors and intestinal neoplasms. Am J Surg 155:526–536

Trede M, Schwall G (1988) The complications of pancreatectomy. Ann Surg 207:39–47

Tulassy Z, Sandor Z, Bodrogi L et al. (1988) An endocrine model for pancreatic cancer. Br Med J 297:1447–1448

Upp JR Jr, Singh P, Townsend CM Jr, Thompson JL (1987) Predicting response to endocrine therapy in human pancreatic cancer with cholecystokinin receptors. Gastroenterology 92:1677 (abstract)

Upp JR Jr, Olson D, Poston GJ et al. (1988) Inhibition of growth of two human pancreatic adenocarcinomas in vivo by somatostatin analogue SMS 201-995. Am J Surg 155:29–35

Warburg O (1956) On the origin of cancer cells. Science 123:309–314

Wicker C, Puigserver A, Rausch U et al. (1985) Multiple level caerulein control of the gene expression of secretory proteins in the rat pancreas. Eur J Biochem 151:461–466

Wilking N, Appelgren L-E, Carlstrom K et al. (1982) The distribution and metabolism of ^{14}C-labelled tamoxifen in spayed female mice. Acta Pharmacol Toxicol 50:161–168

Williams JA, Hootman SR (1986) Stimulus-secretion coupling in pancreatic acinar cells. In: Go VLW et al. (eds) The exocrine pancreas: biology, pathophysiology and disease, Raven Press, New York, pp 123–139

Williams JA (1987) Role of receptors in mediating trophic stimuli in the pancreas. Gut 28:S1:45–49

Yao CZ, Poston GJ, Townsend CM Jr, Thompson JC (1987) Covalent cross linking identification of vasoactive intestinal receptors in human colon and pancreatic cancers and hamster pancreatic cancer. Gastroenterology 92:1702(A) (abstract)

Zalatnai A, Schally AV (1989) Treatment of the N-nitrosobis(2-oxopropyl) amine-induced pancreatic cancer in Syrian golden hamsters with D-Trp-6-LH-RH and somatostatin analogue RC-160 microcapsules. Cancer Res 49:1810–1815

Chapter 5

Chemotherapy in Inoperable Pancreatic Cancer

C. N. Mallinson

Both the low level of operability and the very short median survival of patients with carcinoma of the exocrine pancreas are well known. These observations induce contrasting attitudes. On the one hand the short survival has encouraged the use of non-operative stenting for malignant jaundice to reduce time in hospital, on the other the feeling persists that even a modest increase in survival would be worth having in order to give the patient and the family a little more time.

In spite of increasing efforts in clinical trials and the evolution of new drugs, no cytotoxic regime can be relied upon to increase the length of survival, even in carefully selected patients (Temple and Burkitt 1991). Reports of research in this field are difficult to interpret, usually for two principal reasons: first, the numbers of patients in reported series are usually very small and, second, often the selection of patients makes it difficult to compare the results of one series with another. Although the influence on survival exerted by factors such as age, sex, race, and, in particular, cell differentiation and the extent of spread are comparatively small, it is undeniable that bias can be caused by a preponderance of patients with potentially longer survival in a study of treatment, or inclusion of patients with a poorer prognosis in control groups, (Carter and Comis 1975; Litka and Schein 1986).

Single Agent Chemotherapy

In the 1950s there were few agents with any activity against adenocarcinoma, and they tended to be used singly – a practice which has now come full circle. There are a number of reliably effective agents and others have been shown in occasional trials to have some effect. However, even among the effective agents there are none which have ever been shown consistently to be more than moderately effective.

5-Fluorouracil (5FU)

First described in 1958, this alkylating agent has been widely used as a single agent in the treatment of adenocarcinomas and has been included in almost every multiple-agent regime for carcinoma of the pancreas (Carter and Comis 1975). When used as originally described, by the intravenous route, with a loading course followed by pulses at regular intervals of one to six weeks for 20 to 30 doses, this agent has been recorded as having a response rate of 0–30% in carcinoma of the pancreas. Probably 25% is a reasonable approximation across the board (Carter and Comis 1975).

In the context of Phase II trials, response means the reduction in a measurable dimension of a marker tumour, sustained over a given period, with the appearance of no new disease. Most responses recorded in patients with carcinoma of the pancreas are partial responses. Complete response implies the disappearance of all tumour with no new tumour appearing (Litka and Schein 1986). Obviously this criterion of effectiveness is very much dependent on imaging methods. A further, extremely important criterion of effect is, therfore, the extent to which any treatment can improve the median survial of the group, usually assessed in Phase III clinical trials. The importance of this measure of effectiveness is emphasised by the observation that although 5FU has an effect on creating response, no evaluable study has appeared which shows any effect of 5FU on median survival.

Recently, 5FU has been administered in two ways which have allowed very much higher doses to be given without major side effects, by the portable, constant-infusion pump (Caballero et al. 1985) or by high-dose infusion with folinic acid rescue (Erlichman et al. 1988).

In the second method folinic acid is administered in an infusion over 2 h followed by 5FU at first in a bolus and then in a constant infusion over 22 h. The entire cycle is repeated. Six courses are given at two-week intervals. Very few patients with cancer of the pancreas have been evaluated, and no large series has been reported. However from personal experience it can be said that these high doses are extremely well tolerated and have occasionally produced striking results in other gastrointestinal adenocarcinomas.

Mitomycin-C

This Japanese alkylating agent has also been widely used, often in combination with 5FU but also on its own. It is a more toxic drug than 5FU and latterly has not been included in new regimes although it is an integral part of three of the more promising combination regimes described below.

Streptozotocin (STZ)

STZ is a nitrosourea which is an effective antisecretory and cytotoxic agent in pancreatic endocrine tumours. It is also of considerable interest in exocrine cancer because it has been associated with more complete remissions, used as a single agent, than other drugs. Its value in combination, which is how it is usually used, is discussed below. As a single agent its response rate is low at 12%–15%. Used in anything but the minimum dosage it is extremely emetic. STZ is largely without side effects on bone marrow but it has a dose-dependent nephrotoxic effect which can be reversed or arrested if it is detected early.

Adriamycin (Daunorubicin)

Adriamycin gives a low response rate in pancreatic cancer but has, perhaps slightly mysteriously, been included in several of the more successful multiple regimes.

4-Epirubicin

This analogue of adriamycin has in one well-designed study shown promise as a single agent. The response rate in 41 patients was 24% and although the median survival was not prolonged with the group as a whole (5 months), the responders showed a median survival of 9 months.

Combination Chemotherapy Regimes

The idea of combining two or more agents is to attack the malignant cell by different mechanisms, creating additive cytotoxicity and reducing the dose of each agent to below those which cause serious side effects. Agents are combined which have different toxic effects and have shown activity as single agents. There is no reason to believe that combination with another agent will confer activity on an inactive single agent. However, the possibility that corticosteroids, so consistently useful in lymphoma regimes, could enhance anti-tumour activity in pancreatic cancer has never been tested. The two most widely used combination regimes use similar doses of 5FU and mitomycin-C with the addition of either STZ (SMF) (Wiggans et al. 1978) or adriamycin (FAM) (Smith et al. 1980) respectively. In the reports of these two regimes, the patients treated have been similar in age, sex, tumour-load and general health. In most, but not all, series the response rate was in the region of 30%. In each series the responders showed a distinctly increased survival to 10 or 12 months, which is better than patients with stable disease or non-responders. The non-responders showed no increase over historical controls. The possibility, of course, exists that such potent chemotherapy in patients to whom it is of no benefit could actually be harmful. From these studies another general point emerged, that tumour reduction is very seldom seen in large single masses, but more commonly seen with small multiple metastases, for example in the liver (Smith et al. 1980). This is not surprising but points the way towards better selection of individual patients. The initial results of these regimes have been less satisfactorily reproduced in subsequent trials in other units (Bukowski et al. 1983). Nevertheless the logical step was taken by Bukowski et al. (1982), when they combined all four agents (FAM-STZ) in the treatment of 25 patients, of whom 12 responded (48%) with four complete responses. The mean survival of the whole group was 6.8 months (range 1–23 months) but responders showed a median survival of ten months compared with two months in non-responders. Toxic vomiting was the principal complication but this was controllable. This regime was complicated to administer but has produced the best results of any chemotherapy so far. Its complexity and expense have probably been the main reasons that have prevented it being more widely used.

Streptozotocin was evaluated by Bukowski (1984) in a different way. The 222 patients with carcinoma of the pancreas treated by the South Western Oncology Group (SWOG) included 152 treated with SMF and 70 with MF alone. Twenty four (16%) on SMF and seven (10%) on MF survived for one year. Of these 31 patients, seven survived 18 months, all of whom were on SMF. Thus there is a hint that STZ may be of lasting benefit to a handful of patients. Another point that came out of this study was that 24 of the 31 long-term survivors had metastatic disease at the start of treatment. This implies that the presence of metastases is not necessarily a contraindication to treatment and does not necessarily indicate a short survival, although as a general rule patients with metastases have a shorter survival than those without.

Controlled Studies

It is the nature of Phase II studies that they are preliminary investigations into the effectiveness of agents or regimes in the reduction of tumour size. It is regrettable that very few studies have been carried out using apparently effective regimes in a randomised controlled fashion. Two studies exist, both originating in the south east of England and both showing a modest advantage for treatment over control.

In one small study with 24 patients in each group the treated patients received an initiation course of 5FU, cyclophosphamide, methotrexate and vincristine followed by monthly intravenous 5FU and mitomycin-C (Mallinson et al. 1980). The median survival of treated patients was 11 months and of untreated patients 2.5 months which was obviously and statistically significant. In further studies in which the initiation course was omitted, the median survival was only seven and eight months in the treated group. This was an early study by an unspecialised group of gastroenterologists using a primitive protocol. The possibility exists that bias crept in to influence results in favour of the treated patients or possibly even to the detriment of the untreated patients. The other prospective randomised controlled trial of pharmacotherapy as opposed to cytotoxic therapy was, in addition, double-blind. In this study, tamoxifen was given to the treatment group, with control groups of no treatment and cyproterone acetate (Keating et al. 1989). The median survival in the tamoxifen group was 5.8 months and in the untreated patients two months which was a small but significant difference. A point of interest is that the tamoxifen study was begun when pancreatic cancer cells were believed to have oestrogen binding sites. It now appears that although some surface binding can be demonstrated, true cell-modifying binding is probably insignificant.

Combined Modality Treatment: Chemotherapy and Radiotherapy

In brief, it must be admitted that there is very little evidence that radiotherapy either by external beam or intraoperatively has any effect on survival in advanced pancreatic cancer though the picture is different following resection. Several studies have shown, in the face of careful design and meticulous execution, no advantage for this modality of treatment. An exception is the 1981 report which showed that medium-dose radiotherapy (4000 rads) with 5FU intravenously was more effective than 5FU on its own (GITSG 1981). Since then attempts to improve upon or even equal this result have been made with some success in patients with locally advanced disease. On the face of it it is logical to treat the primary site with radiotherapy since this is resistant as a rule to chemotherapy, and to treat the metastases which are almost invariably present at the time of diagnosis by cytotoxic chemotherapy.

The problem appears to be that while both modalities of treatment are partially effective in some patients, very seldom indeed does either modality completely eradicate cancer cells which then continue to divide and spread after treatment has stopped or even while it continues (Ozaki et al. 1988; Ishikawa et al. 1989).

Endocrine Treatment

In the experimental setting several promising methods exist for maintaining cell lines of pancreatic cancer in vitro. Using such systems, inhibitors of cholecystokinin binding, and somatostatin analogues have been investigated and found to reduce tumour growth (Sternberg et al. 1987; Liebon et al. 1989). So far no significant clinical application has been reported. However, this line of research brings a renewed interest to chemotherapy in the treatment of pancreatic cancer.

Conclusion

Although there is suggestive evidence that a few patients benefit from cytotoxic chemotherapy by an increase in survival at tolerable cost, it is not yet possible to predict which patients will respond and to what extent their survival will be prolonged. It remains to be seen whether the new high-dose regimes for 5FU are more effective than older dose schedules and whether the formidable combination of 5FU, adriamycin, mitomycin-C and streptozotocin does really produce results which justify its use. Advances in endocrine therapy are awaited.

References

Bukowski RM (1984) Characteristics of long-term survivors receiving chemotherapy for pancreatic adenocarcinoma in South-West oncology group studies (abstract) *Proc ASCO* 3:149

Bukowski RM, Schachter LP, Groppe CW, Hewlett JS, Weick JK, Livingston RB (1982) Phase II trial of 5-fluorouracil, mitomycin-C and streptozotocin (FAM-S) in pancreatic cancer. *Cancer* 50:197–200

Bukowski RM, Balcerzak SP, O'Bryan RM, Bonnet JD, Chen TT (1983) Randomized trial of 5-fluorouracil and mitomycin-C with or without streptozotocin for advanced pancreatic cancer. *Cancer* 52:1577–1582

Caballero GA, Ausman RK, Quebbeman EJ (1985) Long term ambulatory continuous intravenous infusion of 5-fluorouracil for treatment of advanced adenocarcinoma. *Cancer Treat Rep* 69:13–15

Carter S, Comis R (1975) Adenocarcinoma of the pancreas. In: Stagnet MJ (ed) Cancer Therapy; Prognostic Factors and Criteria of Response, Raven Press, New York, pp 237–253

Erlichman C, Fine S, Wong A et al. (1988) A randomized trial of 5-fluorouracil and folinic acid in metastatic colon cancer. *J. Clin Oncol* 6:469–475

Gastrointestinal Tumour Study Group (1981) Therapy of locally unresectable pancreatic carcinoma: a randomized comparison of high dose (6000 rads) radiation alone, moderate dose radiation (4000 rads) + 5-fluorouracil and high dose radiation + 5-fluorouracil. *Cancer* 48:1705–1710

Ishikawa O, Ohhigashi H, Teshima T et al. (1989) Clinical and histopathological appraisal of pre-operative irradiation for adenocarcinoma of the pancreatico-duodenal region. *J Surg Oncol* 40:143–151

Keating JJ, Johnson PJ, Cochrane HMC et al. (1989) A prospective randomized controlled trial of tamoxifen and cyproterone acetate in pancreatic carcinoma. *Br J Cancer* 60:789–792

Liebon C, Reilly C, Serrano M, Schally AV (1989) Somatostatin analogues inhibit growth of pancreatic cancer by stimulating tyrosine phosphatase. *Proc Natl Acad Sci USA* 86:2003–2007

Litka PA, Schein PS (1986) Chemotherapy of pancreatic cancer. In: Go VLW et al. (eds) The Exocrine Pancreas, Raven Press, New York, pp 689–697

Mallinson CN, Rake MO, Cocking JB et al. (1980) Chemotherapy in pancreatic cancer. Results of a controlled prospective randomised multi-centre trial. *Br Med J* 281.1589–1591

Ozaki H, Hojok, Kato H, Kinoshita T, Egawa S, Kishi K (1988) Multi-disciplinary treatment for resectable pancreatic cancer. *Int J Pancreatol* 3:249–260

Smith F, Hoth D, Levin B et al. (1980) 5-Fluorouracil, adriamycin and mitomycin-C (FAM) chemotherapy for advanced adenocarcinoma of the pancreas. *Cancer* 46:2014–2018

Sternberg CN, Sordillo PP, Cheng E, Cuang YJ, Niedzwiecki D (1987) Evaluation of an in-vitro model used to assess putative chemotherapeutic agents in pancreatic cancer. *Am J Clin Oncol* 10:219–221

Temple NJ, Burkitt DP (1991) The war on cancer – failure of therapy and research: discussion paper. *Proc R Soc Med* 84:95–98

Wiggans G, Woolley PV, MacDonald JS, Smythe T, Ueno W, Schein PS (1978) Phase II trial of streptozotocin, mitomycin-C and 5-fluorouracil (SMF) in the treatment of advanced pancreatic cancer. *Cancer* 41:387–391

Chapter 6

Surgical Palliation of Pancreatic Cancer

P. Watanapa and R. C. N. Williamson

The Scope of the Problem

Carcinoma of the exocrine pancreas remains a major therapeutic challenge. The global incidence of this cancer has been increasing over the past few decades (Muir et al. 1987; Fontham and Correa 1989; Hirayama 1989), so that in Britain it has become the third most frequent cause of death from gastrointestinal cancer (following large bowel and stomach) (Office of Population Censuses and Surveys 1990). Over 6000 Britons die of this disease each year (Williamson 1988).

Recent advances in both diagnostic and therapeutic means have failed to alter the course and prognosis of pancreatic cancer patients. The vague and often trivial nature of the presenting symptoms, coupled with a lack of effective screening tests, explains the customary delay in diagnosis and the dismal salvage rates that ensue. In the experience of most pancreatic surgeons, only 10%–20% of patients with this cancer have tumours suitable for resection and possible cure by the time the diagnosis is made (Kummerle and Ruckert 1984; Trede 1985; Connolly et al. 1987; Funovics et al. 1989). This figure does not differ greatly from that of some years ago, even though the diagnosis can be established more quickly today than in the past. Thus the great bulk of patients with pancreatic carcinoma, at least 80%, still require some form of palliation.

There are three important objectives for surgical palliation in patients with irresectable pancreatic cancer: (a) to relieve jaundice, and in particular pruritus, (b) to maintain gastric outflow, and (c) to control pain. Since patients with cancer of the pancreatic head usually present with jaundice and/or vomiting, which demand symptomatic relief, a good case can be made for surgical palliation even when preoperative imaging shows that resection is unlikely to be feasible. By contrast, cancers of the body or tail are generally large and irresectable by the time of diagnosis. In such cases, and in the absence of obstructive symptoms laparotomy has little to offer provided that the tumour can be accurately diagnosed (by percutaneous biopsy) and staged without operation.

Biliary Obstruction

Obstructive jaundice is present in 70%–85% of patients with pancreatic cancer at the time of presentation (Trede 1985; Rosemurgy et al. 1989). The incidence reaches 90% if the tumour lies in the pancreatic head but is only 6% in cancers of the body and tail (Reber 1987). A carcinoma of the head can impinge on the bile duct at a relatively early (and potentially curable) stage of its development, whereas a carcinoma of the neck or uncinate process has almost always spread too far by the time it produces jaundice. Although jaundice can be entirely painless in this disease, most patients have at least some degree of pain at the time of presentation (Howard and Jordan 1977).

Therapeutic goals in icteric patients with irresectable cancer are: (a) permanent relief of the symptoms and signs of biliary obstruction and (b) extension of survival by eliminating causes of early death. Relief of biliary obstruction can alleviate jaundice and pruritus, correct metabolic derangements, improve hepatic function, renal function, nutritional health and coagulopathy and generally enhance appetite and well-being. In addition cholangitis, which occurs in about 10% of patients with malignant biliary obstruction, may be prevented or treated by ductal decompression.

There are two ways to relieve jaundice: non-operative stenting and operative bypass. Each has its own advantages and disadvantages. Our preference is to operate on all but the frail and those with very advanced disease for reasons that we shall try to explain below.

Non-operative Stenting

Nowadays external biliary decompression can be performed by means of percutaneous transhepatic biliary drainage (PTBD) with a high rate of technical success (85%–97%) (Joseph et al. 1986; McGrath et al. 1989). Thus adequate decompression of the obstructed biliary system can be achieved but at the cost of an appreciable incidence of complications, both short term and long term. Early complications of PTBD occur in 33%–43% of patients and include cholangitis, haemorrhage, bile duct perforation, haemopneumothorax, electrolyte disorders and catheter malfunction (Devereux and Greco 1986; McGrath et al. 1989). Long-term complications of PTBD occur in up to 86% of patients surviving their initial hospitalisation. These include catheter dislodgement, tube obstruction, cholangitis and sepsis (McGrath et al. 1989). Besides these unacceptably high complication rates, PTBD condemns the patient to the nuisance and discomfort of an external biliary fistula for the rest of his life.

Although PTBD alone has, therefore, fallen into disrepute, endoprostheses have recently been introduced to provide permanent internal drainage of the duct in malignant obstruction without the need for an external catheter. In experienced hands these prostheses can be inserted either by the percutaneous transhepatic route with a 93% success rate or by the endoscopic transpapillary route with a 90% success rate (Table 1). Transhepatic endoprostheses are associated with a lower initial morbidity rate (18% vs 25%) and a shorter hospital stay than surgical bypass (18 vs 25 days), but long-term complications

Table 1. Comparative results between surgical bypass and endoprosthetic stents in patients with malignant obstruction of the common bile duct

	Surgical bypass[a] (n = 345) (ref.2–4, 10–14)[b]		Percutaneous stents (n = 377) (ref. 1,3,5,8,15)		Endoscopic stents (n = 638) (ref. 6–11)	
	Range	Mean	Range	Mean	Range	Mean
30-day mortality rate (%)	0–32	10	7–33	12	8–20	14
Hospital stay (days)	9–27	16	10–18	14	3.5–26	5
Success rate (%)	76–100	92	76–100	93	82–100	90
Early complications (%)	6–56	25	9–67	18	8–30	19
Recurrent jaundice or cholangitis (%)	8–16	10	6–38	26	16–30	26

[a] Only those patients with biliary bypass alone have been included (i.e. not those with combined biliary and duodenal bypass) so as to allow a direct comparison with non-operative stenting.
[b] 1, Mueller et al. (1985); 2, Rosenberg et al. (1985); 3, Bornman et al. (1986); 4, Devereux and Greco (1986); 5, Lammer and Neumayer (1986); 6, Siegel and Snady (1986); 7, Tytgat et al. (1986); 8, Speer et al. (1987); 9, Meduri et al. (1988); 10, Shepherd et al. (1988); 11, Anderson et al. (1989); 12, McGrath et al. (1989); 13, Kahn et al. (1990); 14, Procter and Mauro (1990); 15, Adam et al. (1991).

appear to be commoner (26% vs 10%). Problems comprise catheter obstruction and recurrent jaundice (23%–38%), repeated attacks of cholangitis (10%–38%) and displacement of the prosthesis (6%–10%) (Mueller et al. 1985; Bornman et al. 1986; Speer et al. 1987; Adam 1990; Procter and Mauro 1990).

The advent of self-expanding metallic endoprostheses has opened a new era of percutaneous stenting (Adam et al. 1991). These special endoprostheses are made of a closely woven mesh of stainless steel and are introduced percutaneously through a 7 FG catheter. When the stent is released it achieves a maximal internal diameter of 10 mm, which is much larger than the diameter of a standard plastic endoprosthesis. The small size of the introducing catheter reduces the risk of early complications (such as haemobilia) and allows introduction of the prosthesis in one session, with minimum patient discomfort. The large internal diameter of this stent provides long-term patency and certainly reduces the long-term complications. The success rate is now more than 95% (Adam et al. 1991). The major disadvantages of this type of stent are its high cost and the difficulty in removing or replacing it if it blocks. However, a second stent may be placed in continuity with the first if tumour begins to encroach above the stent.

The technique for endoscopic insertion of a biliary stent through the papilla has now become established. Small stents (5–8 FG) were used initially, but wider channel endoscopes have become available that allow the use of polyethylene or Teflon endoprostheses (stents) with a diameter of up to 12 FG. Most studies since 1986 showed that the endoscopic endoprosthesis is as good as surgical bypass for palliating malignant biliary obstruction in terms of success and 30-day mortality rates. Moreover, the endoprosthesis has three advantages: (a) a low incidence of early major complications; (b) a short hospital stay and (c) avoidance of operation in frail, elderly and high-risk patients. However, endoscopic stents have their own disadvantages. First, 3%–9% of patients successfully stented develop duodenal obstruction and require subsequent surgical bypass (Siegel and Snady 1986; Meduri et al. 1988; Shepherd et al. 1988; Speer and Cotton 1988) and this figure would be greater if all patients were treated non-operatively (see below). Second, late complications, especially recurrent jaundice secondary to prosthesis obstruction of cholangitis, are commoner after endoscopic stenting than surgical bypass (26% vs 10%, Table 1). In fact the incidence exceeds 50% if the patients survive beyond 6 months (Siegel and Snady 1986).

In our view, a permanent endoprosthesis should be preferred to surgical bypass in (a) frail or elderly patients who might not withstand the operation, (b) patients with advanced pancreatic cancer (e.g. those with ascites) but without evidence of impending or established duodenal obstruction and (c) patients whose bilirubin level fails to decrease despite adequate flow through a temporary external drain, because the 30-day mortality rate in such patients is very high (up to 90%) if they are submitted to operation (Ferrucci et al. 1980; Neff et al. 1983). Since the results of percutaneous and endoscopic endoprostheses are generally similar (Table 1), there is no absolute criterion to determine the optimal route. As is true for most interventional techniques, the complication rate for non-operative decompression decreases with experience, so the choice of route in a particular hospital will clearly be influenced by the expertise most readily available. Other things being equal, however, it would seem sensible to stent high (hilar) obstructions from above and low (periampullary) obstructions from below.

Surgical Bypass

At present, surgical bypass remains the standard treatment for patients with irresectable pancreatic cancer in our unit unless they are elderly or frail or have disseminated cancer with a poor expectation of survival. The 30-day mortality rate in recent series averages only 3%, and the success rate exceeds 90% (Table 1). Our justification for laparotomy is as follows. It provides the opportunity to biopsy the lesion, to prove beyond doubt that the tumour is not resectable and to palliate jaundice, vomiting (imminent or future) and pain all at one sitting. Moreover, late complications, notably recurrent jaundice and cholangitis, occur less frequently after surgical bypass than non-operative stenting.

The results of surgical bypass versus laparotomy alone, as culled from eight series between 1971 and 1990, are shown in Table 2. Laparotomy alone was associated with a higher operative mortality rate (29% vs 17%) and shorter survival time (3.7 vs 6.9 months), probably because patients with the most advanced disease were turned down for bypass. The enormous advances in pancreatic imaging mean that there is little or no role for "staging" laparotomy today. Patients with carcinomatosis should be spared a fruitless laparotomy and should be stented to relieve jaundice. Those with less unfavourable disease and those in whom there is even a chance of resection should be submitted to full assessment at laparotomy, and biliary-enteric bypass is then indicated if resection cannot be performed. However, this policy of palliative surgery must carry low morbidity and mortality rates to be justifiable. Thus the operation

Table 2. Operative mortality rate and average survival period following palliative biliary bypass and laparotomy alone

Reference	Total[a]	Biliary bypass	Lapar- otomy	Operative mortality (%)		Mean survival (months)	
				Biliary bypass	Lapar- otomy	Biliary bypass	Lapar- otomy
Pope and Fish (1971)	158	101	49	24 (22)	33 (16)	10.4	8.4
Richards and Sosin (1973)	106	91	15	20 (18)	33 (5)	5.8	3.0
Hertzberg (1974)	169	148	21	13 (19)	43 (9)	6.8	1.6
Knight et al. (1978)	286	153	133	22 (34)	25 (33)	6.7	3.5
Forrest and Longmire (1979)	169	103	66	20 (21)	44 (29)	5.6	3.6
Morrow et al. (1984)	124	76	48	12 (9)	19 (9)	4.0	3.0
Rosenberg et al. (1985)	341	207	134	16 (34)	30 (39)	6.3	2.9
Kahn et al. (1990)	92	66	26	6 (4)	8 (2)	11.3	3.7
Total	1437	945	492	17 (161)	29 (142)	6.9	3.7

Actual numbers of patients are given in parentheses.
[a] Total number of patients undergoing operation, excluding resection.

should be undertaken or at least be supervised by surgeons adequately experienced in techniques of biliary–intestinal anastomosis.

Several different types of surgical bypass procedure are available, using either the common bile duct or the gallbladder on the biliary side and the stomach, duodenum or jejunum on the intestinal side. The commoner techniques are illustrated in Fig. 1.

Cholecystogastrostomy and Choledochogastrostomy

Although these two procedures are still being used in some centres, we do not recommend them. It can be difficult to construct a safe and leak-proof anastomosis between the thick-walled stomach and the thin-walled gallbladder. Moreover, bile gastritis and acid hypersecretion can be troublesome among the survivors.

Cholecystoduodenostomy and Choledochoduodenostomy

The duodenum has also been used to circumvent malignant biliary obstruction. Choledochoduodenostomy, whether side-to-side or end-to-side, is an effective bypass for benign biliary obstructions, such as choledocholithiasis. However, its use in malignant obstruction is severely limited because of the propensity for pancreatic carcinoma to invade and obstruct the duodenum. The anastomosis must inevitably lie close to the tumour mass and is very likely to be compromised by extension of the pancreatic neoplasm. In 48 patients with cancer (37 pancreatic, 11 periampullary), Stuart et al. (1971) undertook choledochoduo-denostomy when the gallbladder was not available and cholecystoduodenostomy when it was. Their mortality rate was 10%, complications occurred in 14.6% and jaundice recurred in 10.4%. In Reber's (1990) experience about a third

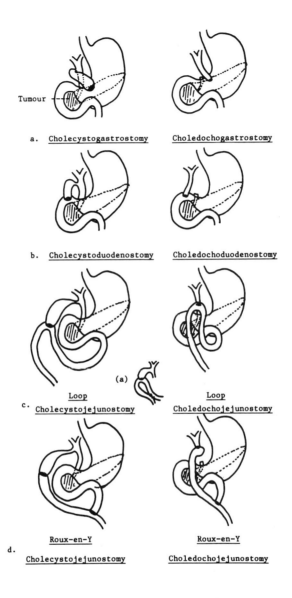

Fig. 1. Various palliative biliary–enteric bypass procedures for irresectable pancreatic carcinoma. Inset to **c** shows modification of loop cholecystojejunostomy by adding enteroenterostomy.

of the 16 patients treated with this operation developed late biliary obstruction.

The accumulated experience with these procedures is shown in Table 3. The mortality rate of cholecystoduodenostomy was similar to that of choledochoduodenostomy (12%), but the mean survival time was shorter (5.2 vs 7.7 months). We do not believe that it is appropriate to use the duodenum to bypass biliary

Table 3. Operative mortality rate and average survival time after cholecystoduodenostomy or choledochoduodenostomy

Reference	Cholecystoduodenostomy			Choledochoduodenostomy		
	No.	Mortality rate (%)	Mean survival time (months)	No.	Mortality rate (%)	Mean survival time (months)
Buckwalter et al. (1965)	34	18 (6)	4.4	44	21 (9)	7.7
Bufkin et al. (1967)	7	—	2.8	3	—	17.0
Richards and Sosin (1973)	21	10 (2)	5.5	12	33 (4)	6.0
Bergstrand et al. (1978)	58	9 (5)	5.7	76	12 (9)	7.4
Sonnenfeld et al. (1986)	6	—	7.2	18	—	7.2
Potts et al. (1990)	—	—	—	60	0	8.0
Total	126	12 (13)	5.2	213	12 (22)	7.7

Actual numbers of patients are given in parentheses.

obstruction secondary to pancreatic cancer because of the risk of recurrent jaundice.

Cholecystojejunostomy and Choledochojejunostomy

These are the most commonly performed procedures nowadays for the relief of obstructive jaundice in pancreatic cancer, at least in the United Kingdom, but argument still surrounds their relative merits. Cholecystojejunostomy is certainly the simplest and most rapid technique for internal biliary decompression (Richards and Sosin 1973; Potts et al. 1990), requiring little or no dissection of the gallbladder or jejunum. Although it maximises the distance between the anastomosis and the tumour, cystic duct encroachment by cancer may lead to recurrent jaundice. This seriously undermines the value of the procedure. The mere presence of a distended gallbladder does not ensure adequate biliary decompression after cholecystojejunostomy, because a partly obstructed gallbladder can contain as much mucus as bile. In at least 10% of patients, the cystic duct runs alongside the common bile duct for some distance before entering it low down near the duodenum, and it is thus at risk of early obstruction by local tumour extension (Sarr and Cameron 1984). Before the gallbladder is selected for the anastomosis, therefore, it is important to ensure that the cystic duct (a) is still patent and (b) enters the common duct at least 2–3 cm above the tumour mass. If this anatomical arrangement cannot easily be verified by direct inspection of the junction between cystic and common bile ducts, cholangiography should be performed by inserting a needle or catheter into the dilated gallbladder. Preoperative endoscopic retrograde cholangiopancreatography (ERCP) is more likely to have displayed the crucial anatomy than PTC.

Uncertainty about cystic duct patency is avoided by routine use of choledochojejunostomy (Fig. 1d), which is our own preference. Table 4 summarises the collected results of these two biliary–enteric bypass procedures in seven series reported between 1965 and 1989. The mortality rates of cholecystojejunostomy and choledochojejunostomy are similar but much too high (mean 21%), and the mean survival times are also similar (5.9 months and 7.6 months). Most recent studies have shown a marked decrease in operative mortality rate following both procedures (8.6% after cholecystojejunostomy and 3.3% after choledochojejunostomy) (McGrath et al. 1989; Rosemurgy et al. 1989). In terms of long-term morbidity, the incidence of recurrent jaundice is generally lower when the common duct is used for decompression (0–17% as compared with 4%–64% following gallbladder–enteric bypass) (Richards and Sosin 1973; Eastman and Kune 1980; Ubhi and Doran 1986).

Another controversial issue in performing biliary–enteric bypass is whether to use a jejunal loop in continuity or a Roux-en-Y type of anastomosis (Fig. 1c, d). Morgenstern and Shore (1970) studied the relative merits of a simple jejunal loop, a loop with an enteroenterostomy and a Roux-en-Y anastomosis in dogs, using either the gallbladder or the bile duct for the upper end of the anastomosis. Cholangitis was most likely to occur with a simple loop (86%), it was not prevented by adding an enteroenterostomy (86%), and it was least likely to occur with a Roux-en-Y anastomosis (43%). Death from ascending cholangitis only occurred with loop anastomoses (14%). Although Roux-en-Y biliary–enteric bypass clearly entails a longer operative time and more anastomoses than a simple loop, it still conveys important benefits: (a) a lower operative mortality rate (Buckwalter et al. 1965; Lee 1984); (b) a better rate

Table 4. Operative mortality rate and mean survival time after cholecystojejunostomy or choledochojejunostomy

Reference	Cholecystojejunostomy			Choledochojejunostomy		
	No.	Mortality rate (%)	Mean survival time (months)	No.	Mortality rate (%)	Mean survival time (months)
Buckwalter et al. (1965)	83	22 (18)	5.3	18	17 (3)	6.6
Richards and Sosin (1973)	26	15 (4)	6.8	5	20 (1)	4.9
Bergstrand et al. (1978)	57	21 (12)	3.6	10	50 (5)	5.3
Brooks et al. (1981)	24	—	6.0	10	—	6.0
Ubhi and Doran (1986)	66	—	7.0	12	—	11.0
Rosemurgy et al. (1989)	22	23 (5)	7.5	15	7 (1)	10.4
McGrath et al. (1989)	36	0	7.0	15	0	7.0
Total	314	21 (39)	5.9	85	21 (10)	7.6

Actual numbers of patients are given in parentheses.

of bilirubin clearance (Bergstrand et al. 1978); and (c) slight prolongation of survival (Buckwalter et al. 1965; Bufkin et al. 1967).

Our own policy is therefore as follows. In patients with reasonable expectation of survival, we prefer to resect the gallbladder, divide the common hepatic duct well above the "leading edge" of the tumour and bring up a Roux loop for end-to-side choledochojejunostomy. The rationale for cholecystectomy is partly to improve access and partly to avoid the risk of infection in an obstructed gallbladder. The rationale for duct transection is to interrupt possible upward spread of carcinoma within or alongside the wall of the duct. In patients found to have unexpectedly advanced cancer at operation in whom survival cannot be anticipated beyond a very few weeks, we perform cholecystojejunostomy so as not to prolong proceedings. However, if this situation can be identified on preoperative imaging, we would prefer to stent such patients and avoid the need for operation altogether.

Gastric Outflow Obstruction

Nausea and vomiting are presenting symptoms in 30%–45% of patients with pancreatic cancer, although actual gastric outflow obstruction occurs in only 5% at the time of diagnosis. Another 21% of patients (range 8%–50%) develop duodenal obstruction at a later stage of the disease. In such patients, the need for a gastrojejunostomy is clear. The question then arises as to whether all patients undergoing palliative laparotomy should be subjected to gastroenterostomy. Table 5 reveals the collected results of patients undergoing biliary bypass with and without gastrojejunostomy. In this review of nearly 1000 patients, adding gastrojejunostomy did not increase the operative mortality rate of biliary bypass (13% with initial gastrojejunostomy versus 16% without). Average survival times in the two groups were approximately the same (6.4 versus 7.2 months). Among 578 patients surviving biliary bypass alone, a mean of 16% (range 6%–44%) required reoperation because of duodenal obstruction, which developed 7.9 months later. The mortality rate of this subsequent gastrojejunostomy was high, up to 50% (average 19%), and survival time after this second operation was only 3.2 months. Thus prophylactic gastrojejunostomy is safe and should probably be performed in any patient who is likely to survive for at least a few weeks.

The main objection to prophylactic gastrojejunostomy is the risk of postoperative complications of delayed gastric emptying (DGE) and upper gastrointestinal bleeding owing to stomal ulceration or biliary gastritis. DGE is defined as the inability to tolerate oral fluids 8 days or more after the operation, leading to prolonged nasogastric intubation and hospital stay. Doberneck and Berndt (1987) were concerned that a gastrojejunostomy might even provoke postoperative DGE. They found a 57% incidence of DGE when duodenal obstruction was present and a 16% incidence when it was not. This complication has now been reported in 10%–30% of patients with irresectable pancreatic carcinoma undergoing gastric bypass (Schantz et al. 1984; Jacobs et al. 1989; Potts et al. 1990), and the incidence of DGE is the same after either

Table 5. Operative mortality rate and mean survival period of patients with and without initial gastrojejunostomy (GJ) at the time of biliary bypass

Reference	Total[a]	Those with initial GJ			Those without initial GJ			Those going on to GJ later				
		No.	Operative mortality (%)	Mean survival (months)	No.	Operative mortality (%)	Mean survival (months)	No.	%[b]	Operative mortality (%)	Mean interval[c] (months)	Mean survival[d] (months)
Richards and Sosin (1973)	91	21	19 (4)	6.5	70	20 (14)	5.5	19/56	34	11 (2)	7.1	3.6
Hertzberg (1974)	148	5	0	6.8	143	13 (18)	6.8	7/125	6	—	—	—
Schantz et al. (1984)	103	46	15 (7)	8.4	57	14 (8)	8.8	6/49	12	16 (1)	8.0	—
Lee (1984)	111	64	11 (7)	—	47	17 (8)	—	3/39	8	—	4.0	—
Rosenberg et al. (1985)	187	47	22 (10)	5.2	140	14 (19)	7.1	18/121	15	6 (1)	9.1	2.5
Uhbi and Doran (1986)	78	42	14 (6)	6.7	36	31 (11)	6.7	11/25	44	—	—	—
La Ferla and Murray (1987)	100	14	14 (2)	—	86	28 (24)	—	8/62	13	—	5.4	2.5
Jacobs et al. (1989)	58	17	18 (3)	4.2	41	7 (3)	9.4	14/38	37	50 (7)	9.8	3.9
Potts et al. (1990)	122	56	0	6.0	66	5 (3)	8.0	7/63	11	—	—	—
Total	998	312	13 (39)	6.4	686	16 (108)	7.2	93/578	16	19 (11)	7.9	3.2

[a] Total number of patients undergoing biliary bypass procedure. [b] Percentage of those surviving initial biliary bypass and undergoing subsequent gastrojejunostomy. [c] Mean interval from biliary to gastric drainage. [d] Mean survival period after second operation (gastrojejunostomy). Actual numbers of patients are given in parentheses.

prophylactic or therapeutic gastrojejunostomy (Jacobs et al. 1989).

The aetiology of DGE is still uncertain. Autonomic denervation may result from malignant involvement of the celiac plexus and inhibition of upper gastrointestinal motility (Meinke et al. 1983). Barkin (1986) showed that 60% of pancreatic cancer patients without duodenal obstruction or electrolyte imbalance had gastric emptying curves more than two standard deviations below normal mean values. Chronic impending obstruction of the duodenum might delay the return of normal gastric motility and explain the high incidence of DGE in patients with preoperative vomiting. In Doberneck's experience of patients with combined biliary and duodenal bypass ($n = 46$), two of 12 (17%) with gastrojejunostomy proximal to the biliary–enteric anastomosis had DGE as opposed to six of 22 (27%) with gastrojejunostomy distal to the biliary–enteric anastomosis (Doberneck and Berndt 1987). Placing the gastroenterostomy proximal to the biliary–enteric anastomosis may reduce the irritant effects of bile on the gastric mucosa.

Most patients with DGE will recover spontaneously after varying periods of nasogastric tube drainage. Total parenteral nutrition should be started early in these malnourished patients while mechanical obstruction is ruled out by radiological contrast studies and/or endoscopy. The return of motility may be hastened by giving prokinetic agents such as metoclopramide, domperidone or cisapride.

Upper gastrointestinal bleeding occurred in 0–17% of patients undergoing gastrojejunostomy in three series (Richards and Sosin 1973; Schantz et al. 1984; Jacobs et al. 1989). Malignant invasion of the gut, pre-existing peptic ulcer disease, biliary gastritis and stress ulceration are all possible aetiological factors; Sarr et al. (1981) found stomal (marginal) ulcers in three of 100 patients. The fact that loop gastrojejunostomy has a slightly higher incidence of gastrointestinal bleeding than Roux-en-Y anastomosis (17% versus 10%) (Kairaluoma et al. 1987) supports the aetiological role of bile gastritis.

In summary, prophylactic gastroenterostomy can relieve incipient obstruction of the descending duodenum, whether mechanical or functional, and avoid the need for reoperation (for vomiting) at a later stage of the disease, but it does prolong the initial operation and may add its own complications. Although we recommend prophylactic Roux-en-Y gastrojejunostomy in all patients with a reasonable expectation of survival, a case could be made to reserve it for those patients whose tumour lies relatively close to the duodenal loop and not in the uncinate process or pancreatic neck. To minimise bile gastritis, we now prefer to place the gastrojejunostomy proximal to the biliary–enteric anastomosis but on the same Roux loop of jejunum (Fig. 2). We have not encountered subsequent cholangitis as a result of food debris entering the bile duct. We do not advocate truncal vagotomy (unless the patient has active duodenal ulcer disease), because this is likely further to delay gastric emptying. H_2 receptor antagonists are given routinely, and agents to stimulate gastric motility are tried in those with gastric atony.

Pain Relief

Pain is a presenting symptom in 70%–90% of pancreatic cancer patients, regardless of the site of the primary lesion, but it is often relatively minor in

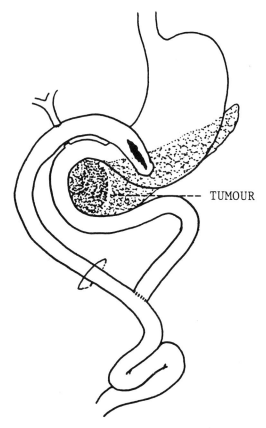

TUMOUR

Fig. 2. Roux-en-Y choledochojejunostomy with gastrojejunostomy (prophylactic or therapeutic). Gastroenterostomy lies proximal to biliary–enteric anastomosis to prevent biliary gastritis and may reduce the incidence of delayed gastric emptying.

degree. Pain seems to be related to the stage of the disease: 65% of those undergoing palliative bypass procedures and more than 85% of those who were unsuitable for any operation had moderate to severe pain (Singh and Reber 1989). Characteristically the pain of advanced pancreatic cancer is perceived deep in the abdominal cavity, in either the periumbilical or epigastric region; it is chronic rather than episodic and it radiates through to the back. Pain may be affected by positional changes, being aggravated by the supine position and relieved by sitting up and leaning forwards.

Since surgical exploration is frequently required in patients with pancreatic cancer, alleviation of pain at the time of operation would seem to be a sensible endeavour. It is those unfortunate patients with deep boring pain radiating to the back who are most in need of an attempt at permanent analgesia. Pancreatic duct decompression over a T-tube into the stomach or jejunum has been tried with some benefit but without dramatic pain relief (Gallitano et al. 1968; Flanigan and Kraft 1978). We have employed intubated pancreaticogastrostomy (Apalakis et al. 1977) in a few selected patients who have troublesome pain together with an irresectable carcinomia of the head and no distant disease.

Dilatation of the pancreatic duct in the body of pancreas may be seen on preoperative imaging (ERCP, CT) and confirmed at operation by palpation, needling and ambigrade ductography (Cooper and Williamson 1983). It is a simple matter to open a short segment of pancreatic duct, insert a T-tube, bring the tube through the stomach to the exterior and then tack the small posterior gastrotomy to the pancreas with a few interrupted sutures. Although gastrointestinal and biliary obstruction may contribute to the pain of pancreatic cancer, less than 10% of the 107 UCLA patients who underwent biliary or gastric bypass reported any noticeable relief from pain thereafter, and even these relapsed within a few weeks or months (Singh and Reber 1989).

Surgical splanchnicectomy involves resection of as much as possible of the greater, lesser and least splanchnic nerves and is a formidable technical exercise. The results of this operation were reviewed in 56 patients who had undergone splanchnicectomy since 1950 (Sadar and Cooperman 1974), some of whom had concurrent bypass procedures. Complete pain relief was achieved in 21 (37%), but pain recurred in six of these. Another 34% were improved but still required analgesics for optimal pain control. As surgical splanchnicectomy offers rather lower success rates than other methods (Sadar and Cooperman 1974) and prolongs the complexity and duration of the operation, it is rarely undertaken nowadays.

Peroperative ablation of the celiac ganglia is a more attractive therapy for the severe pain of pancreatic cancer. It is one of the simplest, most effective and least hazardous means of palliation. In two series totalling 90 patients, 90% experienced initial pain relief and 70%–80% had no further pain up to the time of death (Flanigan and Kraft 1978; Gardner and Solomou 1984). Either 6% phenol or 50% ethanol can be used as the neurolytic agent, but we prefer alcohol which may act more rapidly. After identifying the aorta, the surgeon injects 20–25 ml of the agent on either side, retroperitoneally and close to the vertebral bodies, to infiltrate the celiac ganglia and the splanchnic nerves which run upwards and laterally to pierce the crus of the diaphragm. Fig. 3 demonstrates the relationship of the celiac ganglia to the surrounding structures. Care must be taken to avoid intravascular injection (which can cause convulsions) by repeated aspiration before and during injection. Complications are uncommon but include hypotension and diarrhoea, which may reflect a relative excess of parasympathetic tone. Nausea and vomiting may be improved due to interruption of vagal fibres as they travel through the celiac plexus. In patients unsuitable for operation or those in whom pain recurs, percutaneous celiac plexus block can be carried out under the auspices of a pain clinic.

Radiotherapy may have little or no impact on survival in pancreatic cancer, but it will usually relieve the severe pain of those with irresectable disease. Chemotherapy alone is of doubtful benefit. Recently, combination treatment with radiotherapy and chemotherapy has been employed (following surgical palliation) with some success. Intravenous 5-fluorouracil followed by radiation significantly increased survival time from 8.9 months to 13.5 months in patients with previous (operative) biliary bypass. Nearly 80% (29 of 37) of those with pain at the outset were free of pain upon completion of therapy (Kahn et al. 1990). These promising results merit further study.

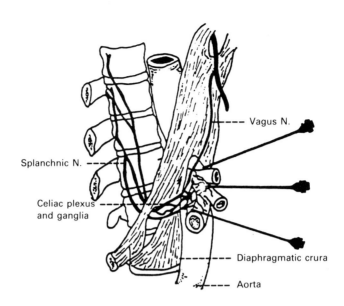

Fig. 3. Relative anatomy of celiac plexus and ganglia to adjacent aorta, vagus nerve and diaphragm. Ethanol or phenol should be injected on each side and in front of the aorta at the origin of celiac artery. Vagal fibres may be interrupted as they travel through the plexus.

Conclusions

We believe that laparotomy is desirable in most patients with irresectable cancer of the pancreatic head. It provides the opportunity to obtain definitive histology, confirm irresectability beyond any doubt, provide permanent biliary and duodenal bypass and address the problem of intractable pain all at one sitting. By contrast, operation offers little or no benefit to patients with cancers of the body or tail of pancreas, unless the tumour appears to be one of the very few which are resectable. Such patients usually die of disseminated malignancy before the tumour obstructs the bile duct or duodenojejunal flexure sufficiently to cause jaundice and vomiting. Laparotomy may still be needed if investigations are equivocal as regards resectability or to provide a tissue diagnosis if adjuvant therapy is planned.

References

Adam A (1990) Percutaneous biliary drainage for malignancy – an expanding field. Clin Radiol 41:225–227
Adam A, Chetty N, Roddie M, Yeung E, Benjamin IS (1991) Self-expandable stainless steel endoprostheses for treatment of malignant bile duct obstruction. AJR 156: 321–325
Andersen JR, Sørensen SM, Kruse A, Rokkjær M, Matzen P (1989) Randomised trial of

endoscopic endoprosthesis versus operative bypass in malignant obstructive jaundice. Gut 30:1132–1135

Apalakis A, Dussault J, Knight M, Smith R (1977) Relief of pain from pancreatic carcinoma. Ann R Coll Surg Engl 59:401–403

Barkin JS, Goldberg RI, Sfakianakis GN, Levi J (1986) Pancreatic carcinoma is associated with delayed gastric emptying. Dig Dis Sci 31:265–267

Bergstrand O, Ahlberg J, Ewerth S, Hellers G, Holmstrom B (1978) A retrospective study of carcinoma of the pancreas with special reference to the results of surgical treatment. Acta Chir Scand Suppl 482:26–28

Bornman PC, Harries-Jones EP, Tobias R, van Stiegmann G, Terblanche J (1986) Prospective controlled trial of transhepatic biliary endoprosthesis versus bypass surgery for incurable carcinoma of head of pancreas. Lancet i:69–71

Brooks DC, Osteen RT, Gray EB Jr, Steele GD Jr, Wilson RE (1981) Evaluation of palliative procedures for pancreatic cancer. Am J Surg 141:430–433

Buckwalter JA, Lawton RL, Tidrick RT (1965) Bypass operations for neoplastic biliary tract obstruction. Am J Surg 109:100–106

Bufkin WJ, Smith PE, Krementz ET (1967) Evaluation of palliative operations for carcinoma of the pancreas. Arch Surg 94:240–242

Connolly MM, Dawson PJ, Michelassi F, Moossa AR, Lowenstein F (1987) Survival in 1001 patients with carcinoma of the pancreas. Ann Surg 206:366–373

Cooper MJ, Williamson RCN (1983) The value of operative pancreatography. Br J Surg 70:577–580

Devereux DF, Greco RS (1986) Biliary enteric bypass for malignant obstruction. Cancer 58:981–984

Doberneck RC, Berndt GA (1987) Delayed gastric emptying after palliative gastrojejunostomy for carcinoma of the pancreas. Arch Surg 122:827–829

Eastman MC, Kune GA (1980) The objectives of palliative surgery in pancreas cancer: a retrospective study of 73 cases. Aust NZ J Surg 50:462–464

Ferrucci JT, Mueller PR, Harbin WP (1980) Percutaneous transhepatic biliary drainage: techniques, results and applications. Radiology 135:1–13

Flanigan DP, Kraft RO (1978) Continuing experience with palliative chemical splanchnicectomy. Arch Surg 113:509–511

Fontham ETH, Correa P (1989) Epidemiology of pancreatic cancer. Surg Clin North Am 69:551–567

Forrest JF, Longmire WP Jr (1979) Carcinoma of the pancreas and periampullary region: a study of 279 patients. Ann Surg 189:129–138

Funovics JM, Karner J, Pratschner T, Fritsch A (1989) Current trends in the management of carcinoma of the pancreatic head. Hepatogastroenterology 36:450–455

Gallitano A, Fransen H, Martin RG (1968) Carcinoma of the pancreas. Results of treatment. Cancer 22:939–944

Gardner AMN, Solomou G (1984) Relief of the pain of unresectable carcinoma of pancreas by chemical splanchnicectomy during laparotomy. Ann R Coll Surg Engl 66:409–411

Hertzberg J (1974) Pancreatico-duodenal resection and bypass-operation in patients with carcinoma of the head of the pancreas, ampulla, and distal end of the common duct. Acta Chir Scand 140:523–527

Hirayama T (1989) Epidemiology of pancreatic cancer in Japan. Jpn J Clin Oncol 19:208–215

Howard JM, Jordan GL Jr (1977) Cancer of the pancreas. Curr Probl Cancer 2:5–52

Jacobs RPM, van der Sluis RF, Wobbes T (1989) Role of gastroenterostomy in the palliative surgical treatment of pancreatic cancer. J Surg Oncol 42:145–149

Joseph PK, Bizer LS, Sprayregen SS, Gliedman ML (1986) Percutaneous transhepatic biliary drainage: results and complications in 81 patients. 255:2763–2767

Kahn PJ, Skornick Y, Inbar M, Kaplan O, Chaichik S, Rozin R (1990) Surgical palliation combined with synchronous therapy in pancreatic carcinoma. Eur J Surg Oncol 16:7–11

Kairaluoma MI, Kiviniemi H, Laitinen S, Stahlberg M (1987) Staplers in palliative bypass surgery for unresectable pancreatic cancer. Pancreas 2:146–151

Knight RW, Scarborough JP, Goss JC (1978) Adenocarcinoma of the pancreas. A ten-year experience. Arch Surg 113:1401–1404

Kummerle F, Ruckert K (1984) Surgical treatment of pancreatic cancer. World J Surg 8:889–894

La Ferla G, Murray WR (1987) Carcinoma of the head of the pancreas: bypass surgery in unresectable disease. Br J Surg 74:212–213

Lammer J, Neumayer K (1986) Biliary drainage endoprostheses: experience with 201 placements. Radiology 159:625–629

Lee YN (1984) Surgery for carcinoma of the pancreas and periampullary structures: complication of resectional and palliative procedures. J Surg Oncol 27:280–285

McGrath PC, McNeill PM, Neifeld JP, Bear HD, Parker GA, Turner MA et al. (1989) Management of biliary obstruction in patients with unresectable carcinoma of the pancreas. Ann Surg 209:284–288

Meduri B, Fritsch J, Calogero G (1988) Pancreatic cancer: palliative endoscopic biliary drainage. Int J Pancreatol 3:S143–S146

Meinke WB, Twomey PL, Guernsey JM, Frey CF, Higgins G, Keehn R (1983) Gastric outlet obstruction after palliative surgery for cancer of head of pancreas. Arch Surg 118:550–553

Morgenstern L, Shore JM (1970) Selection of an optimal procedure for decompression of the obstructed common bile duct. Am J Surg 119:38–44

Morrow M, Hilaris B, Brennan MF (1984) Comparison of conventional surgical resection, radioactive implantation, and bypass procedures for exocrine carcinoma of the pancreas 1975–1980. Ann Surg 199:1–5

Mueller PR, Ferrucci JT, Teplick SK, van Sonnenberg E, Haskin PH et al. (1985) Biliary stent endoprosthesis: analysis of complications in 113 patients. Radiology 156:637–639

Muir C, Waterhouse J, Mack T, Powell J, Whelan S. (1987) Cancer incidence in five continents. Vol V, IARC Sci Publ, Lyon, no. 88

Neff RA, Fankuchen EI, Cooperman AM (1983) The radiological management of malignant biliary obstruction. Clin Radiol 34:143–146

Office of Population Censuses and Surveys (1990) Review of the national cancer registration system. Series MB1: no 17

Pope NA, Fish JC (1971) Palliative surgery for carcinoma of the pancreas. Am J Surg 121:271–272

Potts Jr, Broughan TA, Hermann RE (1990) Palliative operations for pancreatic carcinoma. Am J Surg 159:72–77

Proctor HJ, Mauro M (1990) Biliary diversion for pancreatic carcinoma: matching the methods and the patients. Am J Surg 159:67–71

Reber HA (1987) Palliative operations for pancreatic cancer. In: Howard JM, Jordon GL Jr, Reber HA (eds) Surgical diseases of the pancreas. Lea and Febiger, Philadelphia

Reber HA (1990) Discussion of biliary diversion for pancreatic carcinoma: matching the methods and the patients. Am J Surg 159:77–78

Richards AB, Sosin H (1973) Cancer of the pancreas: the value of radical and palliative surgery. Ann Surg 177:325–331

Rosemurgy AS, Burnett CM, Wasselle JA (1989) A comparison of choledochoenteric bypass and cholecystoenteric bypass in patients with biliary obstruction due to pancreatic cancer. Am Surg 55:55–60

Rosenberg JM, Welch JP, Macaulay WP (1985) Cancer of the head of the pancreas: an institutional review with emphasis on surgical therapy. J Surg Oncol 28:217–221

Sadar ES, Cooperman AM (1974) Bilateral thoracic sympathetic splanchnicectomy in the treatment of intractable pain due to pancreatic carcinoma. Cleve Clin Q 41:185–188

Sarr MG, Cameron JL (1984) Surgical palliation of unresectable carcinoma of the pancreas. World J Surg 8:906–918

Sarr MG, Gladen HE, Beart RW Jr, Van Heerden JA (1981) Role of gastroenterostomy in patients with unresectable carcinoma of the pancreas. Surg Gynecol Obstet 152:597–600

Schantz SP, Schickler W, Evans TK, Coffey RJ (1984) Palliative gastroenterostomy for pancreatic cancer. Am J Surg 147: 793–796

Shepherd HA, Royle G, Ross APR, Diba A, Arthur M, Colin-Jones D (1988) Endoscopic biliary endoprosthesis in the palliation of malignant obstruction of the distal common bile duct: a randomized trial. Br J Surg 75:1166–1168

Siegel JH, Snady H (1986) The significance of endoscopically placed prostheses in the management of biliary obstruction due to carcinoma of the pancreas: results of nonoperative decompression in 277 patients. Am J Gastroenterol 81:634–641

Singh SM, Reber HA (1989) Surgical palliation for pancreatic cancer. Surg Clin North Am 69:599–611

Sonnenfeld T, Nyberg B, Perbeck L (1986) The effect of palliation biliodigestive operations for unresectable pancreatic cancer. Acta Chir Scand Suppl 530:47–50

Speer AG, Cotton PB, Russell RCG, Mason RR, Hatfield ARW, Leung JW et al. (1987) Randomised trial of endoscopic versus percutaneous stent insertion in malignant obstructive jaundice. Lancet ii:57–62

Speer AG, Cotton PB (1988) Endoscopic treatment of pancreatic cancer. Int J Pancreatol 3:S147–S158

Stuart M, Keo T, Hermann RE (1971) Palliation of malignant obstruction of the common bile duct by side to side choledochoduodenostomy. Am J Surg 121:505–509

Trede M (1985) The surgical treatment of pancreatic carcinoma. Surgery 97:28–35

Tytgat GNJ, Bartelsman JFWM, Den Hartog Jager FCA, Huibregtse K, Mathus-Vliegen EMH (1986) Upper intestinal and biliary tract endoprosthesis. Dig Dis Sci 31 (9 Suppl):57S–76S

Ubhi CS, Doran J (1986) Palliation for carcinoma of head of pancreas. Ann R Coll Surg Engl 68:159–162

Williamson RCN (1988) Pancreatic cancer: the greatest oncological challenge. Br Med J 296:445–446

Chapter 7

Endoscopic Palliation of Pancreatic Cancer

A. R. W. Hatfield

Background

In the past the diagnosis of carcinoma of the pancreas, particularly in the presence of jaundice, was often made at exploratory laparotomy and in most patients a biliary and/or gastric bypass would then be performed unless it was possible to perform a radical resection. With the advent of diagnostic endoscopic retrograde cholangiopancreatography (ERCP), ultrasound and CT, the surgeon can achieve a preoperative diagnosis and proceed to planned surgery. In the vast majority of cases this has still meant a surgical biliary bypass and even in the best centres this still carries a substantial 30-day mortality which in various publications has been reported between 5% and 25% (Feduska et al. 1971; Sarr and Cameron 1982). In an attempt to lower the operative mortality of bypass surgery, external transhepatic biliary drainage was performed to lower the serum bilirubin prior to surgery. Controlled trials have shown that there was no difference in the postoperative mortality after surgery whether or not the patients underwent preoperative percutaneous biliary drainage (Hatfield et al. 1982). Transhepatic techniques were developed to allow for internal biliary stenting via the percutaneous route as an alternative to surgery. Such techniques were not without complication and endoscopic endoprosthesis insertion for the palliation of malignant obstructive jaundice was shown to be less dangerous than stenting via the transhepatic route (Speer et al. 1987). Endoscopic stenting has now been widely accepted as the major non-operative technique to palliate obstructive jaundice secondary to carcinoma of the pancreas. It is still not certain whether a period of internal biliary drainage obtained by temporary endoscopic stenting prior to radical pancreatic resection will alter the results of such surgery.

Technique

Insertion of a biliary stent at the time of ERCP should always be considered as a substantial procedure and the patient should be properly prepared. All patients should be adequately hydrated, with intravenous fluids if necessary, and should have received prior intravenous antibiotics which are continued for at least 24 h afterwards. A fall of blood pressure, with or without sepsis, carries as much risk of precipitating the hepatorenal syndrome in a patient undergoing endoscopic stenting as in a patient undergoing major surgery. It is helpful if one is aware of the precise level of obstruction of the biliary tree from good quality ultrasound scanning. This avoids the need to overfill the biliary tree above the level of the stricture (which carries a risk of post-procedure sepsis) but one should always make sure that there is not a second higher level of obstruction at the porta hepatis. Having outlined the level of biliary obstruction it is always advisable to obtain cytological brushings from the stricture which, if positive, may obviate the need for a percutaneous biopsy (Fig. 1a).

A small sphincterotomy, performed prior to the stenting manoeuvre, is helpful as this gives easier access to the biliary tree not only at the time of initial stenting but also later. It is not always essential to perform a sphincterotomy and if there is extensive tumour infiltration at the papilla a sphincterotomy may cause bleeding. If the patient has a coagulation abnormality that cannot be corrected, one can place a stent without a prior sphincterotomy. There is debate as to whether insertion of a stent through an intact papilla may in fact be associated with a greater risk of post-procedure pancreatitis.

After sphincterotomy the stricture is passed with a catheter and guidewire system (Fig. 1b). A dilator of the same size as the stent that is intended to be used can be passed over this system prior to stent insertion. The stent should then be correctly positioned to extend 1.5 – 2 cm above the level of the stricture and about a centimetre beyond the wall of the duodenum which will allow easy retrieval when the time comes for a stent change (Fig. 1c).

It is important to ascertain that the stent is functioning properly. This can be checked immediately by aspirating with the endoscope close up to the stent. One can observe instant decompression of the biliary tree on X-ray screening. Following the procedure the patient can eat and drink normally within an hour. In an elderly frail patient intravenous fluids may be necessary. It is advisable to perform an ultrasound scan at 24 h to confirm satisfactory biliary decompression before the patient is discharged.

Technical Difficulty

There are some patients in whom tumour invasion of the papilla and the duodenum make it extremely difficult to gain access to the biliary tree. In this situation where cannulation has failed, the use of a precut manoeuvre using a needle knife will enhance the success rate of both diagnostic and therapeutic

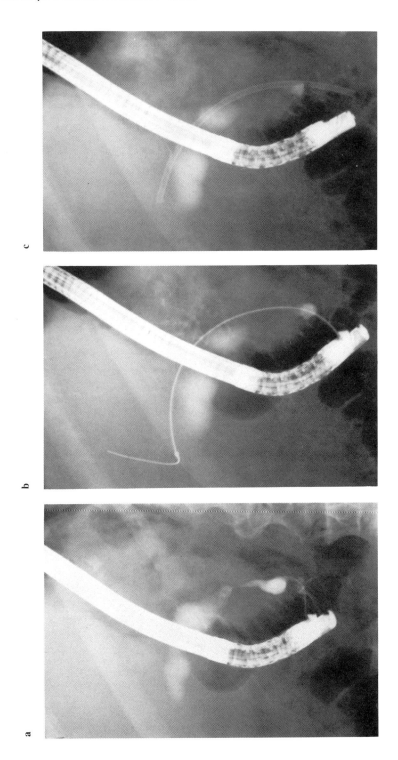

Fig. 1. a An ERCP showing a low malignant stricture in the common bile duct, secondary to pancreatic carcinoma. **b** A catheter and guidewire have been passed through the bile duct stricture, over which a dilator can be passed followed by a stent of the same diameter. **c** The stent has been positioned and the endoscope removed. X-ray contrast can be seen passing down the stent into the duodenum.

manoeuvres. Having made a small longitudinal cut in the area of the papilla, it is usually possible to pass a catheter or guidewire through the apex of this cut and then opacify and cannulate the biliary tree. If performed carefully, this procedure does not carry an undue complication rate.

The other technical problem that occurs in a proportion of patients is a very tight or tortuous stricture that cannot be passed with an endoscopic guidewire. In such patients a combined transhepatic and endoscopic approach can be performed (see Chapter 3) where the obstructed biliary tree is opacified with a percutaneous transhepatic cholangiogram. A radiologist can then pass a catheter and guidewire through the stricture from above and the guidewire can be snared by the endoscopist and pulled up through the endoscope, at the same procedure. The biliary stricture is dilated and stented via the endoscopic route (Dowsett et al. 1989a). This manoeuvre has the advantage that the dilatation and stent insertion are performed endoscopically and the transhepatic manipulation is all done through a small 5FG catheter which minimises any transhepatic bleeding or bile leak.

Stent Size and Material

There is a general feeling among endoscopists that "the larger the stent the better the drainage". This is probably quite correct (Speer et al. 1988). Undoubtedly teflon stents clog less rapidly but the material is a little rigid for routine use as an endoscopic stent in view of the acute angle at the level of the bridge elevator. Polyethylene has proved the most suitable alternative, maintaining some rigidity as well as flexibility. Most major centres now use tapered, straight 10 or 11.5FG stents with a proximal and distal flap to prevent migration and a single proximal side hole.

Stent Occlusion and the Need for Stent Change

Endoscopic stents will gradually clog up as a result of the deposition of a bacterial biofilm on the stent, followed by the adherence of biliary deposits and sludge which eventually occlude the lumen (Speer et al. 1988). Occasional patients suffer frequent or early stent blockage within one or two months. However, most patients will suffer stent occlusion and present with recurrent jaundice and/or biliary sepsis at about five months after initial stent insertion. Some centres routinely replace biliary stents every four to five months. It is my policy to advocate stent change only when the patient actually presents with symptoms. This is preferable as only about 30% of patients with pancreatic cancer survive long enough to present with symptoms of stent blockage. The vast majority succumb from their disease without jaundice and with their original stent in situ. Very occasionally patients will survive for up to a year without jaundice or cholangitis with their original stent in situ. It is likely that the stent has occluded long before in these patients and that bile drains around the side of the stent.

Results of Stenting

There have now been reports and reviews of the success and the advantages of endoscopic stenting from many centres (Cotton 1990). In a series from the Middlesex Hospital of over 400 patients with low malignant bile duct obstruction, the overall success rate of endoscopic drainage was 85% with a low complication rate and a procedure-related mortality rate of only 2% (Dowsett et al. 1989b). The commonest complication following stenting is cholangitis. This can be kept to a minimum by the appropriate use of peri-procedure antibiotics and by ensuring that correct stent positioning and adequate drainage have been achieved on the first attempt. A small number of patients may suffer bleeding and retroperitoneal perforation, mainly as a result of the sphincterotomy performed to position the stent. Pancreatitis occasionally occurs, mainly secondary to the manipulation at the level of the papilla, but is no more common than after diagnostic ERCP. There will always be an associated procedural mortality as many of these patients are extremely frail, elderly and sick at the time of stenting.

There have been very few trials comparing the results of endoscopic stenting against traditional bypass surgery. Shepherd et al. (1988) found no obvious difference in outcome between the two methods of treatment. However, the numbers were small, and it was felt at the time that a larger trial might show advantages in endoscopic stenting, particularly in terms of reducing the 30-day mortality. In a recently completed trial from the Middlesex Hospital, over 200 patients were randomly allocated to bypass surgery or endoscopic stenting as a means of palliating their malignant low bile duct obstruction. All patients were fit for surgery and had a bilirubin of at least 100 μmol/l. Preliminary results (Smith et al. 1989) showed that there was no difference between the two techniques in achieving technically successful drainage, and successful relief of jaundice and itching. There was a significantly lower procedure-related mortality (3% versus 14%), major complication rate (11% versus 29%) and total hospital stay (20 versus 26 days) in the stented patients compared with the surgical group. However, late duodenal obstruction and recurrent jaundice due to stent blockage were more common in the stented group, as one might expect. Despite these early benefits of endoscopic stenting, there was a significant, but unexplained difference in overall survival (median 26 weeks versus 21 weeks) favouring the surgical patients. It is possible that stented patients suffering from low-grade infection from stent blockage might succumb more quickly if this was not recognised and managed with a stent change and this might account for the difference in survival. Larger tumours, over 4 cm, and particularly the presence of distant metastases, were factors that indicated a poor outcome regardless of the method of palliation. From this randomised study, one could infer that endoscopic stenting is more appropriate for those elderly frail patients who seem unfit for surgery, but endoscopic stent insertion in a fit and healthy patient who is unfortunate enough to have a localised but non-resectable tumour might not lead to such good long-term results as a surgical bypass.

New Forms of Stents

Stents with a silver impregnated inner coating and those with antibiotic coatings are being tried at present. These stents may lead to a decrease in bacterial colonisation of the stent in the first few weeks after insertion which could possibly lead to an increase in stent survival. Another extremely interesting development has been the self-expanding metal stent (Wallstent). These stents are made from stainless-steel mesh and are compressed on a catheter delivery system that can be passed down the channel of the endoscope (Fig. 2a). When the stent is released within the bile duct, it expands to a maximum diameter of 10 mm, producing an instant and extremely effective biliary decompression (Fig. 2b). Such stents can be inserted safely and effectively and are associated with an extremely low level of post-procedural sepsis and a prolonged stent patency. Re-admissions for stent blockage are extremely uncommon (Williams et al. 1989). At present these stents are extremely expensive, but the initial cost can be balanced against the avoidance of further re-admission for stent change.

Conclusions

Low bile duct obstruction due to pancreatic carcinoma can be relieved by endoscopic stenting reliably, without major complications, and with a short in-patient stay and a low procedure-related mortality. However, these early benefits of stenting are not reflected in prolonged survival when compared with a similar group of patients undergoing surgical bypass. Clearly both methods of palliation are equally effective, but both have their advantages and disadvantages, and it remains for the clinician to choose the method of palliation in an individual patient. On economic grounds alone, endoscopic stenting, with its short in-patient stay and relatively lower cost, might be preferable. It would seem appropriate to recommend endoscopic stenting for the more elderly and frail patients who represent an increased operative risk, and also in those patients with large tumours, particularly those with distant metastases, who are likely to survive for a shorter period of time. In younger, fit patients, who do not have a resectable tumour, it is reasonable to suggest bypass surgery, based on our current information. However, the newer methods of stenting with self-expanding metal stents offer considerable advantages over conventional stenting and in the years to come might well produce as good results as surgery.

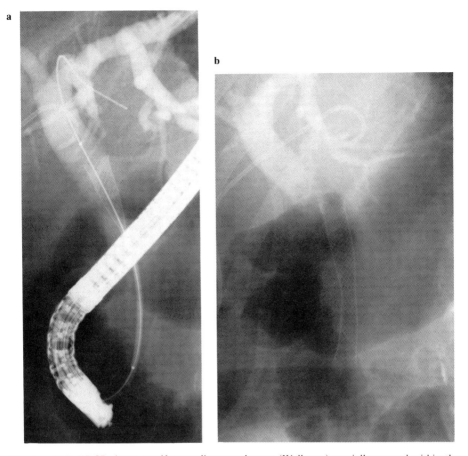

Fig. 2. a This ERCP shows a self-expanding metal stent (Wallstent) partially opened within the bile duct above a low stricture secondary to pancreatic carcinoma. **b** The metal stent has been released and is fully open and the delivery system and endoscope have been removed.

References

Cotton PB (1990) Management of malignant bile duct obstruction. Gastroenterol Hepatol 5:63–77

Dowsett JF, Vaira D, Hatfield ARW et al. (1989a) Endoscopic biliary therapy using the combined percutaneous and endoscopic technique. Gastroenterology 96:1180–1186

Dowsett JF, Williams SJ, Hatfield ARW et al. (1989b) Endoscopic management of low biliary obstruction due to unresectable primary pancreatobiliary malignancy – a review of 463 consecutive cases. Gastroenterology 96:A129

Feduska NJ, Dent TL, Lindenauer SM (1971) Results of palliative operations for carcinoma of the pancreas. Arch Surg 103:330–333

Hatfield ARW, Tobias R, Terblanche J et al. (1982) Preoperative external biliary drainage in obstructive jaundice. A prospective controlled clinical trial. Lancet ii:896–899

Sarr MG, Cameron JL (1982) Surgical management of unresectable carcinoma of the pancreas. Surgery 91:123–133

Shepherd HA, Royle G, Ross AP et al. (1988). Endoscopic biliary endoprosthesis in the palliation of malignant obstruction of the distal common bile duct: a randomised trial. Br J Surg 75:1166–1168

Smith AC, Dowsett JF, Hatfield ARW et al. (1989) A prospective randomised trial of bypass surgery versus endoscopic stenting in patients with malignant obstructive jaundice. Gut 30:A1513

Speer AG, Cotton PB, Russell RCG et al. (1987) Randomised trial of endoscopic versus percutaneous stent insertion in malignant obstructive jaundice. Lancet i:57–62

Speer AG, Cotton RB, Rode J et al. (1988) Biliary stent blockage with bacterial biofilm. Ann Intern Med 108:546–553

Williams SJ, Ainley CC, Smith AC et al. (1989) Self expanding metal stents in the endoscopic palliation of malignant biliary obstruction. Gut 30:A1513

Chapter 8

Why Resect Pancreatic Cancer?

C. D. Johnson

Adenocarcinoma of the pancreas is the third commonest gastrointestinal cancer, after colorectal and gastric adenocarcinoma. In the UK its incidence is steady, whereas that of gastric cancer is falling (Ashton-Key et al. 1991). However, in contrast to gastric and colorectal adenocarcinoma, pancreatic tumours are rarely resectable, and when resected the disease is rarely cured. What then is the justification for resection at all?

There are three arguments to support resection if this is technically feasible. First, patients who undergo resection by expert surgeons live longer than those who do not. Second, palliation is better with a successful resection than with other forms of treatment. Third, resection offers the patient the only chance of cure, however slight. Before considering these arguments in detail, I will outline a practical staging system, and discuss current operative mortality figures.

Staging

Modern imaging should allow accurate preoperative staging, although the final decision on resectability may have to be made at laparotomy. Computed tomography (CT) is the most useful investigation. Arteriography with venous phase films may indicate vascular involvement. Tumours can be classified as follows:

Stage I   Tumour confined to the pancreas
Stage II   Local invasion outside the pancreas or lymph node metastases
Stage III Hepatic, peritoneal or distant metastases

Stage I tumours should always be resected if the patient is fit for surgery. Stage III tumours should not be resected as the anticipated survival is so short. Stage II tumours may well be resectable and if this is technically feasible, resection should be performed.

Operative Mortality

What of those who say that the operative mortality for pancreatectomy is too high to justify its use in treatment of pancreatic carcinoma (Gudjunsson et al. 1978). The mortality of pancreatic resection has fallen dramatically since Gudjunsson et al. compiled their data (Edis et al. 1980; Dunn 1987). Elsewhere in this volume (Chapter 12), Cooper points out the extremely low operative mortality now achieved by some authors: Table 1 gives a fuller list of recent reports. Not all these series refer exclusively to carcinoma of the pancreas, but the message is clear. Resection of the pancreas, particularly of the pancreatic head, can now be achieved with operative mortality and morbidity similar to those reported for resection of the rectum and the stomach, and rather better than several recent reports of oesophageal resection with an operative mortality over 10%.

Carcinoma of the Head of the Pancreas

Postoperative Survival

Most authors now report a two-year survival in the region of 20% (Table 2). If the tumour can be detected at an early stage then the prospects are better.

Table 1. Operative morbidity and mortality following resection of the pancreatic head (Whipple procedure) or total pancreatectomy

Reference	Number of patients	Operative mortality	
		n	%
Sato et al. (1977)[a]	66	5	8
van Heerden (1984)	146	6	4.1
Jones et al. (1985)	87	4	5
Cooper and Williamson (1985)[a]	13	1	8
Grace et al. (1986)	45	1	2
Braasch et al. (1986)[a]	87	2	2
Tsuchiya et al. (1986)	94	4	4
Kairaluoma et al. (1987)	68	6	9
Tashiro et al. (1987)	132	14	10.6
Crist et al. (1987)[a]	47	1	2
Gall (1987)[a]	289	3	1
Cooper et al. (1987)[a]	83	4	4
Ishikawa et al. (1988)	59	6	10
Lygidakis et al. (1989)	78	3	4
Pellegrini et al. (1989)	51	1	2
Trede et al. (1990)	142	0	0
Bradbeer and Johnson (1990)[a]	41	2	45

[a] Includes chronic pancreatitis and other non-adenocarcinoma of pancreas patients.

Trede et al. (1990) report a five-year survival of 25% in patients undergoing what he calls an R_0 resection. By this he means radical resection of the tumour, with macroscopic and microscopic tumour-free resection lines. His figures currently show 12 survivors out of 50 such patients operated on more than five years ago (personal communication). Even for surgeons who have never seen an extended survival after resection for carcinoma of the pancreas, there is an increase in the duration of survival, when compared with patients of similar age and tumour size (Chandiramini et al. 1990).

Adjuvant Therapy

The current interest in adjuvant therapy in association with pancreatic resection is reviewed in detail in Chapter 8. The North American Gastrointestinal Tumour Study Group (1987) reported a doubling of two-year survival from 20% to 40% when adjuvant therapy was given following resection. This therapy consisted of simultaneous radiotherapy and 5-fluorouracil (5-FU). The 5-FU was given in conjunction with radiotherapy as a radiosensitiser and was then continued for two years. There was no apparent difference between patients given 40Gy and those given 60Gy. A multicentre European study is currently underway to compare the effectiveness of adjuvant radiotherapy and 5-FU as a radiosensitiser (without long-term therapy) against systemic chemotherapy alone following surgical resection. Clearly, for patients to obtain the potential benefits of adjuvant therapy, they must first undergo resection.

Quality of Life

It is extremely difficult to obtain factual information about the quality of life of patients with pancreatic cancer. Given that the operation is performed by a competent surgeon with low mortality and morbidity, the time required for recovery from a resection is amply repaid by prolongation of survival. Resection relieves the jaundice, which rarely recurs. The pain of pancreatic cancer is usually due to obstruction of the pancreatic duct. After resection and pancreaticogastric or pancreaticoenteric anastomosis, this obstruction is relieved. In my experience

Table 2. Two-year survival after resection for adenocarcinoma of the head of the pancreas

Reference	Number of patients	Median (months)	% 2-year survivors
Andren-Sandberg and Ihse (1983)	61	14	13
Braasch et al. (1986)	14	18	18
Bradbeer and Johnson (1990)	19	13	22
Dunn (1987)	22	18	21
Edis et al. (1980)	133		29
Ishikawa et al. (1988)	37 (R1)		13[a]
	22 (R2)		38[a]

[a] 3-year survivors.

it is unusual for local recurrence after resection to be painful. The patient's ability to eat and enjoy his food may be impaired by the side effects of any concomitant gastric resection. Nevertheless, removal of the primary tumour generally diminishes gastrointestinal symptoms related to anatomical distortion or ulceration into the gut, and the overall balance is in favour of the patient.

In an area where factual evidence is not available, one must accept the opinion of those with a large experience. Trede (1987) has observed that "the quality of survival in our experience weights the scales in favour of resection".

Possible Cure

Can pancreatic cancer be cured? Some surgeons, from their experience of invariable cancer-related death within three years, would argue that cure is extremely unlikely. Others have seen survival up to five years in 10%–20% of patients and some, who report highly selected series of early tumours, have up to 25% five-year survivors (Trede et al. 1990). One cannot talk of cure in terms of five-year survival because even these patients often ultimately die of recurrent tumour. Nevertheless, there are a few very long-term survivors in the literature and at present the only hope of achieving this outcome lies with resection. It may be that in future more patients will achieve a permanent freedom from recurrence with the addition of adjuvant therapy to resection. What is clear, is that five-year survival without resection is extremely unusual if the histology is unequivocally pancreatic ductal adenocarcinoma.

Carcinoma of the Body of the Pancreas

The same arguments in favour of resection apply to carcinoma of the body of the pancreas as to carcinoma of the head. Unfortunately these tumours are often clinically silent until they have reached an advanced stage and they are rarely resectable at the time of diagnosis. This accounts for the appalling prognosis of carcinoma of the body of the pancreas. Moosa (1982) reviewed the literature over 45 years and found only one case of carcinoma of the body of the pancreas in which the patient survived more than one year after resection. This has led some surgeons to question the value of ever attempting to resect such a tumour.

I recently had the opportunity to review the records of Professor Trede's clinic in Mannheim. Carcinoma of the body of the pancreas was rarely resectable. Only 13 such operations were performed in a total of over 700 cases of pancreatic cancer, of which 105 were in the body or tail. Recently, however, there has been an increased readiness to resect these tumours, as shown by the fact that 11 of these resections were performed in the last three years. This is probably a consequence of earlier diagnosis with widespread use of CT in the investigation of abdominal pain.

Seven of these patients were treated by distal pancreatectomy, with en bloc resection of spleen and in some instances other organs. Six patients required total pancreatectomy for resection of the tumour. Follow-up at more than one year showed four patients dead from recurrent tumour within 12 months. Three others had died, 24, 25 and 40 months after operation. Two patients were alive with recurrence and four patients were tumour free, 13–36 months postoperatively. Median survival for all 13 patients was 24 months.

These remarkable results from a specialist clinic which acts as a tertiary referral centre for a wide area indicate that some tumours of the body of the pancreas, if diagnosed sufficiently early, can be resected with hope of long-term survival.

Conclusion

Resection of exocrine adenocarcinoma of the pancreas is certainly justified if the tumour is operable and the patient is fit for surgery. The operative mortality rate should be in the region of 5%, with an acceptable rate of morbidity. Resection is justified if all the visible disease can be resected, that is all Stage I tumours and some Stage II tumours in which the local invasion or lymph node involvement can be resected with the primary tumour. Finally, the long-term survival of these patients is so poor, even in the best units, that no effort can be spared in the search for an improvement. Patients who undergo resection should be entered into a trial of adjuvant therapy, in the hope that this will improve the outlook for the individual patient. For all these reasons resection is justified if it is performed by a surgeon with experience, expertise and an interest in the management of carcinoma of the pancreas.

References

Andren-Sandberg A, Ihse I (1983) Factors influencing survival after total pancreatectomy in patients with pancreatic cancer. Ann Surg 198:605–610

Ashton-Key M, Hammersley S, Johnson CD (1991) Relative incidence of gastric and pancreatic cancer in England and Wales. Gut 32: A580–A581

Braasch JW, Rossi RL, Watkins E et al. (1986) Pyloric and gastric preserving pancreatic resection. Ann Surg 204:411–418

Bradbeer J, Johnson CD (1990) Pancreaticogastrostomy after pancreaticoduodenectomy. Ann R Coll Surg Engl 72:266–269

Chandiramini VA, Theis BA, Russel RCG (1990) Role of resection in the management of pancreatic cancers. Gut 31:A488

Cooper MJ, Williamson RCN (1985) Conservative pancreatectomy. Br J Surg 72:801–803

Cooper MJ, Williamson RCN, Benjamin IS et al. (1987) Total pancreatectomy for chronic pancreatitis. Br J Surg 74:912–915

Crist DW, Sitzmann JV, Cameron JL (1987) Improved hospital morbidity, mortality and survival after the Whipple procedure. Ann Surg 206:358–373

Dunn E (1987) The impact of technology and improved perioperative management upon survival from carcinoma of the pancreas. Surg Gynecol Obstet 164:237–244

Edis AJ, Kieman PD, Taylor WF (1980) Attempted resection of ductal carcinoma of the pancreas. Review of Mayo Clinic Experience 1951–75. Mayo Clin Proc 55:531–536

Gall FP (1987) Chronische pancreatitis: Chirugische therapie durch resections verfahren. Langenbecks Arch Chir 372:363–368

Gastrointestinal Tumour Study Group (1987) Further evidence of effective adjuvant combined radiation and chemotherapy following curative resection of pancreatic cancer. Cancer 59:2006–2010

Grace PA, Pitt HA, Longmire WP (1986) Pancreatoduodenectomy with pylorus preservation for adenocarcinoma of the head of the pancreas. Br J Surg 73:647–650

Gudjunsson B, Livstone E, Spiro H (1978) Pancreatic cancer: diagnostic accuracy and survival statistics. Cancer 42:2454–2506

Ishikawa O, Ohigashi H, Sasaki Y et al. (1988) Practical usefulness of lymphatic and connective tissue clearance for carcinoma of the pancreas head. Ann Surg 208:215–219

Jones BA, Langer B, Taylor BR, Girotti M (1985) Periampullary tumours. Which ones should be resected? Am J Surg 149:46–52

Kairaluoma MI, Kiviniemi H, Stahlberg M (1987) Pancreatic resection for carcinoma of the pancreas and periampullary region in patients over 70 years of age. Br J Surg 74:116–118

Lygidakis NJ, van der Hyde MN, Houthoff HJ et al. (1989) Resectional surgical procedures for carcinoma of the head of the pancreas. Surg Gynecol Obstet 168:157–165

Moosa AR (1982) Pancreatic cancer. Approach to diagnosis, selection for surgery and choice of operation. Cancer 50:2689–2698

Pellegrini CA, Heck CF, Roper et al. (1989) An analysis of the reduced morbidity and mortality rates after pancreaticoduodenectomy. Arch Surg 124:778–781

Sato T, Saitch Y, Noto N, Matsuno S (1977) Followup studies of radical resection for pancreaticoduodenal cancer. Ann Surg 186:581–588

Tashiro S, Mirata E, Hiraoka T et al. (1987) New techniques for pancreaticojejunostomy using a biological adhesive. Br J Surg 74:392–394

Trede M (1987) Treatment of pancreatic carcinoma: the surgeon's dilemma. Br J Surg 74:79–80

Trede M, Schwall G, Saeger HD (1990) Survival after pancreatoduodenectomy: 118 consecutive resections without operative mortality. Ann Surg 211:447–458

Tsuchiya R, Noda T, Harada N et al. (1986) Collective review of small carcinomas of the pancreas. Ann Surg 203:77–81

Van Heerden JA (1984) Pancreatic resection for carcinoma of the pancreas: Whipple versus total pancreatectomy – an institutional persective. World J Surg 8:880–888

Chapter 9

Adjuvant Therapy After Resection of Pancreatic Cancer

B. Isgar and J. Neoptolemos

Pancreatic cancer affects around 8–12 per 100 000 of the population each year in Europe and North America (Haddock and Carter 1990). It is the fourth commonest cause of cancer death with an overall survival rate of 0.4% (Gudjonsson 1979). Surgery offers the only chance of long-term cure. In the past decade there has been a dramatic improvement in the operative outcome with many series reporting a mortality below 10% (Russell 1990; Trede et al. 1990), whilst resectability rates have improved to 8%–15% and even more in some Japanese institutions (Hiraoka 1990; Tsuchiya et al. 1990). A number of recent studies have indicated long-term survival figures of over 30% (Russell 1990). This may indicate selection of favourable cases or better surgical technique. Alternatively, this may represent an alteration in the biological behaviour of pancreatic cancer at a time when the incidence of the disease has ceased to rise, and may even be in a slight decline (unpublished observations).

Generally speaking, however, survival rates following resection are poor (Russell 1990). In over 250 patients from the West Midlands who underwent resection we found a 5-year survival rate of only 6%. Important determinants of survival are tumour size (more favourable for tumours less than 2 cm), lymph node status, invasion of adjacent structures (Kalser and Ellenberg 1985; Tsuchiya et al. 1990) and residual disease following resection (Hiraoka 1990). Russell (1990) has gone as far as saying that "There is little evidence that larger tumours (>2 cm) of ductal origin are benefited by operation". Small tumours, however, constitute only 5.4% of all pancreatic cancers at the time of diagnosis and the 8 year survival rate is still only 27% (Tsuchiya et al. 1990). Adjuvant therapy therefore has a crucial role to play in the surgical management of pancreatic cancer. The results of surgery are so poor that surgery alone cannnot be justified in many cases, but may be more acceptable with the addition of adjuvant therapy. Even in favourable cases, there is an obvious need for further measures to reduce local and distant tumour recurrence, and adjuvant therapy appears to be the only way to improve survival following resection.

Rationale for Adjuvant Therapy

After surgical resection there are three main patterns of treatment failure which each contribute approximately equal proportions (Bell 1957). These are (a) local recurrence at the site of previous resection, (b) liver metastases from occult metastases undetected at the time of primary resection and (c) local and metastatic disease recurrence.

Adjuvant therapy following resection must therefore be targeted at low-volume residual disease in the area of resection as well as distant micrometastases.

In principle the best means of local control after resection is radiotherapy and for systemic control this is chemotherapy. For a long time pancreatic cancer was believed to be resistant to radiotherapy and chemotherapy. These views are no longer tenable (Arbuck 1990; Dobelbower and Bronn 1990). Considerable impetus has been given to these forms of treatment by the remarkable results now emerging with their use in colorectal cancer (Gastrointestinal Tumour Study Group (GITSG) 1985; Moertel et al. 1990).

The ultimate choice of which adjuvant regimen should be used can only be determined by Phase III (prospectively randomised) trials. The results of Phase III studies in advanced disease provide an important guide as to which regimens should be tested in a resectable disease, with further useful information derived from Phase II (response-seeking) trials.

Sensitivity of Pancreatic Cancer to Chemotherapy

Single Agent Therapy

More than 30 different agents have been tested in pancreatic cancer (Arbuck 1990; Brennan et al. 1989) and of these only 5-fluorouracil (5-FU) achieves a response rate with the lower 95% confidence interval exceeding 20% (Table 1). Despite the considerable interest shown in alkylating agent therapy with isofosfamide the results are disappointing. The Gastrointestinal Tumour Study Group of North America (GITSG, 1989) recently reported on another 30 patients in a Phase II study. Only three partial tumour responses were noted and the median survival was only 11 weeks. Toxicity was considerable despite the use of uroprotection (2-mercaptoethane, mesna) and there were two deaths due to toxicity. Despite some responses having been achieved with single agent regimens, no clinical survival benefit has ever been shown. For this reason, multiple agent regimens have been tested.

Multiple Drug Regimens

Bukowski et al. (1983) showed a higher response rate (34%) with the three-drug regimen of streptozotocin, 5-FU and mitomycin-C than with 5-FU and

Table 1. Response rates for single agent chemotherapy agents in advanced pancreatic cancer

Chemotherapy agent	Number of patients	Response rate (95% confidence interval)
5-Fluorouracil	212	28 ($\pm$6)%
Mitomycin-C	53	21 ($\pm$6)%
Isofosfamide	117	12 ($\pm$6)%
Streptozotocin	27	11 ($\pm$6)%
Doxorubicin	28	7 ($\pm$5)%
Methyl-CCNU	91	4 ($\pm$2)%
BCNU	31	0 %

CCNU = N-(2-chloroethyl)-N-cyclohexyl-N-nitrosourea;
BCNU = 1,3-bis(2-chloroethyl)-1-nitrosourea.
Adapted from Arbuck (1990), with permission.

mitomycin-C (8%) but there was no difference in median survival (18 vs. 17 weeks). The only trial to show a survival benefit with multiple chemotherapy was reported by Mallinson et al. (1980). Patients (n=21) treated with an induction programme of 5-FU, methotrexate, vincristine and cyclophosphamide and then maintained on 5-FU and mitomycin-C survived longer than the control group (n=19; median of 44 vs. 9 weeks). Of the agents used in this trial, only 5-FU has been shown to produce objective responses in pancreatic cancer and only 26 of the patients had had a histological diagnosis. A recent Phase III trial of 172 patients, however, showed no significant differences in median survival between 5-FU alone (4.5 months), 5-FU, doxorubicin and cisplatin (FAP) (4.5 months) and the Mallinson regimen (3.5 months) (Cullinan et al. 1989). There have been numerous Phase III trials of combination drug regimens in pancreatic cancer, none of which have shown any survival advantage over 5-FU alone and they were all associated with higher toxicity (Arbuck 1990). Since no Phase III trial has ever been conducted comparing 5-FU with observation alone the true benefit of 5-FU is not known.

Sensitivity of Pancreatic Cancer to Radiotherapy

External beam radiotherapy (EBRT) to the pancreas has in the past been limited to a dosage of about 40 Gy within 4 weeks because of the critical radiotolerance of surrounding vital organs. This has prompted the development of a variety of techniques to enhance dose delivery while minimising radiation damage (Dobelbower and Bronn 1990). Dobelbower et al. (1980) used precision high dose radiotherapy (60–80 Gy over 7–9 weeks) to treat 40 patients with unresectable cancer. They achieved survival figures similar to that of 31 other patients who had had resection; two of the patients treated with radiotherapy were still alive at 5 years. Similarly Nguyen et al. (1982) showed a 27% 2-year survival rate in 18 patients treated with 60 Gy by EBRT over 6 weeks. Other methods of applying radiotherapy to pancreatic tumours have also been shown to produce a moderate response rate (Dobelbower and Bronn 1990).

Sensitivity of Pancreatic Cancer to Combination Chemoradiotherapy

5-FU may be used not only for cytotoxic therapy following radiotherapy but also as a radiosensitiser during radiotherapy. Moertel et al. (1969) randomised 64 patients to 35– 40 Gy and 5-FU or placebo; those receiving concomitant 5-FU had a prolonged survival time (10.4 vs. 6.3 months; $P<0.05$). These data are supported by a recent study of 40 patients who received 40 Gy with 5-FU in ten split doses; the median survival of these patients (13.5 months bypass group; 8.9 months laparotomy-only group) was significantly better compared to historical control groups (5.4 and 2.7 months respectively; both $P<0.01$) (Kahn et al. 1990).

Tepper et al. (1987) assessed the role of misonidazole in conjunction with a 20 Gy dose of intraoperative electron beam radiotherapy (IOEBRT) in 41 patients with locally advanced disease. In addition, patients received 10 Gy EBRT preoperatively and 40 Gy EBRT postoperatively (variously in conjunction with 5-FU). Although local disease control was better in these patients compared to 22 patients similarly treated but without radiosensitisation (45% vs. 31% at 2 years) there was no survival benefit (median of 12 vs. 16.5 months respectively).

Radiotherapy and Prolonged Chemotherapy

There have been three trials comparing radiotherapy (EBRT) and prolonged treatment with chemotherapy compared to either alone, two of which showed a significant survival benefit for combination therapy (Table 2). The trial which failed to demonstrate such a benefit (Klaassen et al. 1985) has been criticised on three counts. First, patients were entered into the trial with either locally advanced disease or local recurrence. Second, the number of patients who completed radiotherapy was not given. Third, 22% of the patients were considered ineligible or failed to complete the treatment. The two GITSG trials (1981, 1988) avoided these criticisms.

Whilst the survival benefits shown by the Mayo clinic study (Moertel et al. 1969) and the GITSG studies (1981, 1988) are small, they positively point to the type of regimen that is likely to be of benefit in patients who have undergone resection.

Intraoperative Versus External Radiotherapy in Conjunction with Prolonged Chemotherapy

Roldan et al. (1988) reported a considerable improvement of local control using a combination of IOEBRT and EBRT compared to EBRT alone (66%

Table 2. Results of Phase III Trials comparing radiotherapy, chemotherapy and radiotherapy with prolonged chemotherapy in patients with locally advanced pancreatic cancer

Series	Radiotherapy dose (Gy)	Radiosensitiser	Prolonged chemotherapy	Number of patients	Median survival	P
GITSG (1981)	60	—	—	25[a]	5.5	
	40	5-FU	5-FU	83	10.5	< 0.01
	60	5-FU	5-FU	86	10.5	
Klaasen et al.	—	—	5-FU	41	8.2	NS
(1985)	40	5-FU	5-FU	47	8.3	
GITSG (1988)	—	—	SMF	21	8.0	< 0.05
	54	5-FU	SMF	22	10.5	

GITSG = Gastrointestinal Tumour Study Group; 5-FU = 5-fluorouracil; SMF = streptozotocin, mitomycin-C and 5-fluorouracil.
[a] Accrual stopped early because of significantly poor survival compared with other arms.

vs. 20% at 2 years) but no improvement in median survival (12.6 vs. 13.4 months). Sindelar and Kinsella (1986a) in a Phase III trial compared IOEBRT, EBRT and immediate and prolonged 5-FU with EBRT and immediate and prolonged 5-FU in 32 patients. Although patients who had received IOEBRT and EBRT had a prolonged time to local disease progression compared to the EBRT alone group, the median survival time was the same (8 months). Similar results have been reported when the radiosensitising agent used was misonidazole (Sindelar 1988). On balance IOEBRT appears to enhance local tumour control (Dobelbower and Bronn 1990).

Hepatic Artery 5-FU Infusion in Conjunction with Hepatic and Pancreatic Radiotherapy

Since occult liver metastases are an important reason for determining long-term survival in pancreatic cancer, one approach has been the delivery of 5-FU by selective arterial catheterisation to the liver for 2 weeks prior to liver irradiation (20 Gy) and pancreatic irradiation (50–60 Gy) (Wiley et al. 1988). The median survival in 17 out of 21 patients who completed this study was 50 weeks. Overt liver metastases occurred in only 6%. Local tumour bed recurrence occured in 70% and was inversely correlated with the time dose fraction (TDF) value. Effective local control was equivalent to a dose of 50 Gy given in fraction sizes of 2 Gy each.

Adjuvant Therapies in Conjunction with Pancreatic Resection

Preoperative Radiotherapy

Preoperative radiotherapy may be used to increase the chance of resection in a locally advanced cancer. Pilepich and Miller (1980) treated 17 patients with

40–50 Gy. Tumour assessment six weeks later revealed progression in five patients and further treatment was not considered. One patient who had developed cardiovascular disease was also offered further treatment. Resection was possible in six of the remaining 11 patients, of whom two survived for at least 5 years.

More recently Ishikawa et al. (1989) reported that 10 out of 12 patients were able to undergo resection following preoperative irradiation with 50 Gy. Weese et al. (1990) gave 50.4 Gy preoperatively with a continuous infusion of 5-FU and mitomycin-C to 13 patients; resection was then possible in six. One patient died at 7 months from myocardial infarction but the remaining five were alive and free of recurrence at 9–38 months.

Postoperative Radiotherapy and Prolonged 5-Fluorouracil Following Standard Pancreatic Resection

In 1985, the GITSG reported the results of a Phase III trial in which 21 patients who had received 40 Gy by EBRT and i.v. 5-FU (500 mg/M^2 body surface area during EBRT and then weekly for two years) were compared with 22 control patients (Kalser and Ellenberg 1985). The disease-free median

Table 3. Patient profile and survival data for patients in the two GITSG studies of postoperative radiotherapy and 5-FU following pancreatic cancer resection (Kalser and Ellenberg 1985; GITSG 1987)

Variable	Randomised control	Randomised treatment	Registered to treatment
Number	22	21	20
Patient variable			
Men	59%	62%	50%
> 60 years	41%	62%	50%
ECOG[a] 0 or 1	50%	59%	53%
Tumour variable			
Head of pancreas	95%	95%	97%
Contiguous invasion	36%	38%	46%
Nodal involvement	28%	29%	27%
Pancreatectomy			
Whipple's	72%	62%	80%
Total	28%	38%	20%
Survival at 2 years			
All patients	18%	43%	43%
ECOG 0 or 1	18%	54%	46%
Disease-free survival at 2 years			
All patients	14%	48%	32%
ECOG 0 or 1	9%	54%	38%

[a] Eastern Cooperative Oncology Group Performance Status.
Adapted from GITSG (1987), with permission.

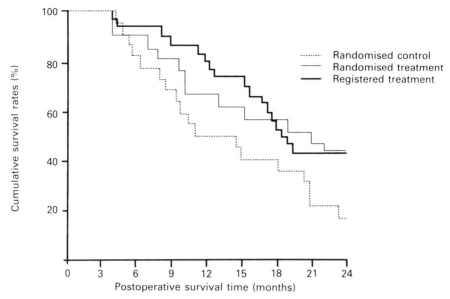

Fig. 1. Actuarial survival times for the two GITSG studies of postoperative radiotherapy and 5-FU. Modified from GITSG (1987), with permission.

survival was greater in the treated group (11 vs. 9 months, $P=0.04$). The 2-year survival rate was also greater in the treated group (42% vs. 15%, $P=0.03$). Local recurrence occured in 71% of the treated group compared with 86% in the control group. Of particular interest is that hepatic metastases occurred in 50% of the control group compared to only 32% in the treatment group.

Two important prognostic indicators, independent of treatment emerged from this study; these were the extent of tumour at the time of resection and the initial performance status.

This trial was criticised on three counts. First, the minimum accrual target was 100 patients (50 in each arm with a 90% power to detect a doubling of survival time at the 0.05 level, one-sided test) yet only 43 patients were recruited. Second, the accrual period was exceptionally long (February 1974 to May 1982), and third, there were eleven contributing institutions – a disproportionately large number compared to the final number of patients recruited. This gives an average of 0.49 patients recruited per institution per year.

In view of these criticisms, the GITSG recruited a further 30 patients into the treatment arm over a period of 28 months (GITSG 1987). The patient profile, disease-free survival and overall survival (Table 3, Fig. 1) were identical to those previously reported.

Intraoperative Versus Postoperative Radiotherapy

Sindelar and Kinsella (1986b) reported on a Phase III trial of IOEBRT (20 Gy) versus postoperative EBRT (50 Gy) in 32 patients. The postoperative mortality was high (28%) but this did not differ between the groups. All the EBRT patients had local recurrence within 12 months compared to 20% in the IOEBRT group. Although disease-free survival was extended in the IOEBRT treated patients, the survival time was identical to those treated by EBRT.

These data support the view that IOEBRT provides effective local control but has little influence in altering the effects of distant micrometastases. This study made no mention of the use of radiosensitisers.

Intraoperative Radiotherapy and Extended Radical Resection

Recently Hiraoka (1990) reported on the experience of pancreatic surgery and IOEBRT at Kumamoto University Medical School, Japan (Table 4). The use of a stardard resection and standard IOEBRT (30 Gy of 8 MeV to a 6–8 cm diameter field) failed to produce any improvement over resection alone (all patients were dead within 2 years). Although better local control was obtained with extended radical resection (involving a complete en bloc, central lymph node clearance from the diaphragm to the inferior mesenteric artery) none of the patients survived beyond 3.2 years. The extended radical operation was then combined with an extended IOEBRT treatment (30 Gy of 9 MeV given to include the whole of the lymphadenectomy field) resulting in a 29% actuarial 5-year survival rate for the 16 patients so treated ($P<0.01$, Fig. 2).

In order to treat hepatic micrometastases Ozaki et al. (1988, 1990) combined extended radical resection and 30 Gy IOEBRT with intraoperative hepatic

Table 4. Details of patients treated by pancreatic resection and intraoperative radiotherapy (IOEBRT) at Kumamoto University Medical School, 1966–1989

Period	Resection	IOEBRT	Number of patients	Number of males	Mean age (years)	Tumour stage[a]				Complete tumour clearance
						I	II	III	IV	
1966–75	Standard	Standard	19	14	61.2	2	5	7	5	11 (58%)
1976–81	Standard	Standard	15	8	63.6	0	3	9	3	9 (60%)
1982–83	Extended	None	9	5	66.8	0	1	3	5	9 (60%)
1984–89	Extended	Extended	16	11	58.0	0	2	11	3	12 (75%)

[a] According to the classification of the Japanese Pancreatic Society (1982).
Adapted from Hiraoka (1990), with permission.

artery or portal vein infusion of mitomycin-C. This agent was continued systemicly after surgery. The 3-year survival rate in 16 patients so treated was 53% compared to 10% previously treated at the same institution by extended radical resection alone.

Conclusions and Future Prospects

The long-term results of surgery for pancreatic ductal adenocarcinoma remain devastatingly poor. There is now considerable evidence that these cancers are

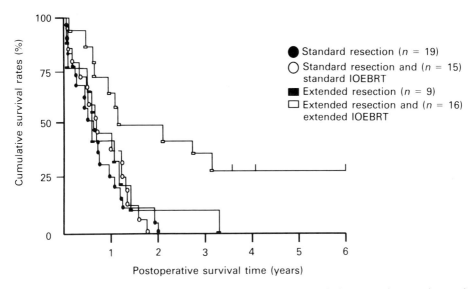

Fig. 2. Actuarial survival times comparing standard and extended pancreatic resection and intraoperative radiotherapy (IOEBRT) at Kumamoto University Medical School. Modified from Hiraoka (1990), with permission.

sensitive to chemotherapy and radiotherapy. Because the pattern of treatment failure is both local and systemic an improvement in survival is only possible by a combination of local and systemic adjuvant therapy. It is both surprising and distressing that only three prospective randomised trials have ever been performed to compare resection alone with some form of adjuvant therapy (Kalser and Ellenberg 1985; Sindelar and Kinsella 1986a,b). Whilst the results of postoperative radiotherapy and prolonged 5-FU have shown statistically significant results (Kalser and Ellenberg 1985; GITSG 1987) we urgently need confirmation of these putative benefits by a major prospective randomised trial which achieves target accrual within 2–3 years.

There are continued developments both with regard to improved delivery techniques for radiotherapy (Dobelbower and Bronn 1990) and methods of improving the cytotoxicity of 5-FU (Arbuck 1990). The current practice of surgeons who remove large pancreatic tumours without giving consideration to adjuvant treatment is now indefensible. Equally unacceptable is the 0.05% resection rate found among general surgeons treating nearly 10 000 patients with pancreatic cancer in the West Midlands, England (unpublished observation). We believe that all patients with potentially operable pancreatic cancer should be considered for surgery. If resection is possible the patient should be entered into a formal study of adjuvant and combination therapy. Single agents with no proven benefit, such as isofosfamide, should not be used.

The development of new adjuvant forms of therapy in North America and Japan is encouraging but several Phase III trials are now urgently required. The need for a European Pancreatic Cancer Trials Organisation to promote. such trials is self evident.

References

Arbuck SG (1990) Chemotherapy for pancreatic cancer. Clin Gastroenterol 4:953–968
Bell ET (1957) Carcinoma of the pancreas. I. A clinical and pathologic study of 609 necropsied cases II. The relation of carcinoma of the pancreas to diabetes mellitus. Am J Pathol 33:449–453
Brennan MF, Kinsella T, Friedman M (1989) Cancer of the pancreas. In: Devita VT, Helman S, Rosenberg SA (eds) Cancer principles and practice of oncology, 3rd edn. JB Lippincott, Philadelphia, pp. 800–835
Bukowski RM, Balcerzak SP, O'Bryan RM, Bonnet JD, Chen TT (1983) Randomized trial of 5-fluorouracil and mitomycin with or without streptozotocin for advanced pancreatic cancer. A South West Oncology Study Group Study. Cancer 52:1577–1582
Cullinan S, Moertel C, Wieand H (1989) A Phase III evaluation of drug combinations in the therapy of advanced pancreatic cancer. Proc Am Soc Clin Oncol 8:124
Dobelbower RR, Bronn DG (1990) Radiotherapy in the treatment of pancreatic cancer. Clin Gastroenterol 4:969–983
Dobelbower RR, Borgelt BB, Strubler KA, Kutcher GJ, Suntharalingam N (1980) Precision radiotherapy for cancer of the pancreas: technique and results. Int J Radiat Oncol Biol Phys 6:1127–1133
Gastrointestinal Tumour Study Group (1981) Therapy of locally unresectable pancreatic carcinoma: a randomized comparison of high dose (6000 rads) radiation alone, moderate dose radiation (4000 rads + 5-fluorouracil) and high dose radiation and 5-fluorouracil. Cancer 189:1705–1710
Gastrointestinal Tumour Study Group (1985) Prolongation of the disease-free interval in surgically treated rectal carcinoma. N Engl J Med 312:1465–1472
Gastrointestinal Tumour Study Group (1987) Further evidence of effective adjuvant combined radiation and chemotherapy following curative resection of pancreatic cancer. Cancer 59:2006–2010
Gastrointestinal Tumour Study Group (1988) Treatment of locally unresectable carcinoma of the pancreas: comparison of combined-modality therapy (chemotherapy plus radiotherapy) to chemotherapy alone. J Natl Cancer Inst 80:751–755
Gastrointestinal Tumour Study Group (1989) Isofosfamide is an inactive substance in the treatment of pancreatic carcinoma. Cancer 64:2010–2013
Gudjonsson B (1979) Cancer of the pancreas. Fifty years of surgery. Cancer 9:2284–2303
Haddock G, Carter DC (1990) Aetiology of pancreatic cancer. Br J Surg 77:1159–1166
Hiraoka T (1990) Extended radical resection of cancer of the pancreas with intra-operative radiotherapy. Clin Gastroenterol 4:985–993
Ishikawa O, Ohhigashi H, Teshima T et al. (1989) Clinical and histopathological appraisal of pre-operative irradiation for adenocarcinoma of the pancreatoduodenal region. J Surg Oncol 40:143–151
Japanese Pancreatic Society (1982) General rules for surgical and pathological studies in cancer of the pancreas, 2nd edn (in Japanese). Kanchona Publishing, Tokyo
Kahn PJ, Skornick Y, Inbar M, Kaplan O, Chaichik S, Rozin R (1990) Surgical palliation combined with synchronous therapy in pancreatic carcinoma. Eur J Surg Oncol 16:7–11
Kalser MH, Ellenberg SS (1985) Pancreatic cancer. Adjuvant combined radiation and chemotherapy following curative resection. Arch Surg 12:899–903
Klaassen DJ, MacIntyre JM, Catton GE, Engstrom PF, Moertel CG (1985) Treatment of locally unresectable cancer of the stomach and pancreas: a randomized comparison of 5-fluorouracil alone with radiation plus concurrent and maintenance 5-fluorouracil. An Eastern Cooperative Oncology Group Study. J Clin Oncol 3:373–378
Mallinson CN, Rake MO, Locking JB et al. (1980) Chemotherapy in pancreatic cancer: results of a controlled prospective randomised, multicentre trial. Br Med J 281:1589–1591
Moertel CG, Childs DS, Reitermeier RJ, Colby MY, Holbrook MA (1969) Combined 5-fluorouracil and supervoltage radiation therapy of locally unresectable gastrointestinal cancer. Lancet ii:865–867
Moertel CG, Fleming TR, McDonald JS et al. (1990) Levamisole and fluorouracil for adjuvant therapy of resected colon carcinoma. N Engl J Med 332:352–358
Nguyen TD, Bugat R, Combes PF (1982) Post operative irradiation of carcinoma of the head of the pancreas area. Cancer 50:53–56
Ozaki H, Hojo K, Kato H (1988) Multidisciplinary treatment for resectable pancreatic cancer. Int J Pancreatol 3:249–260

Ozaki H, Ignoshita T, Kosuge T, Egawa S, Kishi K (1990) Effectiveness of multimodality treatment for resectable pancreatic cancer. Int J Pancreatol 7:195–200

Pilepich MV, Miller HH (1980) Pre-operative irradiation in carcinoma of the pancreas. Cancer 46:1945–1949

Roldan GE, Gunderson LL, Nagorney DM et al. (1988) External beam versus intraoperative and external beam irradiation for locally advanced pancreatic cancer. Cancer 61:1110–1116

Russell RCG (1990) Surgical resection for cancer of the pancreas. Clin Gastroenterol 4:889–916

Sindelar WF (1988) Intraoperative radiotherapy in carcinoma of the stomach and pancreas. Recent Results Cancer Res 110:226–243

Sindelar WF, Kinsella TJ (1986a) Randomized trial of intraoperative radiotherapy in unresectable carcinoma of the pancreas (Abstract). Int J Radiat Oncol Biol Phys 12 (suppl 1):148–149

Sindelar WF, Kinsella TJ (1986b) Randomized trial of intraoperative radiotherapy in resected carcinoma of the pancreas (Abstract). Int J Radiat Oncol Biol Phys 12 (suppl 1):148

Tepper JE, Shipley WU, Warshaw AL, Nardi GL, Wood WC, Orlow EL (1987) The role of misonidazole combined with intraoperative radiation therapy in the treatment of pancreatic carcinoma. J Clin Oncol 5:579–784

Trede M, Schwall G, Saeger HD (1990) Survival after pancreatoduodenectomy. 118 resections without an operative mortality. Ann Surg 211:447–458

Tsuchiya R, Tsunoda T, Ishida T, Saitoh Y (1990) Resection for cancer of the pancreas – the Japanese experience. Clin Gastroenterol 4:931–939

Weese JL, Nussbaum ML, Paul AR (1990) Increased resectability of locally advanced pancreatic and periampullary carcinoma with neoadjuvant chemoradiotherapy. Int J Pancreatol 7:177–185

Wiley AL, Wirtanen GW, Ramirez G, Shahabi S (1988) Treatment of probable subclinical liver metastases and gross pancreatic carcinoma with hepatic artery 5-fluorouracil infusion and radiation therapy. Acta Oncol 27:337–381

Section C

Surgical Techniques

Chapter 10

Operative Pancreatography

P. Watanapa and R. C. N. Williamson

Historical Development

Doubilet first undertook operative pancreatography in 1947 and published the results four years later (Doubilet and Mulholland 1951). He stated that the procedure was both safe and an essential adjunct to pancreatic surgery, an opinion with which we and others concur (Nardi and Acosta 1966; Berni et al. 1982; Cooper and Williamson 1983). The subsequent development of endoscopic retrograde cholangiopancreatography (ERCP) lessened its appeal, since information about the ductal tree then became available in advance of operation.

There is a small risk of acute pancreatitis following injection of contrast medium into the pancreatic duct whether endoscopic retrograde pancreatography (ERP) or on-table pancreatography (OTP) is performed. In 1958 Pollock reported two deaths and a third case of severe postoperative pancreatitis among 11 patients having OTP and concluded that the technique was not only dangerous but also of limited value. However, Trapnell et al. (1966) pioneered a new method of transduodenal pancreatography in an autopsy study in Philadelphia. In 40 of 45 cadavers studied (42 adults, three infants), the pancreatic duct was entered without the additional use of sphincterotomy and the ductal system was clearly outlined by serial radiographs after slow injection of 70% sodium diatrizoate (Hypaque) (Trapnell et al. 1966; Trapnell 1967). Howard and Short (1969) applied this technique to man in 26 patients without a single case of pancreatitis developing. They advocated OTP as a safe and informative procedure.

The advantages of ERP include its technical simplicity in dexterous hands and the fact that information about the biliary and pancreatic ductal trees can be used to plan the operation. Yet ductography may be incomplete by this route, especially in patients with chronic pancreatitis in whom precise anatomical knowledge is required by the surgeon. Concomitant duodenitis, papillary fibrosis and pancreatic ductal strictures hamper ERP in a substantial number of cases. More recently, modern CT scanners have given useful information about the calibre of the pancreatic duct, and preoperative pancreatography can now be obtained percutaneously under computed tomography (CT) or ultrasound control (Haaga et al. 1979; Lees and Heron 1987; Matter et al. 1987). These techniques are not generally available and may only be successful if the main pancreatic duct is dilated (Lees and Heron 1987). By contrast, OTP is simple to perform, requires no specialised apparatus, can provide more information than ERCP and is a very safe investigation.

Indications

Chronic Pancreatitis

This is the commonest indication for OTP (56% in our series). Full ductography is needed to show the extent of ductal ectasia and the site of any strictures in the main pancreatic duct, information of crucial importance in selecting patients for resection or drainage of the pancreas. Longitudinal pancreaticojejunostomy is the safest and simplest operation for chronic pancreatitis and provides good long-term pain relief, but it is only applicable to the minority of patients with a dilated main duct (Cooper and Williamson 1984; Cuilleret and Guillemin 1990). Otherwise, pancreatic resection is preferred, but here too OTP is invaluable for delineating ductal anatomy in the proximal or distal remnant after partial pancreatectomy.

Recurrent Acute Pancreatitis

Patients with one or more attacks of "idiopathic" acute pancreatitis require ERCP particularly to look for surgically remediable causes such as pancreas divisum, periampullary tumour and ductal stricture. In pancreas divisum it is usually difficult and often impossible to cannulate the accessory papilla to opacify the isolated dorsal duct, and this may necessitate an operative (transduodenal) approach.

Pancreatic Pseudocyst

Pseudocysts only communicated with the main pancreatic duct in about a quarter of our patients with acute or chronic pancreatitis who were submitted to on-table cystography (5 of 21 patients). The absence of such a communication indicates that drainage of the cyst alone may be inadequate, at least in chronic pancreatitis.

Other Conditions

1. A few patients with suspected chronic pancreatitis in whom ERP is either unobtainable or inadequate may require OTP as part of a "diagnostic"

laparotomy. In our experience *pancreas divisum* has been the commonest indication among those with obscure pain.

2. Although OTP plays little role in the diagnosis of *pancreatic carcinoma*, a few patients with an irresectable cancer of the head and neck may be suitable for an intubated pancreaticogastrostomy in an attempt to relieve severe back pain (Apalakis et al. 1977). OTP is useful to confirm the presence of a dilated duct before incision into the gland.

3. Successful treatment of *pancreatic trauma* depends on early recognition of the injury, identification of the site of ductal injury and an appropriate operation to control pancreatic secretions. In a 10-year experience of 54 patients with pancreatic trauma, OTP reduced the major pancreatic complications in those with suspected injury to the proximal duct from 55% to 15% (Berni et al. 1982).

Technique

Operative pancreatograms can be obtained by several different routes (Fig. 1) (Cooper and Williamson 1983; Desa and Williamson 1990).

Retrograde Pancreatography

This is carried out either via a transduodenal approach to the major or minor papilla or via the duct in the neck of the pancreas following a proximal resection. We generally "cover" retrograde ductography in patients with a functioning pancreas by giving an intravenous injection of aprotinin (Trasylol 1×10^6 units) to prevent postoperative acute pancreatitis.

From the Major Papilla

The orifice of the main pancreatic duct is consistently located on the lower lip of the major pancreatic papilla and can usually be cannulated with a 4 or 6 FG umbilical catheter, with or without prior sphincteroplasty. In most instances, the catheter enters the pancreatic duct at the first attempt, and a flow of clear pancreatic juice appears. The catheter is then advanced for 2–3 cm. If sphincteroplasty has been performed, the cannulated orifice is occluded with Babcock's forceps to prevent reflux of contrast material. The first radiograph is obtained after introducing 1–2 ml of contrast medium under gentle pressure. This radiograph should be developed and reviewed before any further injection is made, unless an image intensifier is available to monitor injection. A dilated ductal system may require much more contrast to obtain adequate filling. Care must be taken not to over-distend the ductal tree, since this can precipitate acute pancreatitis (Pollock 1958).

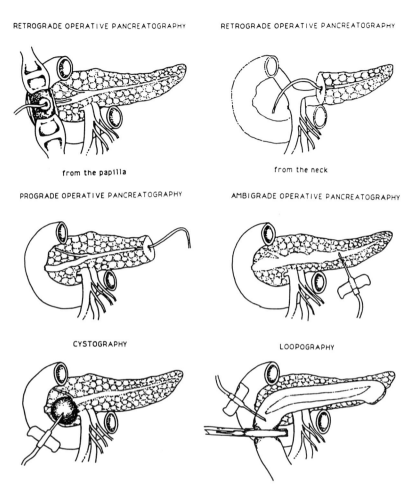

RETROGRADE OPERATIVE PANCREATOGRAPHY   RETROGRADE OPERATIVE PANCREATOGRAPHY

from the papilla   from the neck

PROGRADE OPERATIVE PANCREATOGRAPHY   AMBIGRADE OPERATIVE PANCREATOGRAPHY

CYSTOGRAPHY   LOOPOGRAPHY

Fig. 1. Various types of on-table pancreatography.

From the Minor Papilla

The accessory duct of Santorini, when patent, enters the posteromedial aspect of the descending duodenum about 2 cm proximal to the major papilla. Identification of the minor papilla can be very difficult but is greatly facilitated by giving an intravenous injection of secretin (1unit/kg). Pancreatic juice will flow copiously from the papilla within 30–60 s of the injection, and cannulation can then be performed using a 3 or 4 FG umbilical (or ureteric) catheter.

From the Neck

This simple technique should be carried out following proximal pancreatectomy in every patient with chronic pancreatitis, unless recent and complete distal ductograms are available. The transected duct is cannulated with a 4, 6 or 8 FG umbilical catheter (depending on the size of the duct), and the catheter is sutured in place to prevent leakage of the contrast material. Marked ductal ectasia or a "chain of lakes" appearance is an indication to consider side-to-side pancreaticojejunostomy after opening up the distal duct.

Prograde Pancreatography

This is obtained via the duct in the neck or body of the pancreas after a distal resection. The normal main pancreatic duct is 2–3 mm in diameter at this site and will accept a 5 FG umbilical catheter, which is sutured in place to prevent leakage of contrast. Usually 5–10 ml or more of contrast can be introduced easily (in chronic pancreatitis), and serial radiographs will confirm free flow of the contrast into the duodenum. Since contrast can virtually always escape into the duodenum, the risk of pancreatitis is very low provided that contrast is instilled gently.

Ambigrade Pancreatography

In chronic pancreatitis or an obstructing carcinoma of the head of the gland, the dilated pancreatic duct may be palpable as a softish cord rather like a vein in the antecubital fossa. Such a duct can easily be entered using a 23 FG scalp vein ("butterfly") needle. After removal of a few ml of pancreatic juice, contrast is introduced as necessary to fill the dilated duct system. This examination is usually the prelude to a duct drainage procedure.

Pancreatic Cystography

Pancreatic (pseudo-) cysts can be localised by inspection or palpation and entered by direct needle puncture. Cyst contents are aspirated, and similar volumes of contrast are instilled. If the cyst is large, a Foley catheter may be inserted through a small incision. The balloon is inflated to occlude the defect and enough contrast material is injected to delineate the cyst and demonstrate any communication with the duct system.

Loopography

Opacification of the main pancreatic duct can be obtained in patients with previous pancreaticojejunostomy by clamping the Roux loop just distal to the anastomosis and injecting contrast medium into the jejunum above this point.

Contrast Material

Diatrizoate (Hypaque, Urografin), iohexol (Omnipaque) and ioxaglate (Hexabrix) are the three contrast media commonly employed in pancreatography.

Diatrizoate is an ionic monomer with high osmolality and low viscosity, and iohexol is a non-ionic monomer with lower osmolality and high viscosity. Ioxaglate is an ionic dimer, with lower osmolality but higher viscosity than diatrizoate. Absorption of diatrizoate and iohexol into portal and systemic venous blood and lymph is similar whether escape of the medium through the papilla is free or impaired. However, diatrizoate escapes more rapidly if drainage is unimpeded (probably because of its low viscosity), hence our preference for iohexol which produces a clearer ductogram. Ioxaglate concentration rises more slowly in systemic plasma and lymph and falls more slowly in portal plasma than diatrizoate and iohexol, suggesting that it is absorbed over a longer period (Saari 1989). In experimental pancreatography the absorption of contrast medium occurs mainly during injection and varies markedly between individuals (Saari et al. 1988), suggesting that changes in intraductal pressure and flow are more important than the type of contrast medium used.

Three factors may explain the acute pancreatitis that can follow retrograde pancreatography:

1. Excess filling pressure ruptures the small intralobular ducts (Pollock 1958)
2. Chemical irritation results from the particular contrast medium employed
3. Manipulation of the pancreatic papilla produces oedema and obstructs outflow from the pancreatic duct

Gentle instillation of contrast, which has already been emphasised, may be the single most important step to prevent pancreatitis. The delayed absorption of ioxaglate may make it less desirable than diatrizoate or iohexol (Kivisaari 1979; Saari 1989) although several studies have reported no difference in the incidence of acute pancreatitis using contrast media of high or low osmolality (Hamilton et al. 1982; Hannigan et al. 1985; Makela and Dean 1986). We used diatrizoate in the early 1980s but have switched to iohexol because of the denser ductogram obtained. The incidence of postoperative pancreatitis has been negligible with either agent.

Personal Experience

Between August 1977 and August 1989, we performed 124 OTPs during 117 operative procedures in 112 patients treated at the Bristol Royal Infirmary and Hammersmith Hospital. Chronic pancreatitis was the commonest indication for OTP (63 patients, 56%), followed by recurrent acute pancreatitis in 18 patients (16%), including five with pancreas divisum (Table 1). There were five failures to obtain a ductogram (4%), resulting from a tiny duct (two cases), a tight stricture, an obstructing stone and extravasation of contrast through the major papilla. The 98 successful ductograms included 45 retrograde examinations, 32 prograde, 20 ambigrade and one ascending loopogram. It is difficult to define the upper limit of normal for the calibre of the pancreatic duct. After correction for magnification, Axon et al. (1984) suggested values of up to 6.5 mm in the head, 5 mm in the body and 3 mm in the tail. In

Table 1. Indications for on-table pancreatography among 112 patients

Indication	Number of patients	%
Chronic pancreatitis	63	56
Recurrent acute pancreatitis	18	16
Obscure abdominal pain		
Post cholecystectomy	8	7
Pancreas divisum	9	8
Papillary fibrosis	3	3
Acute pancreatitis with pseudocysts	6	5.5
Carcinoma of pancreas	5	4.5
Total	112	100

practice, dilatation is usually apparent when these dimensions are exceeded or when one section of the duct is wider than the rest of an apparently normal calibre duct. Of the 98 ductograms, ductal dilatation was shown in 37 and some degree of ductal stenosis in 10. In chronic pancreatitis ERP tends to over-diagnose ductal strictures, presumably because of inadequate filling.

Table 2 demonstrates the findings of OTP in our 63 patients with chronic pancreatitis. Again duct dilatation was the commonest finding, with or without associated stricture. We seldom demonstrated clear-cut stones in the main pancreatic duct unlike Lees and Heron (1987) who found stones in five of 12 patients with chronic pancreatitis using percutaneous pancreatography. Some degree of ductal dilatation was found in every patient receiving ambigrade pancreatography, because this method was selected when we could palpate the duct.

There was a 73% (61 of 84) success rate for visualisation of the main pancreatic duct at ERCP. Of the 23 patients with failed endoscopic pancreatography, OTP was invaluable in all but one technical failure, showing normal ducts in 12, dilated ducts in nine and ductal communication with a pseudocyst (by cystography) in one. Only 17 of 30 patients with complete visualisation of the main pancreatic duct on ERCP had matching appearances on OTP. Among the remaining 13, seven patients with a "stricture" on ERCP had a normal duct (one) or dilated ducts (six) beyond that point, and three with "dilated" ducts on ERCP actually had normal ducts; in the other three

Table 2. Pancreatographic findings in 63 patients with chronic pancreatitis

Type of pancreatography	Dilated MPD	Small or normal MPD	Stenosis	Ductal stone
Retrograde	9	10	3	1
Prograde	8	9	4	1
Ambigrade	15	—	3	—
Total	32 (51%)	19 (30%)	10 (16%)	2 (3%)

MPD, main pancreatic duct.

patients on-table ductography was not obtained because of technical failure or because cystography was performed instead. Lees and Heron (1987) had a similar experience: among 16 patients undergoing ERCP for preoperative evaluation of duct anatomy, there were eight failures (two patients with previous gastric surgery and six with pancreas divisum). In the remaining eight the results were inconclusive. It must, therefore, be stressed that ERCP is not always successful and that the results obtained may be unreliable in chronic pancreatitis.

Conclusions

From the surgical standpoint OTP is valuable in tailoring the operation to the ductal pathology in that particular patient (Keddie and Nardi 1965; Nardi and Acosta 1966; Ham and Yeo 1976). In our own experience, OTP resulted in a change of operative plan in 35 patients; 19 had additional procedures and 16 had altered procedures (Desa and Williamson 1990).

The only potential complication of OTP is postoperative acute pancreatitis. Collected results from six series of 261 patients undergoing OTP provide only two instances (0.85%) of this complication (Keddie and Nardi 1965; Nardi and Acosta 1966; Howard and Short 1969; Ham and Yeo 1976; Scott et al. 1984; Desa and Williamson 1990). Gentle instillation of contrast medium and perhaps the prophylactic use of aprotinin may help to explain this low incidence, which compares with an incidence of up to 7% after ERP (Bilbao et al. 1976).

In conclusion, OTP is a safe and invaluable adjunct in the surgery of pancreatic disease, especially chronic pancreatitis, pancreas divisum and pseudocyst. It provides more information than ERCP and quite often results in modification of the operative procedure.

References

Apalakis A, Dussault J, Knight M, Smith R (1977) Relief of pain from pancreatic carcinoma. Ann R Coll Surg Engl 59:401–403

Axon ART, Classen M, Cotton PB, Cremer M, Freeny PC, Lees WR (1984) Pancreatography in chronic pancreatitis: international definitions. Gut 25:1107–1112

Berni CA, Bandyk DF, Oreskovich MR, Carrico CJ (1982) Role of intraoperative pancreatography in patients with injury to the pancreas. Am J Surg 143:602–605

Bilbao MK, Dotten CT, Lee TG, Katon RM (1976) Complications of endoscopic retrograde cholangiopancreatography (ERCP). A study of 10 000 cases. Gastroenterology 70:314–320

Cooper MJ, Williamson RCN (1983) The value of operative pancreatography. Br J Surg 70:577–580

Cooper MJ, Williamson RCN (1984) Drainage operations in chronic pancreatitis. Br J Surg 71:761–766

Cuilleret J, Guillemin G (1990) Surgical management of chronic pancreatitis on the continent of Europe. World J Surg 14:11–18

Desa LA, Williamson RCN (1990) On-table pancreatography: importance in planning operative strategy. Br J Surg 77:1145–1150

Doubilet H, Mulholland JH (1951) Intubation of the pancreatic duct in the human. Proc Soc Exp Biol Med 76:113–114

Haaga JR, Highman LM, Cooperman AV, Owens FJ (1979) Percutaneous CT-guided pancreatography and pseudocystography. AJR 132:829–830

Ham JM, Yeo BW (1976) Operative pancreatography. Aust NZ J Surg 46:387–390

Hamilton I, Lintott DJ, Rothwell J, Axon ATR (1982) Metrizamine as contrast medium in endoscopic retrograde cholangiopancreatography. Clin Radiol 33:293–295

Hannigan BF, Keeling PWN, Slavin B, Thompson RPH (1985) Hyperamylasaemia after ERCP with ionic and non-ionic contrast media. Gastrointes Endosc 31:109–110

Howard JH, Short WF (1969) An evaluation of pancreatography in suspected pancreatic disease. Surg Gynecol Obstet 129:319–324

Keddie N, Nardi GL (1965) Pancreatography: a safe and effective technic. Am J Surg 110:863–865

Kivisaari L (1979) Contrast absorption and pancreatic inflammation following experimental ERCP. Invest Radiol 14:943–947

Lees WR, Heron CW (1987) US-guided percutaneous pancreatography: experience in 75 patients. Radiology 165:809–813

Makela P, Dean PB (1986) Frequency of hyperamylasemia after ERCP with iohexol. Eur J Radiol 6:303–304

Matter D, Bret PM, Bretagnolle M, Valette PJ, Fond A (1987) Pancreatic duct: us-guided percutaneous opacification. Radiology 163:635–636

Nardi GL, Acosta JM (1966) Papillitis as a cause of pancreatitis and abdominal pain: role of evocative test, operative pancreatography and histologic evaluation. Ann Surg 164:611–618

Pollock A (1958) Pancreatography in the diagnosis of chronic relapsing pancreatitis. Surg Gynecol Obstet 407:765–770

Saari A, Standertskjold-Nordenstam CG, Karonen SL, Schroder T, Kivisaari L (1988) The pharmacokinetics of a contrast medium in experimental pancreatography. ROFO 148:694–698

Saari A (1989) Pharmacokinetics of three contrast media in experimental pancreatography. Acta Radiol 30:81–86

Scott HW, Neblett WW, O'Neill JA, Sawyers JL, Avant GS, Starnes VA (1984) Longitudinal pancreaticojejunostomy in chronic relapsing pancreatitis with onset in childhood. Ann Surg 199:610–622

Trapnell JE, Howard JM, Brewster J (1966) Transduodenal pancreatography: an improved technique. Surgery 60:1112–1119

Trapnell JE (1967) Pancreatography – a reassessment. Br J Surg 54:934–939

Chapter 11

Distal Pancreatectomy in Chronic Pancreatitis

M. C. Aldridge and R. C. N. Williamson

Surgical Techniques in Chronic Pancreatitis

In the absence of specific, effective medical treatment, patients with chronic pancreatitis are often referred for surgical management of their disease. It is one of the most difficult conditions the abdominal surgeon may be called upon to treat, requiring clinical skill in patient selection and technical skill to overcome the surgical problems associated with a severely diseased gland. Despite these difficulties, unrelenting pain, pseudocyst formation and bile duct obstruction often demand a surgical approach in this relatively young group of patients.

Recent advances in the surgical management of chronic pancreatitis include much better imaging of the pancreas (by computed tomography (CT), ultrasound and endoscopic retrograde cholangiopancreatography (ERCP)) and the lower morbidity and mortality rates that stem from improved operative techniques in pancreatic resection along with better preoperative and postoperative care. It is our own experience that poor results are largely confined to those patients who are already addicted to opiate analgesics and those who resume alcohol abuse.

If there is dilatation of the main pancreatic duct (7 mm or more), longitudinal pancreaticojejunostomy is probably the optimal procedure as it can relieve pain without sacrificing pancreatic function. If there is no evidence of duct dilatation on CT, ultrasound or ERCP, the surgical procedures for the relief of pain are limited to resection of part or all of the pancreas. If preoperative ductography is incomplete, the surgeon should employ on-table pancreatography (see Chapter 10).

The decision whether to proceed with pancreatic resection relies upon careful assessment of the severity of pancreatic pain, the risk of developing diabetes and the likelihood of successful postoperative analgesia. Certainly when the patient has had several hospital admissions for pain control, has lost a significant time from work and is taking regular narcotics, resection should be strongly considered. It is important to assess the patient's personality in terms of drug and alcohol dependence, compliance with therapy and ability to manage pancreatic exocrine and endocrine insufficiency. Since diabetes occurs in 40% of patients with chronic pancreatitis even in the absence of treatment (Ammann et al. 1984), incidence of postoperative diabetes should be compared with that in patients treated medically or by duct decompression rather than with the incidence in the population at large.

In the patient who still has some endocrine or exocrine function and in whom the disease can be localised to either the head or to the body and tail of the gland, partial resection is indicated with preservation of the more normal segment of the pancreas. The decision as to which is the more normal half of the gland is taken following examination by CT, ultrasound and ERCP for the distribution of calcification, ductal strictures and inflammation. This decision is often far from easy. If lateralisation of the disease can be determined in this way, the indications for resection outlined above can be relaxed a little with acceptance of a lesser degree of preoperative disability.

Sometimes in patients with generalised pancreatitis, especially when disease is maximal in the head, partial pancreatectomy may be accompanied by ductal drainage in the retained gland in preference to total removal of the pancreas.

Indications for Distal Pancreatectomy

Specific indications for distal pancreatectomy include:

1. Disease predominantly affecting the body and tail of the pancreas
2. Severe disease of the body and tail with duct obstruction at the level of the pancreatic neck
3. A pseudocyst in the body or tail of the pancreas.

Conventionally, splenectomy is performed at the same time as distal pancreatectomy because of the close relationship between the splenic vessels and the body of the pancreas. The spleen, however, serves an important immunological function (Cooper and Williamson 1984; Billar et al. 1988; Aldridge et al. 1989) and is worthy of preservation if this can be achieved safely. Spleen-preserving or conservative distal pancreatectomy (Cooper and Williamson 1985) was first described by the French surgeon Mallet-Guy (Mallet-Guy and Vachon 1943), who advocated the technique for distal resection in patients with chronic pancreatitis. The technique is now regaining popularity amongst pancreatic surgeons (Cooper and Williamson 1985; Warshaw 1988; Scott-Conner and Dawson 1989). We have recently shown that this technique is possible in over 40% of patients coming to distal pancreatectomy for a variety of pancreatic diseases including chronic pancreatitis (Aldridge et al. 1990). It is particularly indicated in those patients with chronic pancreatitis in whom the gland has undergone sclerosis and atrophy and has "shrunk away" from the splenic vessels, leaving a dissection plane between the vessels and the pancreatic parenchyma. If there is either gross calcification or inflammation, a pseudocyst or splenic vein thrombosis, conservative distal pancreatectomy is contraindicated and conventional resection with splenectomy should be performed.

Surgical Techniques

Conservative Distal Pancreatectomy

The decision as to whether the spleen can be preserved during distal pancreatectomy for chronic pancreatitis must finally be made at operation, and often only after a trial dissection, although preoperative imaging may show features such as pseudocyst, splenic vein thrombosis or extensive calcification which make conservation unlikely. We perform routine preoperative angiography (Appleton et al. 1989).

The abdomen is explored through a bilateral subcostal or "high gable" incision, and a full laparotomy is carried out. The lesser sac is entered by division of the grastrocolic omentum outside the epiploic arcade, and the posterior wall of the stomach is mobilised from the anterior surface of the pancreas. A retractor is placed within the lesser sac to keep the stomach out of the operating field, and the pancreas is examined throughout its length. The extent and distribution of the inflammatory process are assessed and compared with preoperative imaging to confirm that distal resection is the most appropriate procedure. Direct measurement of pancreatic parenchymal pressures using a perfused needle connected to a transducer may be helpful to assess the distribution of inflammation and fibrosis within the pancreas. Our early experience with this technique suggests that higher pressures are obtained in the more severely diseased areas of the pancreas (Jalleh et al. 1991).

Once the decision has been made to perform a distal resection, the dissection may proceed in one of two ways, either prograde or retrograde. In the prograde dissection, the tail of the pancreas is mobilised within the lesser sac and the gland is slowly peeled off the splenic vessels in a left to right direction, using fine ligatures or diathermy to secure the many arterial and venous branches that enter the posterior surface of the pancreas (Fig. 1a). While this technique is useful for performing a 20%–30% distal pancreatectomy (for example for small neuroendocrine tumours in the tail), it is a difficult exercise in the patient with chronic pancreatitis. We have now largely abandoned the prograde dissection in favour of the alternative technique of retrograde dissection, which commences at the level of the neck or proximal body of the pancreas (depending on the extent of the planned resection). A plane is carefully developed between the pancreas in front and either the splenic vein or superior mesenteric and portal veins behind. Once 2–3 cm of pancreas has been freed, a Kocher's director is placed behind the neck of the pancreas to protect the vein, and the pancreas is divided between stay sutures. Retrograde dissection now proceeds from right to left towards the spleen, securing the pancreatic branches of the splenic artery and vein as before (Fig. 1b). The splenic vessels can often be seen grooving the posterior surface of the pancreas.

If the splenic artery is damaged during this dissection, it can be safely ligated away from the splenic hilum and the spleen will retain its vascular supply from the vasa brevia and gastroepiploic vessels. Indeed, in the technique described by Warshaw (1988), the splenic artery and vein are deliberately ligated and divided within the splenic hilum. Even though scintigraphy may be normal and there may be no haematological evidence of hyposplenism after this procedure,

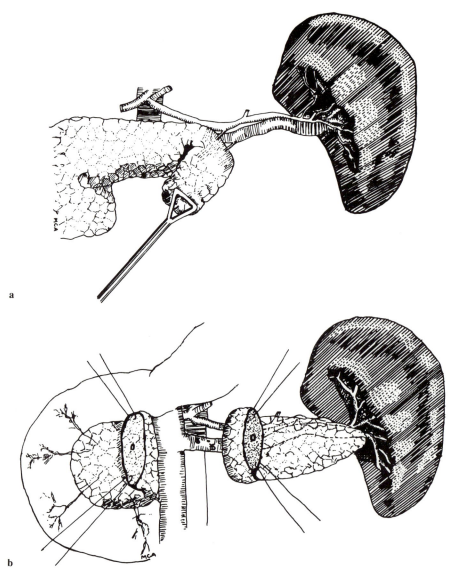

Fig. 1. a Conservative distal pancreatectomy. The tail of the pancreas has been elevated from the splenic vessels and the dissection proceeds in a left to right or prograde direction. The pancreatic branches can be seen and ligated as they appear. **b** The pancreatic neck has been divided at an early stage and the distal pancreas is 'peeled' backwards towards the spleen. The pancreatic branches are ligated as they appear and the dissection proceeds in a right to left or retrograde direction.

it is unknown whether immunological function remains normal once the main vessels are divided, so we prefer to preserve the splenic artery and vein where possible.

If there has been no clear image of the proximal pancreatic duct on preoperative ERCP there is an opportunity to perform prograde pancreatography (Desa and Williamson 1990) before the transected duct is under-run and the pancreatic stump is oversewn with 3/0 silk sutures. If the pancreatogram shows a dilated duct with stones or a stricture in the head of the pancreas and poor flow of contrast into the duodenum, the duct is slit open for several centimetres and an onlay pancreaticojejunostomy is performed. The spleen is inspected before closing the abdomen and two soft silicone drains are placed in the pancreatic bed.

It is convenient to record the extent of the distal pancreatectomy in terms of the percentage of the gland removed (Fig. 2). A 30% resection (caudal pancreatectomy) is done when the gland is divided at the junction between its body and tail; a 50% resection (hemipancreatectomy) when the gland is divided along the front of the portal vein; a 70% resection when the gland is divided at the level of the gastroduodenal artery and a 95% resection (subtotal pancreatectomy) when only a thin rim of pancreas is retained within the duodenal loop.

Conventional Distal Pancreatectomy with Splenectomy

The abdomen and pancreas are explored as described above. In conventional distal pancreatectomy, the spleen is mobilised as the first step and the spleen

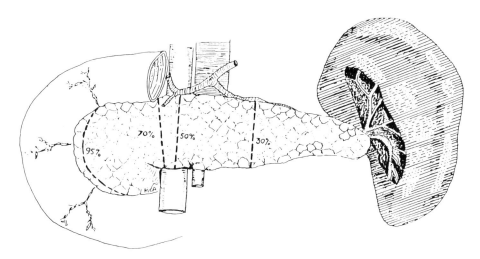

Fig. 2. Various types of distal pancreatectomy. In a 30% resection (caudal pancreatectomy) the pancreas is divided at the junction between its body and tail. In a 50% resection (hemipancreatectomy) the gland is divided along the front of the portal vein. In a 70% resection, the gland is divided at the level of the gastroduodenal artery. In a 95% resection (subtotal pancreatectomy) only a thin rim of pancreas is retained within the duodenal loop.

and distal pancreas are lifted forwards out of the pancreatic bed. The spleen can either be removed at this stage (which may be convenient if the capsule is torn) or left attached to be resected *en bloc* with the distal pancreas. In the patient with chronic pancreatitis, the posterior plane of dissection between the tail and body of the pancreas and its cocoon of inflammatory scar tissue needs to be developed by sharp dissection, and this manoeuvre can be particularly difficult if a pseudocyst is present. Subsequently, the splenic vein is gently separated from the pancreas and ligated to the left of its junction with the superior mesenteric vein. The inferior mesenteric vein enters close to the origin of the portal vein and can almost always be preserved. The splenic artery is doubly ligated as it gains the superior border of the proximal body of pancreas. The gland is then transected at an appropriate site and oversewn as before unless an onlay pancreaticojejunostomy is indicated.

Results of Distal Pancreatectomy for Chronic Pancreatitis

Over the last 12 years, we have undertaken distal pancreatectomy in 46 patients with chronic pancreatitis, mainly associated with alcohol abuse. These patients comprised 31 men and 15 women with ages ranging between 17 and 75 years (median 38 years). In 12 patients, a conservative resection was performed, preserving the spleen, while the remaining 34 patients underwent conventional distal pancreatectomy with splenectomy.

The 12 patients who underwent conservative distal pancreatectomy comprised seven men and five women with ages ranging between 17 and 72 years (median 36 years). The indication for pancreatic resection in all these patients was severe abdominal pain and in addition four patients had a pseudocyst in either the body or tail of pancreas, two patients had strictures of the pancreatic duct and one patient had papillary stenosis.

The extent of distal resection ranged between 30% and 70% (median 50%). In two patients the splenic artery had to be ligated because of bleeding. Division of the artery was carried out close to the point of pancreatic transection, or well away from the splenic hilum, and the spleen appeared viable and was not removed. Postoperative haematological screening showed no thrombocytopenia or Howell Jolly bodies (i.e. no evidence of hyposplenism), and radionuclide scans showed normal uptake of isotope by the spleen.

Postoperative complications occurred in two patients (17%) but there were no deaths. Both patients developed a pancreatic fistula which presented via abdominal drains and in both cases the fistula closed spontaneously after 21 and 35 days, respectively. One of these patients later developed a partial rupture of a false aneurysm of the splenic artery requiring emergency laparotomy and splenectomy.

Eight of the 12 patients have had pain relief and only one patient has required a completion total pancreatectomy.

The 34 patients who underwent conventional distal pancreatectomy comprised 24 men and 10 women with ages ranging between 20 and 75 years (median 39 years). In five of these patients, conventional resection was performed after an attempt at conservative resection had failed. In four of these five, dissection of the splenic vessels from the pancreas had to be abandoned because they were too adherent to a severely inflamed and scarred gland, whereas in the fifth the pancreatic tail actually lay posterior to the vessels at the splenic hilum making further dissection impossible.

The indication for pancreatic resection in these patients was severe, recurrent abdominal pain. In addition, 11 patients had pseudocysts in either the body or tail of pancreas and in four of these distal pancreatectomy was undertaken urgently because of recurrent gastrointestinal haemorrhage. In three, the source of bleeding was found to be a false aneurysm of either the splenic or pancreatoduodenal artery in the wall of the pseudocyst and the remaining patient had recurrent bleeding following a cystgastrostomy.

The extent of distal resection ranged between 30% and 70% (median 60%). In 30 patients the transected pancreatic duct was under-run and the pancreatic stump oversewn while in four an onlay pancreaticojejunostomy was performed using a Roux loop.

Postoperative complications occurred in eight patients (23%) but there were no deaths. Three patients had to be re-operated because of reactive haemorrhage. In three patients a peripancreatic collection was detected on ultrasound and all three collections were successfully drained percutaneously under radiological control. Two patients developed a gastrointestinal fistula (one gastric, one colonic).

Of the 34 patients 20 have had pain relief and five (15%) have gone on to have completion total pancreatectomy.

Management of the Pancreatic Stump

This is an unresolved problem. Pancreatic leaks occurred in two of our patients following conservative distal pancreatectomy and in three patients following conventional resection. They appeared either as peripancreatic collections seen on ultrasound or as a pancreatic fistula presenting via an abdominal drain. Those with a collection had pain and fever whereas those with a fistula were symptom free. Collections were successfully treated by percutaneous drainage under radiological control, but the two pancreatic fistulas prolonged hospital stay by 3–4 weeks. Several other patients with an uneventful recovery had high concentrations of amylase detected from abdominal drains.

Our preferred technique for dealing with the stump of the transected pancreas is to find and ligate the pancreatic duct and then to oversew the stump with non-absorbable sutures, placing two abdominal drains down to the pancreatic bed. If, however, prograde pancreatography shows a dilated duct with stones or stricture in the head, we open the proximal pancreatic duct and perform an onlay pancreaticojejunostomy.

Routine drainage into a Roux-en-Y loop of jejunum has been recommended by some surgeons (DuVal 1954; Longmire et al. 1956; Leger 1958), but Shankar et al. (1990) from the Middlesex Hospital have shown in a large retrospective study that lateral pancreaticojejunostomy confers no benefit in terms of reducing the incidence of pancreatic fistula. Their overall incidence of pancreatic fistula was 4%, a figure identical to ours (5/113 versus 2/46). Since Roux-en-Y pancreaticojejunostomy adds to the length of the operation and does not reliably prevent the problem of leakage, it should probably be reserved for those with a dilated duct and/or stricture in the head of pancreas.

Stapling of the pancreatic remnant has become popular among surgeons in the United States in recent years and has been shown to be accompanied by a low postoperative morbidity (Patcher et al. 1979; Anderson et al. 1980; Fitzgibbons et al. 1982; Lansing et al. 1983; Scott-Conner and Dawson 1989). More recently, Cuschieri has described a technique of pancreatic 'banding' (Sadek et al. 1988). In this, double silk ligatures are passed around the pancreas and tied on either side of the proposed site of pancreatic transection to achieve complete haemostasis. Following division of the parenchyma, the pancreatic duct is suture ligated and the raw surface of the pancreas is covered with adjacent fat from the transverse mesocolon. The incidence of pancreatic fistula with this technique, however, was 9%. With regard to our own pancreatic fistula rate of 4%, it is conceivable that the use of two silicone tube drains might actually encourage fistula formation. It might be better to leave either only a single small drain (if the spleen is removed) or no drain at all, accepting that a peripancreatic collection could be successfully treated by percutaneous drainage.

References

Aldridge MC, Cheslyn-Curtis S, Chadwick SJD, Dudley HAF (1989) Splenic reticuloendothelial function following surgery (abstract). Br J Surg 76:647

Aldridge MC, Cooper MJ, Williamson RCN (1990) Splenic preservation during distal pancreatectomy for pancreatic disease (abstract). HPB Surg 2 (Suppl):258

Ammann RW, Akovbiantz A, Largiader F, Schueler G (1984) Course and outcome of chronic pancreatitis: longitudinal study of a mixed medical-surgical series of 245 patients. Gastroenterology 86:820–828

Anderson DK, Bolman RM III, Moyan JA Jr (1980) Management of penetrating pancreatic injuries: subtotal pancreatectomy using the Auto Suture stapler. J Trauma 20:347–349

Appleton GVN, Bathhurst NCG, Virjee J, Cooper MJ, Williamson RCN (1989) The value of angiography in the surgical management of pancreatic disease. Ann R Coll Surg Engl 71:92–96

Billar TR, West MA, Hyland BJ, Simmons RL (1988) Splenectomy alters Kupffer cell response to endotoxin. Arch Surg 123:327–332

Cooper MJ, Williamson RCN (1984) Splenectomy: indications, hazards and alternatives. B J Surg 71:173–180

Cooper MJ, Williamson RCN (1985) Conservative pancreatectomy. Br J Surg 72:801–803

Desa LA, Williamson RCN (1990) On-table pancreatography: importance in planning operative strategy. Br J Surg 77:1145–1150

DuVal MK (1954) Caudal pancreato-jejunostomy for chronic relapsing pancreatitis. Ann Surg 140:775–785

Fitzgibbons TJ, Yellin AE, Maruyama MM, Donovan AJ (1982) Management of the transected pancreas following distal pancreatectomy. Surg Gynecol Obstet 154:225–231

Jalleh RP, Aslam M, Williamson RCN (1991) Raised pancreatic tissue pressures in chronic pancreatitis (SRS abstract). Br J Surg 78:754

Lansing PB, Browder IW, Harkness SO, Kitahama A (1983) Staple closure of the pancreas. Am Surg 49:214–217

Leger L (1958) Technique de la pancréato-jéjunostomie après pancréatectomie gauche pour pancréatite chronique. J Chir Paris 76:93–115

Longmire WP, Jordan PH, Briggs JD (1956) Experience with the resection of the pancreas in the treatment of chronic relapsing pancreatitis. Ann Surg 144:681–695

Mallet-Guy P, Vachon A (1943) Pancréatites chroniques gauches. Masson. Édit Paris

Patcher HL, Pennington R, Chassin J, Spencer FC (1979) Simplified distal pancreatectomy with the Auto Suture stapler: preliminary clinical observations. Surgery 85:166–170

Sadek S, Holdsworth R, Cuschieri A. (1988) Experience with pancreatic banding: results of a simple technique for dealing with the pancreatic remnant after distal partial pancreatectomy. Br J Surg 75:486–487

Scott-Conner CEH, Dawson DL (1989) Technical considerations in distal pancreatectomy with splenic preservation. Surg Gynecol Obstet 168:451–453

Shankar S, Theis B, Russell RCG (1990) Management of the stump of the pancreas after distal pancreatic resection. Br J Surg 77:541–544

Warshaw AL (1988) Conservation of the spleen with distal pancreatectomy. Arch Surg 123:550–553

.

Chapter 12

Resection of the Pancreatic Head

M. J. Cooper

Introduction

Resection of the head of the pancreas is one of the most challenging operations in abdominal surgery; an often difficult dissection is followed by a complex reconstruction. Proximal pancreatectomy, as first described by Whipple et al. (1935), was a conservative operation removing only a limited portion of the pancreas and a short segment of the duodenum. The problem of the pancreatic duct was solved by ligation and reimplantation was not attempted. When the procedure had been proved feasible, it entered a radical phase and within two years Brunschwig (1937) developed an operation involving resection of the entire duodenum and a Polya-type gastric anastomosis. The subsequent high incidence of anastomotic ulceration (17%) that followed this procedure led to more extensive gastric resections, and hemigastrectomy became an integral part of any pancreatoduodenectomy (Warren et al. 1962). Although a wide clearance may be important in the treatment of pancreatic cancer, it is unnecessary if the resection is performed for localised neoplasia or benign disease. Watson (1944) performed the first pylorus-preserving pancreatoduodenectomy but this option was ignored, although the patient survived for 15 years. The procedure was revived in 1978 by Traverso and Longmire for benign disease and is now also widely used in the treatment of localised malignancy (Braasch et al. 1984; Cooper and Williamson 1985). More recently, newer procedures have been described which aim to remove the head of the pancreas without the loss of the duodenum and hence maintain gastrointestinal continuity (Beger et al. 1985; Frey and Smith 1987; Lambert et al. 1987).

Indications

Resection of the head of the pancreas is the operation of choice for periampullary malignancy; this operation offers the only hope of cure. Localised tumours of the ampulla of Vater, bile duct or duodenum can be resected with a 25% chance of 5-year survival (Ihse and Larsson 1980). The role of resection in the treatment of adenocarcinoma of the pancreas is still unclear as 5-year survival remains poor (<5%) (Edis et al. 1980; Matsuno and Sato 1986; Smith 1989; Trede et al. 1990). However, in selected patients it offers the possibility of cure, and recent trends of specialisation have led to dramatic reductions in morbidity and mortality (Edis et al. 1980; Smith 1989; Trede et al. 1990) such that pancreatoduodenectomy can also be considered in some patients as a good palliative procedure.

Resection in chronic pancreatitis is almost always for the relief of pain. Although bypass procedures are preferable, (Warshaw et al. 1980; Prinz and Greenlee 1981), if pain becomes intolerable and the ducts are small, resection will provide good relief of pain in about 75% of patients (Lambert et al. 1987; Williamson and Cooper 1987). Occasionally, despite all the modern imaging techniques, resection may be undertaken without a definite diagnosis of neoplasia or inflammatory disease, as the two can co-exist.

Surgical Anatomy

The pancreas is a retroperitoneal structure extending transversly across the back of the abdomen. It consists of a head, a narrow neck, a body and a tail. The uncinate process is derived from the head and projects behind the superior mesenteric and portal veins where it is in intimate contact with the superior mesenteric artery as it arises from the aorta. Anteriorly the pancreas is separated from the stomach by the lesser sac. The common bile duct traverses the head of the pancreas in a groove that is palpable posteriorly to join the major pancreatic duct at the ampulla of Vater. The minor duct enters the duodenum 2 cm proximal to the major papilla.

The pancreatic head and duodenal loop share a common arterial supply derived from the gastroduodenal and superior mesenteric arteries via the anterior and posterior pancreaticoduodenal arcades (Fig. 1). Until recently therefore, it has been considered that total resection of the head of the pancreas also requires removal of the major part of the duodenum. There are many arterial anomalies in this region which must be carefully observed and some surgeons continue to perform arteriography to map these out prior to operation (Mackie et al. 1979; Appleton et al. 1989). The hepatic artery lies along the top of the gland and can be injured at this point. In up to 25% of the population the right or even the common hepatic artery is a branch of the superior mesenteric artery (Mackie et al. 1979). In this situation it provides the arterial supply to the head of the pancreas and must be recognised to prevent accidental hepatic artery damage.

Behind the neck of the pancreas the superior and inferior mesenteric and the splenic veins coalesce to form the portal vein. There are no anterior tributaries from pancreas to the great veins which enables dissection and division of the pancreas at this point. There are a variable number of tributaries entering on the right lateral and posterior aspects of the main vein; the superior and inferior pancreatic veins are the largest and most constant.

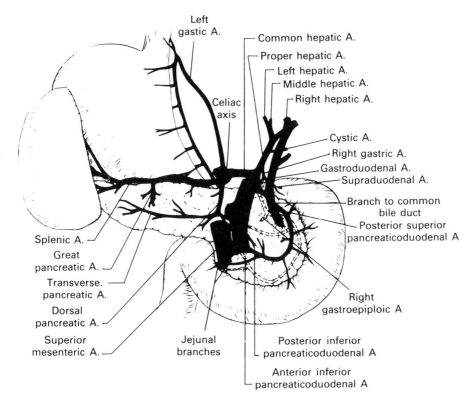

Fig. 1. Diagram demonstrating the major arteries in the region of the pancreas and those supplying the gland itself.

Technique

Although it is now 56 years since the original report by Whipple et al. (1935) there remain many controversies over technique. I shall first describe our technique for a pylorus-preserving proximal pancreatoduodenectomy and then discuss some of the problems.

The incision of choice is a bilateral subcostal or "high gable" which gives excellent visualisation of the upper abdomen as well as permitting a full laparotomy. In operations for malignant disease a search must be made for evidence of metastatic spread. If this is found, the resection should usually be abandoned in favour of a palliative bypass. The initial part of the subsequent dissection is then an assessment of resectability. The head of the pancreas is fully mobilised by Kocher's manoeuvre; this can be carried round from the bile duct along the third part of the duodenum to the superior mesenteric vein. It may be necessary at this point to mobilise the hepatic flexure of the colon and reflect it downward to expose fully the third part of the duodenum. The gastrocolic omentum is opened widely taking great care not to damage the gastroepiploic arcade. The middle colic vein can be traced down to identify the superior mesenteric vein and a plane is developed behind the neck of the pancreas, anterior to the portal vein. A finger can then be gently inserted to ensure that the vein is free of tumour. Superiorly the free edge of the lesser omentum is dissected to reveal the common bile duct, the hepatic artery and the portal vein; the vein usually lies between and behind the other structures and a finger can be inserted from above to confirm that the plane is truly free of tumour. Up to this point the resection can be abandoned if it seems appropriate. Although part or all of the retropancreatic portal vein can be removed, the operation in these cases is certain to be palliative and is probably unjustified.

The first part of the duodenum is dissected off the head of the pancreas so that it can be divided 2–5 cm distal to the pylorus (Fig. 2). Ideally the gastroduodenal artery should be preserved but this is not always feasible in the presence of chronic pancreatitis . We have found no problems with viability if the gastroduodenal artery is divided, but division might affect motility which is often slow after this procedure.

After division of the duodenum, the stomach can then be swung to the left out of the way. The gall bladder is usually removed (always if diseased) and the bile duct is divided. The ligament of Treitz is taken down and the fourth and remaining third part of the duodenum are fully mobilised. The pancreas is then divided with a soft clamp on the body side which can be removed as the small vessels are controlled with diathermy or sutures.

The head is mobilised to the right by division of the vascular tributaries as they are encountered. The most serious potential problem during this part of

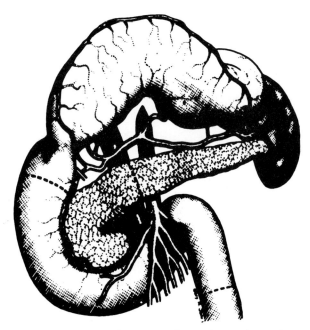

Fig. 2. Pylorus-preserving pancreatoduodenectomy: lines of resection. The pancreatic neck, duodenum and upper jejunum are divided as indicated. In this case only the superior pancreaticoduodenal artery has been divided, the main gastroduodenal artery being preserved. (From Cooper and Williamson (1985), with permission.)

the dissection is injury to the major veins. Vascular clamps should always be immediately available during this procedure and can be placed across the vein to control haemorrhage. The injury should be repaired with a 5/0 prolene suture.

Division of the portal vein tributaries, and traction of the pancreatic head to the right exposes the uncinate process, the mesentery of which is mobilised from behind the portal vein and divided between clamps. Great care must be taken here not to damage the superior mesenteric artery or any associated anomalous arteries as traction easily disturbs the anatomy. With a hand lying behind the Kockerised pancreas as the dissection proceeds, the superior mesenteric artery can be felt at the tip of the fingers. In patients with chronic pancreatitis particularly, leaving a rim of pancreas on the portal vein causes no harm and is preferable to any risk of vascular injury. Lastly the first part of the jejunum is pulled through into the supracolic compartment and divided. The specimen may now be removed.

Reconstruction

There are a number of techniques for reconstruction mostly involving variations of the pancreatic anastomosis. Our chosen method is to bring the jejunum via the retrocolic route and to perform an end-to-end pancreatico-jejunostomy. For this anastomosis the pancreas has to be mobilised off the splenic vein so that the proximal 3–4 cm of the body is accessible all round.

A posterior layer of non-absorbable sutures is placed between the pancreas 2–3 cm from the transected end and the jejunal serosa. These are placed and then tied when all have been inserted, leaving clips on the superior and inferior sutures. If the duct is small the inner layer approximates the ends of the pancreas and jejunum. With a large duct it may be possible to open it anteriorly giving a wide orifice which can then be anastomosed mucosa-to-mucosa, using absorbable sutures. The anterior layer is then completed with interrupted sutures invaginating the end of the pancreas into the jejunum. If the duct is small a stent can be placed (size 4–6 French) to drain the pancreatic juice; this is then removed at 10–12 days once the anastomosis has healed.

Next, an end-to-side choledochojejunostomy is fashioned far enough away from the pancreatic anastomosis to avoid tension (Fig. 3). The bile duct is usually large and a single layer anastomosis can be performed with vicryl. A T-tube is usually placed across the anastomosis with the lower end in the jejunal loop. This protects not only the biliary anastomosis but also decompresses the Roux-loop. The T-tube also permits radiology of this area if a leak is suspected. The loop is hitched gently to the liver capsule to prevent tension on the anastomoses.

Lastly, an end-to-side duodenojejunostomy is constructed 40 cm distal to the biliary anastomosis using two layers of 2/0 vicryl (Fig. 4). Since gastroparesis is common after this operation it is our policy routinely to place a feeding jejunostomy in the first retrocolic loop of jejunum. Nutrition can normally be commenced by this route within 48 h of the operation and built up over a few

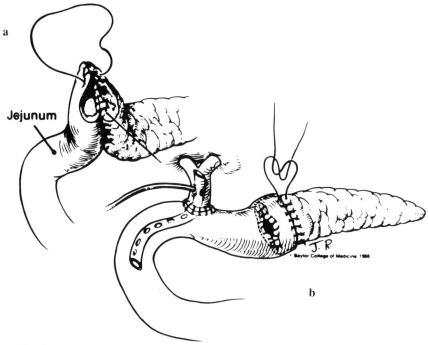

Fig. 3. The first step in reconstruction is an end-to-end pancreaticojejunostomy. **a**, the posterior pancreas to serosa and pancreas to jejunal wall sutures have been placed; the anterior now is in progress. **b** shows the position after invagination of the pancreas into the end of the jejunum. (From Jordan (1989), with permission.)

days. Rarely do we need to use parenteral nutrition even if complications arise or gastroparesis is prolonged. Drains are placed in the area of dissection before the abdomen is closed. Tube or sump drains are used as they are unlikely to block and produce a defined track should a leak occur.

Alternative Techniques

Gastrectomy

The conventional "Whipple" operation includes a 50% gastrectomy to improve nodal clearance and reduce the risk of peptic ulceration. For many surgeons it remains the standard procedure. It differs from the above description only in that the first structure to be divided is the midstomach which is then folded out of the way, the remaining structures are then divided as previously described. Reconstruction is completed by a Polya-type gastrojejunostomy (Fig. 5). Fear of marginal ulceration leads many surgeons to add a truncal vagotomy. The incidence of ulceration is very variable and H_2 receptor antagonists offer an alternative means of therapy or prophylaxis against marginal ulceration.

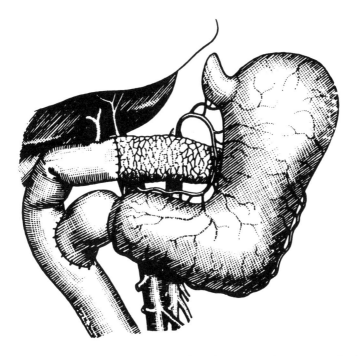

Fig. 4. The final configuration at the completion of a pylorus-preserving pancreatoduodenectomy. The duodenojejunostomy is the last and most anterior anastomosis. (From Cooper and Williamson (1985), with permission.)

End-to-side Pancreaticojejunostomy

An alternative method of anastomosis is to close the end of the jejunal Roux loop and anastomose the pancreas to the side (Fig. 6). A posterior row of non-absorbable sutures is placed first to join the edge of the pancreas to the jejunal serosa. A stab incision is then made in the jejunum, and the duct is anastomosed in a mucosa-to-mucosa fashion with a fine absorbable suture. The anterior layer can then be completed. Many surgeons stent this anastomosis with a tube brought to the exterior but others have not done so with equally good results (Kingsnorth 1989).

Pancreaticogastrostomy

If convenient the pancreas can be joined to the posterior wall of the stomach. A transgastric stent is placed in the pancreatic duct and the edge of the pancreas is sutured to the gastric serosa. No attempt is made to approximate mucosa. This simple technique appears to be well tolerated and successful. Alternatively, pancreaticogastrostomy with mucosal anastomosis also gives good results (Fig. 7; Bradbeer and Johnson 1990).

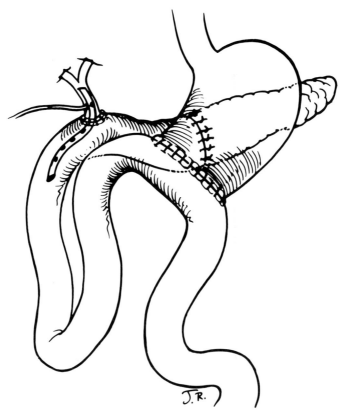

Fig. 5. The alternative configuration after a standard "Whipple" resection completed by a gastrojejunostomy (From Jordan (1989), with permission.)

Duodenum Preserving

In patients with chronic pancreatitis several operations have been described which remove the head of the pancreas without resection of the duodenum. Beger et al. (1985) described a technique for resection of the pancreatic head which involves transection of the gland at the neck with exposure of the portal vein, and then excision of the head of the gland within the pancreatic capsule. If necessary, fibrotic tissue around the bile duct can be incised to open the bile duct into the cavity formed by excision of the pancreatic head. The pancreas is reconstructed with a loop of jejunum anastomosed end-to-end to the transected pancreatic neck. A side-to-side anastomosis is made to the rim of the pancreatic capsule in the duodenal loop. This procedure leaves a bowl-shaped layer of pancreas and capsule anastomosed to the jejunal loop. Any pancreatic secretion, and bile if the duct has been opened, therefore drains into the jejunal loop. Beger commends this procedure because of the good digestive and endocrine function that is observed with duodenal preservation, and because he finds good results for pain relief on long-term follow-up (Beger and Buchler 1990).

A similar operation (Frey and Smith 1987) involves coring out the head of

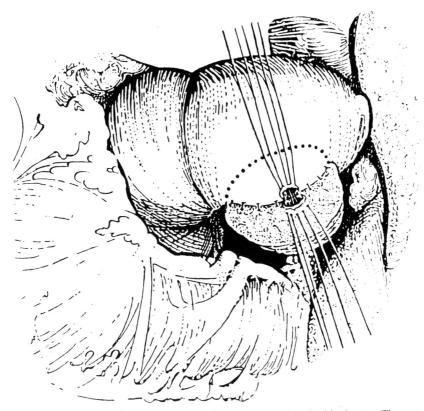

Fig. 6. The technique of end-to-side pancreaticojejunostomy as described in the text. The posterior edge to serosa stitch has been completed. A mucosa-to-mucosa stitch is in progress. (From Kingsnorth (1989), with permission.)

the gland leaving a thin rim of tissue posteriorly. A 4–5 mm rim is preserved within the duodenal loop to ensure a blood supply to the duodenum; to complete the procedure a Roux loop is sewn over the defect to drain the cavity into the gut. Lambert et al. (1987) have taken these options one step further by taking all the pancreatic tissue from the duodenal loop during a total pancreatectomy. They have ultimately had no problems with duodenal viability but have electively ventilated all patients postoperatively for 12–24 h to maintain arterial oxygen. Postoperative gastric stasis has also been invariably prolonged.

Morbidity and Mortality

In the initial reports of pancreatoduodenectomy, complications were the rule and a mortality rate of over 30% was usual. With increasing specialisation and the readiness of surgeons to refer patients to those with the appropriate skills,

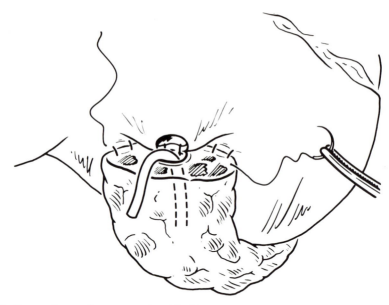

Fig. 7. Pancreaticogastric anastomosis with direct duct to mucosa apposition. The capsule is sutured to the gastric serosa. Interrupted sutures approximate the gastric and pancreatic duct mucosae. A 4 F polyethylene tube serves as a stent during insertion of these sutures. The anastomosis is completed by an anterior serosal suture. (From Bradbeer and Johnson (1990), with permission.)

major changes have taken place over the last two decades. Many series have now been published with mortality rates well under 10% (Table 1). Complications, however, continue to occur.

Haemorrhage

This is the commonest intraoperative complication, which can be reduced by careful preoperative attention to clotting status. At the time of surgery bleeding may occur from the major peripancreatic vessels, but this should be controllable by application of vascular clamps. Haemorrhage also occurs postoperatively,

Table 1. Recent operative mortality rates after pancreatoduodenectomy including total pancreatectomy

Reference	Year	No. of patients	Operative mortality (%)
Crist et al.	1987	47	2.1
Gall	1987	289	1
Cooper et al.	1987	83	4.3
Lygidakis et al.	1989	78	3.8
Pellegrini et al.	1989	51	2
Trede et al.	1990	142	0

often within 24–48 h due to unrecognised injury at the time of surgery; this requires prompt re-exploration. Bleeding may also complicate fistula formation or a local abscess. The gastroduodenal or splenic artery may be involved with haemorrhage occurring a week or so after the resection. This is a major complication and haemorrhage is said to account for 20% of deaths. Early re-operation is essential if haemorrhage occurs. Completion pancreatectomy may be necessary to visualise the area and adequately control the bleeding.

Fistula

Fistula formation due to anastomotic leakage used to cause many deaths and has made many surgeons afraid of pancreaticojejunostomy. However, if adequate drainage is instituted at the time of resection most fistulas can be controlled without the need for operative intervention. Adequate fluid replacement and control of sepsis should allow the fistula to close.

The use of somatostatin and total parenteral nutrition will aid recovery in a high output fistula. If surgery is required then often the only option is a completion pancreatectomy.

Gastric Stasis

This occurs in up to 50% of patients after the pylorus-preserving resection. Initially stasis was thought to be secondary to duodenal ischaemia, but recent evidence points to vagal disruption as the most likely cause. It can usually be managed conservatively with patience and motility agents, but occasionally re-operation is necessary to perform hemigastrectomy. Gastric emptying is not in fact normal after a standard pancreaticoduodenectomy, but obstruction and delay are usually less severe than after pylorus preservation.

Other

Many of the patients are elderly so that the full range of complications that may arise after all surgical operations can occur. Hepatic and/or renal failure are uncommon but may cause around 5% of deaths. It is worth mentioning to the patient preoperatively that the jaundice may initially increase after surgery and often takes a few weeks to clear. Pancreatitis in the remnant is also uncommon and rarely severe.

Mortality

The mortality rate from pancreatoduodenectomy has been decreasing steadily in published series. Occasional pancreatectomists who perform this operation perhaps once every few years will have a high complication rate and inevitable mortality. The impressive figures published by Trede et al. (1990) are an inspiration to others: by January 1990 they reported 142 consecutive operations over a 5-year period with no deaths. Many other large series now report mortality under 5% (Table 1) and this must now be considered the acceptable rate for surgeons who wish to operate in this area.

Conclusion

Pancreatoduodenectomy is a major operation which has become a safer procedure since it was first described over 50 years ago. With increasing specialisation the mortality rate will continue to fall. All cases should be referred to specialist centres. The place of this operation in the treatment of chronic pancreatitis and periampullary neoplasia is now well established. Its role in the treatment of pancreatic cancer is changing as the procedure becomes safer, but it remains undefined.

References

Appleton GV, Cooper MJ, Bathurst NCG et al. (1989) The value of angiography in the surgical management of pancreatic disease. Ann R Coll Surg Engl 71:92–96

Beger HG, Buchler M (1990) Duodenum preserving resection of the head of the pancreas in chronic pancreatitis with inflammatory mass in the head. World J Surg 14:83–87

Beger HG, Krantzberger W, Biltner R et al. (1985) Duodenum-preserving resection of the head of the pancreas in patients with severe chronic pancreatitis. Surgery 97:467

Braasch JW, Ganglian J, Rossi RL (1984) Pancreatoduodenectomy with preservation of the pylorus. World J Surg 8:900–905

Bradbeer JW, Johnson CD (1990) Pancreaticogastrostomy after pancreaticoduodenectomy. Ann R Coll Surg Engl 72:266–269

Brunschwig A (1937) Resection of the head of pancreas and duodenum for carcinoma – pancreatoduodenectomy. Surg Gynecol Obstet 65:681–684

Cooper MJ, Williamson RCN (1985) Conservative pancreatectomy. Br J Surg 72:801–803

Cooper MJ, Williamson RCN, Benjamin IS et al. (1987) Total pancreatectomy for chronic pancreatitis. Br J Surg 74:912–915

Crist DW, Sitzmann JV, Cameron JL (1987) Improved hospital morbidity, mortality and survival after the Whipple procedure. Ann Surg 206:358–373

Edis AJ, Kiernan PD, Taylor WF (1980) Attempted resection of ductal carcinoma of the pancreas. Review of Mayo Clinic experience, 1951–1975. Mayo Clin Proc 55:531–536

Frey CF, Smith GJ (1987) Description and rationale of a new operation for chronic pancreatitis. Pancreas 2:701–708

Gall FP (1987) Chronische pancreatitis; Chirurgische therapie durch resektions verfahren. Langenbecks Arch Chir 372:363–368

Ihse I, Larsson J (1980) Periampullary lesions. In: Preece PE, Cuschieri A, Rosin RD (eds) Cancer of the bile ducts and pancreas. Saunders, London, pp 83–91

Jordan GL Jr (1989) Pancreatic resection for pancreatic cancer. Surg Clin North Am 69:581

Kingsnorth AN (1989) Duct to mucosa isolated Roux loop pancreaticojejunostomy as an improved anastomosis after resection of the pancreas. Surg Gynecol Obstet 169:451–453

Lambert MA, Linehan IP, Russel RCG (1987) Duodenum preserving total pancreatectomy for end stage chronic pancreatitis. Br J Surg 74:35–39

Lygidakis NJ, Van der Hyde MN, Houthoff HJ et al. (1989) Resectional surgical procedures for carcinoma of the head of the pancreas. Surg Gynecol Obstet 168:157–165

Mackie CR, Noble HG, Cooper MJ et al. (1979) Preoperative evaluation of angiography in the diagnosis and management of patients suspected of having pancreatic cancer. Ann Surg 189:11–17

Matsuno S, Sato T (1986) Surgical treatment for carcinoma of the pancreas. Am J Surg 152:499–504

Pellingrini CA, Heck CF, Raper S et al. (1989) An analysis of the reduced morbidity and mortality rates after pancreaticoduodenectomy. Arch Surg 124:778–781

Prinz RA, Greenlee HB (1981) Pancreatic duct drainage in 100 patients with chronic pancreatitis. Ann Sur 194:313–320

Smith RC (1989) Major pancreatic resection. Aust NZ J Surg 59:783–789

Traverso LW, Longmire WP Jr (1978) Preservation of the pylorus in pancreaticoduodenectomy. Surg Gynecol Obstet 146:959–962

Trede M, Schwall G, Saeger HD (1990) Survival after pancreatoduodenectomy. 118 consecutive resections without operative mortality. Ann Surg 211:447–458

Warren AW, Cattel RB, Blackburn JP, Nora PF (1962) A long-term appraisal of pancreaticoduodenal resection for periampullary carcinoma. Ann Surg 155:653–662

Warshaw AL, Popp JW, Schapiro RH (1980) Long-term patency, pancreatic function, and pain relief after lateral pancreaticojejunostomy for chronic pancreatitis. Gastroenterology 79:289–293

Watson K (1944) Carcinoma of the ampulla of Vater. Successful radical resection. Br J Surg 31:368–372

Whipple AO, Parsons WB, Mullins CR (1935) Treatment of carcinoma of the ampulla of Vater. Ann Surg 102:763–779

Williamson RCN, Cooper MJ (1987) Pancreatic resections. Br J Surg 74:807–812

Section D

Normal and Abnormal Exocrine Pancreatic Secretion

Chapter 13

Cellular Secretory Mechanisms

R. Laugier

Electrophysiology of the Cell Membrane

Electrophysiology gives us direct information concerning the transport of electrolytes across the cellular membrane. These ion transports can be studied using two types of electrophysiological techniques: whole cell studies and the patch clamp technique.

The whole cell technique is based on measurement of the membrane potential and resistance through the tip of a microelectrode inside the living cell; it gives general information on the electrical currents which are generated in both directions by ions travelling across the membrane, but only the final electrical result can be recorded. The precise origin of each individual current is very difficult to determine. The patch clamp technique which has been developed more recently consists of electrical clamp recordings of individual patches of cellular membrane; each current generated by each type of ion can be detected and analysed. This technique provides us with more direct evidence of the electrical phenomena. These electrical changes induced by secretagogues also vary according to the species studied.

In mouse and rat, stimulants of protein secretion such as acetylcholine (ACh), cholecystokinin–pancreozymin (CCK), pentagastrin (PG) or bombesin induce a sustained depolarisation (decrease of the cell electronegativity with respect to the external medium) associated with a reduction of the membrane resistance (Petersen and Findlay 1987). The patch clamp technique has allowed the correlation of these electrical changes with the activation of one single type of ion channel. These channels are calcium (Ca^{2+})-activated, voltage-insensitive and permeable to monovalent cations only (Maruyama and Petersen 1982a,b; Petersen and Findlay 1987). They are equally permeable to sodium and potassium and their opening is not influenced by changes of membrane potential. In the basal state, this type of ion channel is closed, due to the low resting intracellular free calcium concentration $[Ca^{2+}]_i$. Elevation of $[Ca^{2+}]_i$ is caused by, and occurs during, a short or sustained stimulation with secretagogues. This is followed by ion channel opening (Laugier and Petersen 1980a; Maruyama and Petersen 1982a; Ochs et al. 1985). Moreover, these ion channels can be activated by CCK or ACh applied to the cell membrane, outside the electrically isolated patch of membrane from which electrical recordings are made. This demonstrates that these stimulants activate ion channels by means of an internal messenger and not directly on the external surface of the cell membrane (Maruyama and Petersen 1982b).

Thus, when intracellular free calcium concentration rises, ion channels open up, allowing sodium and chloride influx as well as potassium efflux, all events which seem to be associated with protein exocytosis (Petersen and Findlay 1987).

In the pig, CCK and ACh evoke a membrane hyperpolarisation associated with a reduction of membrane resistance (Pearson et al. 1984). In that species, the dominant ion channel is a Ca^{2+}-activated and voltage-sensitive channel, selectively permeable to potassium and virtually impermeable to sodium (Maruyama and Petersen 1984). In contrast to the mouse pancreatic cell, this channel is not completely closed in the basal state, but the probability that it will be in the open state nevertheless remains low; it is markedly activated by CCK, which augments intracellular free calcium concentration (Susuki et al. 1985). Thus, this potassium-selective channel allows, as it opens up, a massive potassium efflux which explains the decrease in membrane resistance and cell hyperpolarisation. In this species, non-selective cation channels have not been found.

In the guinea-pig, agonists which release intracellular calcium evoke a biphasic change in membrane potential which consists of an initial depolarisation, followed by a prolonged hyperpolarisation with membrane potential reduction (Davison and Pearson 1981). In fact, the initial depolarisation (as in mouse or rat pancreas) is related to a non-selective cation channel activated by calcium whereas hyperpolarisation is related to activation of potassium-selective channels by Ca^{2+} (Susuki and Petersen 1988). Two types of potassium-selective channels are present on the guinea-pig pancreatic cell membrane: one which has a high conductance (160 pS) and another predominant channel of low conductance (30 pS) (Susuki and Petersen 1988). In that species also, filling the cell interior with a solution containing ethylene glycol-bis-(β-aminoethyl ether) tetra-acetic acid (EGTA) abolishes the electrical response of the cell membrane to pentagastrin; this is a strong argument which favours the role of Ca^{2+} as a second messenger in this species (Susuki and Petersen 1988) as it is in the mouse pancreatic acinar cell (Laugier and Petersen 1980b).

Only one patch-clamp study has been performed on human pancreatic acinar cell membrane (Petersen et al. 1985). It confirms that ACh evokes a large potassium efflux which is followed by a reuptake of potassium into the pancreatic cell. Two types of potassium channels have been found: a high conductance channel (250 pS) which is activated by Ca^{2+} and a second channel with a lower conductance (50 pS): this latter seems to be much less important in human pancreatic cells than in guinea-pig pancreatic cells where it is predominant. Potassium channels are Ca^{2+} sensitive. When $[Ca^{2+}]_i$ rises in the cell, potassium is allowed to move out of the cell; thereafter it is taken up again by an ADP-driven sodium–potassium pump and a sodium–potassium two chloride cotransporter (Petersen 1970; Petersen and Maruyama 1984).

Finally, ACh, CCK or bombesin evoke electrical alterations only when they are applied on the external surface of the basolateral membrane (Petersen et al. 1981). There is an unavoidable delay of 300 ms between application of agonist to the receptor and the electrical changes; this delay could be explained by the fact that the activation of the receptor does not itself directly induce the electrical changes. These changes occur on any patch of membrane, even if it has no direct contact with the agonist, underlining the need for a second messenger. Considering the regulation of the ion channels, and taking into account their calcium sensitivity, it appears that calcium is most likely to be this second messenger.

Of course, this does not demonstrate that $[Ca^{2+}]_i$ is the only second messenger to be released by secretagogue agonist receptor activation. After receptor activation, calcium initially originates directly inside the cell, but enters from outside the cell when stimulation is sustained (Laugier and Petersen 1980a).

Stimulus–Secretion Coupling

Until recently, agonists capable of in vitro stimulation of pancreatic secretion were separated into two groups: those, such as secretin, VIP and helodermin, which act through cyclic adenosine monophosphate (cAMP) and those which release intracellular calcium such as ACh, CCK, pentagastrin, bombesin and tachykinins. However, recent data have emerged that change our understanding of stimulus–secretion coupling, in such a way that this division might be irrelevant in the future (Bruzzone 1990).

Material of Receptors

Stimulus–secretion coupling includes the initial interaction between a hormone and its specific target on the outside surface of the cell membrane, that is, the receptor.

The molecular structure of receptors is still mostly unknown with the exception of muscarinic receptors (Bonner et al. 1988). Five subtypes of muscarinic receptors have been described (m1–m5); they have a common topological orientation within the plasma membrane. The precise physiological role of these various subtypes has yet to be elucidated (Bonner et al. 1988).

Receptors Mobilising Cyclic AMP

In most species, such as guinea-pig, two types of receptor can modulate the release of cAMP: high-affinity VIP-preferring receptors and low-affinity secretin-preferring receptors (Robberecht et al. 1976; Rosselin 1986).

For several peptides (VIP, helodermin, peptide histidine isoleucine, secretin) it has been demonstrated that their ability to stimulate amylase release is closely correlated with their ability to occupy the high-affinity VIP-preferring receptors (Zhou et al. 1989). In contrast, those peptides that bind to secretin-preferring receptors increase cAMP without any major stimulation of enzyme secretion (Gardner and Jensen 1987).

Both these receptors consist of five subunits (Gilman 1984). One is located on the external aspect of the plasma membrane and is responsible for specificity of reaction with the agonist (Rs). A second subunit bears a specificity for an antagonist messenger (Ri). These two subunits are each coupled with a corresponding subunit (Gs and Gi), which are represented by G-proteins (guanitidyl-phosphate proteins) (Ross 1989). Finally, the fifth subunit, which bears the catalytic activity responsible for cAMP formation, collects stimulation and inhibitory information together from the two G-proteins. The catalytic subunit, which is located on the inside of the plasma membrane can be activated directly by forskoline whereas Gs and Gi are directly activated by cholera toxin and *Bordetella pertussis* toxin, respectively (Gilman 1984). G-proteins may also control vesicular transport between intracellular compartments and may be involved in the exocytic process of secretion (Gomperts 1990; Rothman and Orci 1990).

Receptors Mobilising Intracellular Calcium (Ca^{2+})

Carbachol, ACh, CCK, CCK derivatives (and probably tachykinin) all induce changes in membrane ion permeability and reduction of membrane resistance together with a marked secretion of proteins. These changes are associated with an increase of free calcium concentration, as demonstrated by electrophysiology (Petersen et al. 1981). This is why those agonists were thought to act exclusively through an increase of intracellular calcium. In fact, activation of these receptors induces a second series of consequences which lead to alterations of membrane phospholipid metabolism.

Alterations of Calcium Concentration

Changes in calcium concentration are well understood because with the ion-selective microprobe it is possible to measure directly calcium concentration within the cell: in the resting state, intracellular calcium concentration $[Ca^{2+}]_i$ averages 100 mm (Muallem 1989). Maximal stimulation with an agonist induces a very fast and large peak of $[Ca^{2+}]_i$, which is followed by oscillations at a lower value, the frequency of which seems, at least, as important as their amplitude (Bruzzone 1990). Ochs et al. (1985) have suggested that only oscillations above 280 mm would be able to promote secretion. At the beginning of the stimulation, calcium originates from an intracellular pool located either in the endoplasmic reticulum, or in a distinct organelle (Stolze and Schulz 1980). These authors called this pool the "trigger-calcium-pool". Membrane permeability to calcium is very low in the basal state (thus accounting for the very slow exchange with extracellular calcium). Permeability is enhanced by receptor agonist activation (Muallem et al. 1988a). The membrane of the trigger calcium pool becomes more permeable to calcium which can move both into the cytosol and also outside the cell (Imamura and Schulz 1985; Pandol et al. 1987). This explains the initial rise of $[Ca^{2+}]_i$. Later on, during sustained stimulation, intracytoplasmic calcium returns almost to resting levels, albeit with oscillations (Bruzzone et al. 1986). During that period of sustained stimulation, the agonist-sensitive calcium pool partially reloads with extracellular calcium; this reloading is dependent on external calcium (Laugier and Petersen 1980b; Muallem et al. 1988a; Tsunoda et al. 1990). Reloading of the pool takes place by a rapid decrease of calcium permeability of the membrane pool at the end of agonist stimulation, which leads to trapping of calcium in the pool itself (Muallem et al. 1988b).

Besides calcium movements, agonist receptor activation induces hydrolysis of phosphatidylinositol 4,5-biphosphate (PI2) to form inositol 1,4,5-triphosphate (IP3) and diacylglycerol (DG) (Williams and Hootman 1986). Moreover, it has been shown that breakdown of PI2 by a phosphodiesterase (phospholipase C) into IP3 is responsible for the release of calcium from the intracellular pool (Berridge and Irvine 1984; Merritt et al. 1986) whereas DG activates the protein kinase C system (Kikkawa and Nishizuka 1986). It is now accepted that IP3 is the calcium mobilising messenger, as first proposed by Berridge and Irvine (1984).

IP3 is responsible for the release of calcium from the non-mitochondrial pool (Berridge and Irvine 1989), the increase of IP3 being a prerequisite to change of $[Ca^{2+}]_i$ and not the consequence (Pandol et al. 1985). Guanitidinyl triphosphate is also involved in the transfer of calcium from an IP3-insensitive pool to an IP3-sensitive store (Ghosh et al. 1989).

In summary, it can be argued (Rasmussen 1986) that all second-messengers act in a sequential manner: IP3, released from IP2 induces an early increase in $[Ca^{2+}]_i$ which is responsible for the initial secretory response. Sustained secretion follows the increase of protein kinase C, which is released by DG (Rasmussen et al. 1987).

It has also been reported that caerulein may stimulate amylase secretion independently of changes in $[Ca^{2+}]_i$ (Bruzzone et al. 1988). In that respect the system represented by protein kinase C may be the mechanism underlying calcium-independent secretion, and calcium would no longer act as a true second messenger (Bruzzone 1990). It should nevertheless be noted that protein kinase C-induced secretion is greatly enhanced by the presence (rather than by the increase) of $[Ca^{2+}]_i$ which suggests that calcium may act as a cofactor of protein kinase C (Bruzzone 1990).

Relationships between alterations of $[Ca^{2+}]_i$ and the rise in IP3 appear, in fact, to be even more complex: secretin has been shown to enhance both cyclic AMP and IP3 production (Trimble et al. 1987). It is not absolutely proven that release of internal calcium can only occur as a consequence of a rise in IP3. Saluja et al. (1989) have shown that a new CCK analogue is able to increase $[Ca^{2+}]_i$ with no detectable increase in IP3. It is not clear whether this represents a lack of detection or a true effect. DG formed from phosphatidyl 4,5-biphosphate also has a role in stimulus–secretion coupling: it increases the affinity of protein kinase C for calcium (Kikkawa and Nishizuka 1986) and is responsible for the sustained amylase discharge which is induced by 12-O-tetradecanolyphorbol, 13-acetate (TPA) independently of changes in calcium (Pandol et al. 1989).

Finally, some links exist between the membrane phospholipid pathway and the G-proteins released by cAMP receptors: phospholipase C, activated by DG, is also modulated by guanine nucleotides (Gp) (Cockcroft 1987).

Export of Secretory Proteins

In fact, our understanding of intracellular secretory protein transport and exocytosis has not advanced greatly in recent years. It seems nevertheless clear that protein kinase C is involved, not only in regulation of receptor affinity ion channel conductance, but also in the process of exocytosis (Kikkawa et al. 1989). Molecular cloning of protein kinase C has allowed the identification of several isoenzymes, the physiological properties of which are still mainly unknown (Kikkawa et al. 1989).

Ion conductance of zymogen granule membranes may be of crucial importance: agonists, probably through protein kinase changes, have been proven to be responsible for an increase in chloride conductance associated with an increased potassium permeability. It is thus highly probable that swelling of zymogen granules, which occurs after membrane fusion at the apical pole of the cell, is due to a large ion influx into the granules (Gasser et al. 1988). This phenomenon also implies that influx of ions and consequently of fluid across the membrane would facilitate the flushing out of enzymes into the acinar lumen and would also provide the amounts of fluid known to be associated with protein secretion.

References

Berridge M, Irvine R (1984) Inositol trisphosphate, a novel second messenger in cellular signal transduction. Nature 312:315–321

Berridge M, Irvine R (1989) Inositol phosphates and cell signalling. Nature 341:197–205

Bonner T, Young A, Brann M, Buckley N (1988) Cloning and expression of the human and rat m5 muscarinic acetylcholine genes. Neuron 1:403–410

Bruzzone R (1990) The molecular basis of enzyme secretion. Gastroenterology 99:1157–1176

Bruzzone R, Pozzan T, Wollheim C (1986) Caerulein and carboamylcholine stimulate pancreatic amylase release at resting cytosolic free Ca^{2+}. Biochem J 235:139–143

Bruzzone R, Regazzi R, Wollheim C (1988) Caerulein causes translocation of protein kinase C in rat acini without increasing cytosolic free Ca^{2+}. Am J Physiol G33–G39

Cockcroft S (1987) Polyphosphoinositide phosphodiesterase: regulation by a novel guanine nucleotide binding protein Gp. Trends Biochem Sci 12:75–78

Davison J, Pearson G (1981) Electrophysiological studies on guinea-pig pancreatic acinar cells. J Physiol (Lond) 310:44P

Gardner J, Jensen R (1987) Secretagogue receptors on pancreatic acinar cells. In: Johnson LR (ed) Physiology of the gastrointestinal tract, 2nd edn. Raven Press, New York, pp 1109–1189

Gasser K, di Domenico J, Hopfer U (1988) Secretagogues activate chloride transport pathways in pancreatic zymogen granules. Am J Physiol 254:G93–G99

Ghosh T, Mullaney J, Tarazi F, Gill D (1989) GTP-activated communication between distinct inositol 1,4,5-trisphosphate-sensitive and -insensitive calcium pools. Nature 340:236–239

Gilman A (1984) Guanine nucleotide-binding regulatory proteins and dual control of adenylate cyclase. J Clin Invest 73:1–4

Gomperts B (1990) GE: a GTP-binding protein mediating exocytosis. Annu Rev Physiol 52:591–606

Imamura K, Schulz I (1985) Phosphorylated intermediate of $(Ca^{2+}-K^+)$-stimulated Mg^{2+} dependent transport ATPase in endoplasmic reticulum from rat pancreatic acinar cells. J Biol Chem 260:11339–11347

Kikkawa U, Nishizuka Y (1986) The role of protein kinase C in transmembrane signalling. Annu Rev Cell Biol 2:149–178

Kikkawa U, Kishimoto A, Nishizuka Y (1989) The protein kinase C family: heterogeneity and its implications. Annu Rev Biochem 58:31–44

Laugier R, Petersen OH (1980a) Pancreatic acinar cells: electrophysiological evidence for stimulant-evoked increase in membrane calcium permeability in the mouse. J Physiol (Lond) 303:61–72

Laugier R, Petersen OH (1980b) Effects of intracellular EGTA injection on stimulant-evoked membrane potential and resistance changes in pancreatic acinar cells. Pflügers Arch 286:147–152

Maruyama Y, Petersen OH (1982a) Single-channel currents in isolated patches of plasma membrane from basal surface of pancreatic acini. Nature 299:159–161

Maruyama Y, Petersen OH (1982b) Cholecystokinin activation of single-channel currents is mediated by internal messenger in pancreatic acinar cells. Nature 300:61–63

Maruyama Y, Petersen OH (1984) Control of K^+ conductance by cholecystokinin and Ca^{2+} in single pancreatic acinar cells studied by the patch-clamp technique. J Membr Biol 79:293–300

Merritt J, Taylor C, Rubin R, Putney J (1986) Evidence suggesting that a novel guanine nucleotide regulatory protein couples receptors to phospholipases C in exocrine pancreas. Biochem J 236:337–343

Muallem S (1989) Calcium transport pathways of pancreatic acinar cells. Annu Rev Physiol 51:83–105

Muallem S, Schoeffield M, Fimmel C, Pandol S (1988a) Agonist-sensitive calcium pool in the pancreatic acinar cell. I. Permeability properties. Am J Physiol 255:G221–G228

Muallem S, Schoeffield M, Fimmel C, Pandol S (1988b) Agonist-sensitive calcium pool in the pancreatic acinar cell. II. Characterization of reloading. Am J Physiol 255:G229–G235

Ochs D, Korenbrot J, Williams J (1985) Relationship between agonist-induced changes in the concentration of free-intracellular calcium and the secretion of amylase by pancreatic acini. Am J Physiol 249:G389–G398

Pandol S, Thomas M, Schoeffield M, Sachs G, Muallem S (1985) Role of calcium in cholecystokinin-stimulated phosphoinositide breakdown in exocrine pancreas. Am J Physiol 248:G551–G560

Pandol S, Schoeffield M, Fimmel C, Muallem S (1987) The agonist-sensitive pool in the pancreatic acinar cell. Activation of plasma membrane Ca^{2+} influx mechanism. J Biol Chem 262:16963–16968

Pandol S, Rodriguez G, Muallem S, Mendius K (1989) Characteristics of intracellular calcium changes required for augmentation of phorbol ester-stimulated pancreatic enzyme secretion. Cell Calcium 10:255–262

Pearson G, Flanagan P, Petersen OH (1984) Neural and hormonal control of membrane conductance in the pig pancreatic acinar cell. Am J Physiol 247:G520–G526

Petersen OH (1970) Some factors influencing stimulation-induced release of potassium from the cat submandibular gland to fluid perfused through the gland. J Physiol (Lond) 208:431–437

Petersen OH, Findlay I (1987) Electrophysiology of the pancreas. Physiol Rev 67:1054–1116

Petersen OH, Maruyama Y (1984) Calcium-activated potassium channels and their role in secretion. Nature 307:693–696

Petersen OH, Iwatsuki N, Philpott H et al. (1981) Membrane potential and conductance changes evoked by hormones and neurotransmitters in mammalian exocrine gland cells. Methods Cell Biol 31:513–530

Petersen OH, Findlay I, Iwatsuki N et al. (1985) Human pancreatic acinar cells: studies of stimulus–secretion coupling. Gastroenterology 89:109–117

Rasmussen H (1986) The calcium messenger system. N Engl J Med 314:1164–1170

Rasmussen H, Takuwa Y, Park S (1987) Protein kinase C in the regulation of smooth muscle contractions. FASEB J 1:177–185

Robberecht P, Conlon T, Gardner J (1976) Interaction of porcine vasoactive intestinal peptide with dispersed acinar cells from the guinea-pig: structural requirements for effects of VIP and secretin on cellular cyclic AMP. J Biol Chem 251:4635–4639

Ross E (1989) Signal sorting and amplification through Ca-protein-coupled receptors. Neuron 3:141–152

Rosselin G (1986) The receptors of the VIP family peptides (VIP, Secretin, GRF, PHI, PHM, GIP, glucagon and oxyntomodulin) specificities and identy. Peptides 7 suppl 1:89–100

Rothman J, Orci L (1990) Movement of proteins through the Golgi stack: a molecular dissection of vesicular transport. FASEB J 4:1460–1468

Saluja A, Powers R, Steer M (1989) Inositol trisphosphate independent increase of intracellular free calcium and amylase secretion in pancreatic acini. Biochem Biophys Res Commun 164:8–13

Stolze H, Schulz I (1980) Effect of atropine, ouabain, antimycin A and A-23187 on "trigger Ca^{2+} pool" in exocrine pancreas. Am J Physiol 238:G338–G348

Susuki K, Petersen OH (1988) Patch-clamp study of single-channel and whole-cell K$^+$ currents in guinea-pig pancreatic acinar cells. Am J Physiol 255:G275–285

Susuki K, Petersen C, Petersen OH (1985) Hormonal activation of single K$^+$ channels via internal messenger in isolated pancreatic acinar cells. FEBS Lett 192:307–312

Trimble E, Bruzzone R, Biden T, Meehan C, Andreu R (1987) Secretin stimulates cyclic AMP and inositol trisphosphate production in rat pancreatic acinar tissue by two fully independent mechanisms. Proc Natl Acad Sci USA 84:3146–3150

Tsunoda Y, Stuenkel E, Williams J (1990) Characterization of sustained (Ca^{2+}) increase in pancreatic acinar cells and its relation to amylase secretion. Am J Physiol 259:G792–G801

Williams J, Hootman S (1986) Stimulus-secretion coupling in pancreatic acinar cells. In: Go L, Gardner J, Brooks F, Lebenthal E, Dimagno E, Scheele G (eds) The exocrine pancreas, Raven Press, New York, pp 123–139

Zhou Z, Gardner J, Jensen R (1989) Interaction of peptides related to VIP and secretin with guinea-pig pancreatic acini. Am J Physiol 256:G283–G290

Chapter 14

Alcohol and Exocrine Pancreatic Secretion

C. D. Johnson

Chronic ingestion of alcohol (ethanol) is clearly implicated in the pathogenesis of chronic pancreatitis. The effects of ethanol on pancreatic secretion are complex and vary with the circumstances. These effects have been investigated most fully in man and in the dog, with studies covering three different circumstances: first, bolus administration of ethanol in normal subjects; second, the modifications of the response to physiological stimuli after chronic administration; and third, the alterations to the response to a bolus following chronic administration.

Acute Administration

Intravenous injection of ethanol during stimulation with secretin, or secretin and CCK inhibits pancreatic secretion (Mott et al. 1972). This inhibition may be related to release of pancreatic polypeptide (Staub et al. 1981) although the duration of inhibition appeared to last longer than the increased release of pancreatic polypeptide.

In the dog the response to a meal can be inhibited by intragastric ethanol (Tiscornia et al. 1977). The inhibitory effect of alcohol is abolished by prior inhibition with atropine or pentolinium (Tiscornia et al. 1973, 1975). These agents produce a profound inhibition of pancreatic secretion, so it is perhaps not surprising that secretion cannot be depressed further. It is difficult to study the effect of atropine or pentolinium after the administration of alcohol, because the effect of alcohol appears to be related to rising blood levels (Noel-Jorand and Sarles 1983). After administration of ethanol in such a way as to achieve steady blood levels, pancreatic secretion is no different from control responses.

The inhibitory effects of intravenous ethanol are centrally mediated, as they are abolished by vagotomy (Tiscornia et al. 1973). There appears to be a complex interaction with other central nervous system processes. The observation of an inhibitory effect was made in dogs allowed access to the open air. When our kennel was converted to be fully enclosed, and lit by artificial light, the inhibitory effect of ethanol was lost. Instead there was stimulation at all doses. This stimulation was lost when the dogs were kept in the open air for four weeks (Sarles et al. 1984).

Subsequently it was possible to demonstrate both inhibition and stimulation in the same animals, according to the dose of ethanol used. Stimulation occurred maximally at low doses of ethanol and inhibition was greatest at high doses (Fig. 1, Noel-Jorand and Sarles 1983). Both these effects were abolished by atropine and pentolinium. These complexities of the response, which are dependent on the conditions of housing and the dose of alcohol used, emphasise the difficulties of determining what is the pathological effect in man.

Pancreatic Responses After Chronic Ingestion of Ethanol

Chronic alcoholic men produce greater amounts of enzymes or protein in pure pancreatic juice after hormonal stimulation, when compared to non-alcoholic controls (Renner et al. 1978; Rinderknecht et al. 1979). Basal protein concentration is higher in alcoholic men than in non-drinking controls (Planche et al. 1982).

Similar effects are seen in the dog after two years of alcohol feeding. The

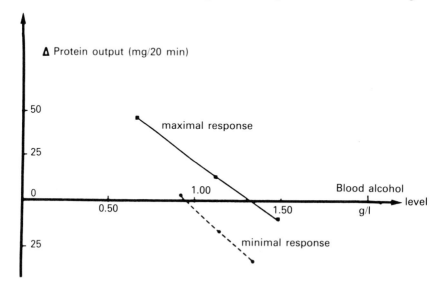

Fig. 1. Response to various doses of ethanol i.v. plotted against corresponding blood ethanol concentration. The upper line represents the greatest 20 min protein output, the lower line the lowest 20 min output, expressed as changes from the stable level of response to a continuous infusion of secretin. (From Noel-Jorand and Sarles 1983, with permission.)

response to hormonal stimulation is increased in these animals (Tiscornia et al. 1974). In dogs, as in man, chronic ingestion of alcohol leads to increased protein concentration in the basal secretion (Noel-Jorand et al. 1981; Roblez-Diaz et al. 1985).

Response to Ethanol After Long-term Consumption

The inhibitory effect of intravenous ethanol is abolished in chronic alcoholic men (Planche et al. 1982). In the chronic alcoholic dog, acute administration of alcohol stimulates pancreatic secretion by an atropine-sensitive mechanism (Sarles et al. 1977) when given during hormonal stimulation.

Although acute administration of ethanol reduces pancreatic secretion after a meat meal in non-alcoholic dogs, chronic administration of ethanol reverses this effect, with potentiation of both fluid and protein output (Roblez-Diaz et al. 1985). One possible explanation for the increased responses to a meal with alcohol in chronic alcoholic dogs could be the disappearance of an inhibitory reflex in these animals; the inhibition produced by acute alcohol administration is also lost after chronic ingestion.

Vagal Efferent Activity

Basal pancreatic secretion is cholinergically mediated, so the reduced fluid output and relatively lesser reduction in protein output in basal secretion could well reflect changes in vagal activity. Basal pancreatic secretion is cyclical and appears to be integrated with migrating motor complexes in the gut (Magee and Naruse 1983; Chen et al. 1983; Mossner et al. 1989). Intravenous administration of ethanol inhibits the appearance of the migrating motor complex (Angel et al. 1980).

Centrally mediated vagal stimulation with 2-deoxyglucose (2DG) leads to an increase of pancreatic protein and fluid output. The appearance of the fluid response was delayed after chronic ethanol administration (Fig. 2) (Schmidt et al. 1984). This suggests that some at least of the vagal efferent effects to the pancreas have been modified by long-term ethanol administration. It is possible that the lesion responsible for these changes in vagal response could be similar to the peripheral neuropathy which is commonly seen in alcoholic patients. Duncan et al. (1980) demonstrated impaired vagal cardiorespiratory reflexes in chronic alcoholics. Alcoholic neuropathy may also affect the splanchnic nerves and celiac ganglia. Degeneration of the sympathetic trunk was reported in an alcoholic patient many years ago (Novak and Victor 1974). We found a reduction of the early part of the fluid response to 2DG after celiac ganglionectomy (Johnson et al. 1989) which was very like the loss of fluid secretion seen in chronic alcoholic dogs (Fig. 3). Vagal fibres traverse the celiac ganglia so the precise pathway of this effect cannot be defined.

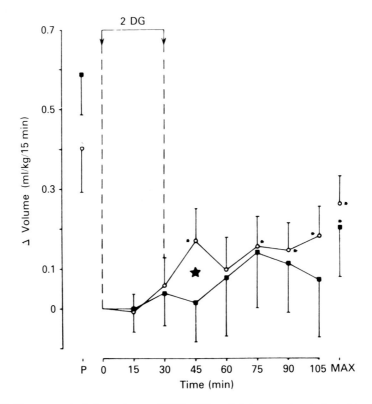

Fig. 2. Fluid response to 2-deoxyglucose (2DG) (100 mg/kg) in normal and alcohol-treated dogs. (From Schmidt et al. 1984, with permission.)

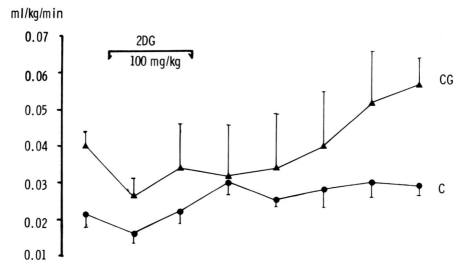

Fig. 3. Fluid response to 2-deoxyglucose (2DG) (100 mg/kg) in normal dogs (C) and after celiac ganglionectomy (CG).

Inhibitory Reflexes

The effects of alcohol on the pancreas are summarised in Table 1. Basal secretion is reduced by chronic alcohol consumption, although fluid is affected more than protein output so the net effect is increased concentration of protein. The reduction in response to vagal stimulation is consistent with this. The general pattern of the effect on exogenous hormone responses and response to a meal is of increased sensitivity, or loss of an inhibitory effect.

Schmidt et al. (1982a,b) examined these changes in greater detail. Hormone-stimulated fluid output was increased in dogs treated with alcohol but the slope of the dose–response curve to secretin was not changed. Low-dose atropine had no effect on the increased fluid output.

Caerulein-stimulated secretion was more complex. Fluid output after caerulein was increased in normal dogs given atropine. A similar increase in fluid response to caerulein was seen after nine months' alcohol feeding. This increased fluid output was not altered by atropine. In contrast the enhancement of protein output by atropine was reduced by chronic ethanol administration. Schmidt et al. (1982a,b) postulate a neural inhibitory effect which is diminished by long-term ethanol feeding. Pancreatic polypeptide is one candidate for the mediation of this effect, particularly as release of this peptide is reduced in chronic alcoholic men (Staub et al. 1981).

Intrapancreatic Changes

There is evidence for a change in the balance of neural input to the pancreas from changes in the pancreas itself. Histochemical studies of the pancreas after prolonged administration of alcohol have shown evidence for increased cholinergic activity. In the dog acetylcholinesterase content was reduced after prolonged alcohol treatment, and in both the dog and the rat increased amounts of cholineacetyltransferase have been found (Celener et al. 1977; Perec et al. 1979).

The functional effects of ethanol directly on the pancreas have been studied in mouse acinar cells (Berger et al. 1985). Ethanol depolarised the acinar cells

Table 1. Summary of effect of alcohol on pancreatic responses. Chronic exposure refers to chronic alcoholic men, or dogs given 2g/kg/day. Effects of ethanol on other stimuli were tested at various doses given as a bolus

| | Effect of ethanol on response to stimulus | | Response to stimulus after chronic ethanol exposure |
	Normal	After chronic exposure	
Exogenous hormones	↓ (↑)	↑	↑
Meal	↓	↑	↓
Vagal stimulation			↓
Basal secretion			↓

directly but this effect was masked by a higher dose of ethanol acting through nicotinic ganglia. This inhibitory effect was resistant to cholinergic and adrenergic blockage but was able to block the response to locally applied acetylcholine.

Summary

The effects of ethanol on pancreatic responses are summarised in Table 1, but this is an over-simplification. In normal animals and in man acute ingestion or administration of alcohol produces counteracting effects, with inhibition predominating at high doses but with stimulation of pancreatic secretion becoming obvious at lower doses in certain conditions. In man, the inhibitory effects are predominant. After chronic ingestion of alcohol, a bolus will stimulate pancreatic secretion although basal secretion is reduced. Inhibitory reflexes are lost during adaptation to alcohol and this correlates with increased cholinergic activity in the pancreas. It is possible that the loss of inhibition in the pancreas seen after chronic administration of alcohol could be related to an autonomic neuropathy. The increased protein concentration, particularly that seen in basal secretion, predisposes to the formation of protein precipitates which are the initiating event in chronic pancreatitis.

References

Angel F, Sava P, Cremer F, Lambert A, Grenier JF (1980) Modifications de la motricite intestinale apres injection intraveineuse d'alcool. CR Soc Biol (Paris) 174:192–198
Berger Z, Laugier R, Sarles H (1985) Effect of alcohol on mouse pancreatic acinar cells: an electrophysiological study. Digestion 32:165–166
Celener D, Lechene de la Porte P, Tiscornia O, Sarles H (1977) Histochemical studies of cholinergic activities in exocrine pancreas of dogs. Modification related to chronic alcoholism. Biomedicine 27:161–165
Chen MH, Joffe SN, Magee DF, Murphy RF, Naruse S (1983) Cyclic changes of plasma pancreatic polypeptide and pancreatic secretion in fasting dogs. J Physiol (Lond) 341:453–461
Duncan G, Johnson RH, Lambie DG, Whiteside EA (1980) Evidence of vagal neuropathy in chronic alcoholics. Lancet ii:1053–1057
Johnson CD, Devaux MA, Sarles H (1989) Pancreatic exocrine responses to secretin, 2-deoxyglucose, a meal and ethanol after coeliac ganglionectomy in the conscious dog. Gut 30:1765–1770
Magee DF, Naruse S (1983) Neural control of periodic secretion of the pancreas and stomach in fasting dogs. J Physiol (Lond) 344:153–160
Mossner J, Wresky HP, Kestel W, Zeek J, Regner U, Fischbach W (1989) Influence of treatment with pancreatic extracts on pancreatic enzyme secretion. Gut 30:1143–1149
Mott C, Sarles H, Tiscornia O, Gullo L (1972) Inhibitory action of alcohol on human exocrine pancreatic secretion. Am J Dig Dis 17:902–910
Noel-Jorand MC, Sarles H (1983) Simultaneous mechanisms on exocrine pancreatic secretion initiated by alcohol in the conscious dog. Dig Dis Sci 28:879–888
Noel-Jorand MC, Colomb E, Astier JP, Sarles H (1981) Pancreatic basal secretion in alcohol-fed and normal dogs. Dig Dis Sci 26:783–789

Novak DJ, Victor M (1974) The vagus and sympathetic nerves in alcoholic neuropathy. Arch Neurol 30:273–284

Perec CJ, Celener D, Tiscornia OM, Barati C (1979) Effects of chronic ethanol administration on the autonomic innervation of salivary glands, pancreas and heart. Am J Gastroenterol 72:46–50

Planche NE, Palasciano G, Meullenet J, Laugier R, Sarles H (1982) Effects of intravenous alcohol on pancreatic and biliary secretions in man. Dig Dis Sci 27:449–453

Renner IG, Rinderknecht H, Douglas AP (1978) Profiles of pure pancreatic secretions in patients with acute pancreatitis. Gastroenterology 75:1090–1098

Rinderknecht H, Renner IG, Kayoma HH (1979) Lysozomal enzymes in pure pancreatic juice from normal healthy volunteers and chronic alcoholics. Dig Dis Sci 24:108–116

Roblez-Diaz G, Devaux MA, Sarles H (1985) Effect of acute and chronic oral administration of ethanol on canine exocrine pancreatic secretion. Digestion 32:77–85

Sarles H, Tiscornia O, Palasciano G (1977) Chronic alcoholism and canine exocrine pancreas secretion. Gastroenterology 72:238–243

Sarles H, Johnson CD, Devaux MA, Noel-Jorand M-C, Roblez-Diaz G, Schmidt D (1984) Influence of environmental conditions on exocrine pancreatic response to intravenous injection of ethanol or 2-deoxyglucose in the dog. Dig Dis Sci 29:19–25

Schmidt DN, Sarles H, Devaux MA (1982a) Early increased pancreatic secretory capacity during alcohol adaptation in the dog. Scand J Gastroenterol 17:49–55

Schmidt DN, Devaux MA, Biedzinski TM, Sarles H (1982b) Disappearance of an inhibitory factor of exocrine pancreas secretion in chronic alcoholic dogs. Scand J Gastroenterol 17:761–768

Schmidt DN, Johnson CD, Devaux MA, Sarles H (1984) Pancreatic responses to 2-deoxyglucose: effect of chronic ethanol feeding. Eur J Clin Invest 14:111–115

Staub JL, Sarles H, Chayvialle JA, Descos F, Lassmann V, Vague P (1981) Relationship between intravenous ethanol, alcohol induced inhibition of pancreatic secretion and plasma concentration of immunoreactive polypeptide, vasoactive intestinal peptide and somatostatin in man. Regul Pept 2:61–68

Tiscornia OM, Hage G, Palasciano G, Brasca AP, Devaux MA, Sarles H (1973) The effects of pentolinium and vagotomy on the inhibition of canine exocrine pancreatic secretion by intravenous ethanol. Biomedicine 18:159–163

Tiscornia O, Palasciano G, Sarles H (1974) Effects of chronic ethanol administration on canine exocrine pancreatic secretion. Digestion 11: 172–182

Tiscornia OM, Palasciano G, Sarles H (1975) Atropine and exocrine pancreatic secretion in alcohol fed dogs. Am J Gastroenterol 63:33–36

Tiscornia OM, Levesque D, Sarles H et al. (1977) Canine exocrine pancreatic secretory changes induced by an intragastric ethanol test meal. Am J Gastroenterol 67:121–130

Chronic Pancreatitis

Chapter 15

Classification of Chronic Pancreatitis

M. Sarner

Classification exercises can shed light on the basic questions of diagnosis, prognosis and therapy. In this chapter the history of attempts at classification in respect of chronic pancreatitis is traced, definitions and gradings of severity are mentioned and pathological and investigatory procedures on which these classifications have been based are described. A classification of chronic pancreatitis is offered, together with examples and some unanswered questions. The adoption of an acceptable classification with agreed criteria will permit a universal language for the physician and an ability to compare data worldwide.

History

At least four attempts have been made by international groups to classify inflammatory pancreatic disease. The first was from Marseille in 1963 and was morphologically based (Sarles 1965). It made the crucial distinction between the reversibility of the acute lesions of acute pancreatitis and the non-reversible and possibly progressive lesions of chronic pancreatitis. These varieties of pancreatitis were distinguished both in terms of aetiology and age at presentation (acute pancreatitis: gall stones and older patients; chronic pancreatitis: alcoholism and younger patients) and the notion that acute pancreatitis could lead to chronic pancreatitis was laid to rest. At this meeting of pancreatologists, the basic histopathologies were clearly laid out and chronic pancreatitis was defined by its lesions. These consist of an irregular sclerosis (fibrosis), with distortion and loss of exocrine parenchyma which could be focal, segmental or diffuse and are associated with variable degrees of dilatation or constriction of segments of the ducts. The chief value of this meeting was to distinguish between the reversibility of acute pancreatitis and the irreversibility of lesions of chronic pancreatitis, but its histopathological (morphological) basis meant that it had serious inadequacies as a clinical classification. However, it altered people's ways of thinking and stood for 20 years while the technologies moved on. The next stage was an attempt at a more clinically based classification, together with some efforts at severity grading (Sarner and Cotton, 1984). This had become possible because of the advent of new imaging modalities (endoscopic retrograde cholangiopancreatography (ECRP), ultrasound, computed tomography (CT)) and increasing experience with function testing. Tests of pancreatic function have remained poor discriminators for determining severity of disease, but imaging had become remarkably valuable and the endoscopists produced a grading of severity based on ERCP findings which is still used, albeit with modifications (Axon 1989). This Cambridge classification was useful at the bedside but was imprecise since it proved difficult to define irreversibility – either functional or morphological – and good histopathological correlation with the various imaging and function modalities was not available. A detected abnormality reflects one aspect of the disease at the time of the study, but the present and future balance between repair and regeneration or fibrosis and destruction is difficult to determine. Furthermore, the concept of a scarred but normally functioning gland was difficult to include in this classification.

In the meantime, a body of knowledge in terms of pathology, aetiology, and molecular mechanisms was beginning to accummulate and a second Marseille symposium was held in 1984 (Gyr et al. 1984), at which the new data were reviewed and a more integrated classification was produced. Apart from noting that, exceptionally, acute pancreatitis could cause chronic pancreatitis (due to postinflammatory stricture of the main pancreatic duct), the most valuable contribution of this symposium was to distinguish chronic "obstructive" pancreatitis due to obstruction of the main pancreatic duct from other causes of chronic pancreatitis.

The most recent international attempt at classification was in 1988 in Rome (Sarles et al. 1989a). A group of gastroenterologists, surgeons and pathologists, hoped that a statistical analysis of morphometric, morphological and epidemiological data, based on a knowledge of molecular pathology, would provide an encompassing classification which would be clinically usable and reflect the state of the art. Here chronic pancreatitis was defined by the presence of chronic inflammatory lesions, characterised by the destruction of exocrine parenchyma and fibrosis and, in the late stages, the destruction of endocrine parenchyma. Chronic pancreatitis is frequently complicated during its early stages by attacks of acute pancreatitis which are responsible for the recurrent pain which may represent the clinical symptoms. After some years exocrine (steatorrhoea) and endocrine (diabetes) insufficiency develop and acute attacks decrease and disappear. The disease is characterised morphologically by an irregular, lobular, patchy distribution of lesions of differing intensity in neighbouring lobules. Intraductal protein precipitates or plugs are always found and, in the later stages, calcified precipitates together with atrophy and stenosis of the ducts are particularly frequent. Areas of acute pancreatitis, cysts and pseudocysts are frequently associated and the structural and functional changes usually progress even if the primary cause of the disease is eliminated. Different types of chronic pancreatitis were described, including chronic obstructive pancreatitis, chronic calcifying pancreatitis and various forms of fibrotic pancreatic disease, the latter causing some difficulty in classification. The participants pointed out that it could be difficult to distinguish between acute (reversible) or chronic (irreversible) pancreatic disease at the clinical level, particularly if the clinician has only the history and physical signs to work with. Aetiology (alcohol or gall stones) might be helpful, as may the various imaging techniques, but it may be only after long follow-up – more than 10 years – that a diagnosis of chronic pancreatitis emerges as insufficiency develops.

Since that time several reviews have appeared in respect of classification of pancreatic inflammatory disease but no new international symposium has taken place.

Definition

Chronic pancreatitis is defined by the presence of lesions of chronic inflammation with the loss of exocrine parenchyma, irreversible fibrosis and possible subsequent destruction of endocrine tissue. It may be complicated initially by attacks of acute pancreatitis but after some years signs of exocrine and endocrine insufficiency will appear and the acute attacks may relent. Different types of chronic pancreatitis may be described, for example: chronic calcifying pancreatitis (alcohol related or tropical), hereditary pancreatitis and obstructive pancreatitis.

In chronic calcifying pancreatitis, a common pathological mechanism for several aetiologies is thought to be central (Sarles et al. 1989b). The precipitation of protein within the duct and the formation of a plug in contact with ductal epithelium is associated with duct cell atrophy and loss of basement membrane. Periductal fibrosis with stricture occurs and exocrine tissue upstream from the stricture disappears. The epithelial lesion allows a transudation of protein and calcium-rich interstitial fluid which presumably allows increasing deposition of calcium. Calcium precipitation is also favoured by abnormalities of secretion, or precipitation of the pancreatic stone protein (PSP, lithostathine) (Sarles et al. 1990). Thus the protein precipitate is the basic lesion, common to the various aetiologies of chronic pancreatitis, and suggests a new definition of chronic pancreatitis – an inflammatory condition of the pancreas in which there is an intraductal precipitate of protein leading to luminal obstruction which eventually causes an irreversible destruction of exocrine parenchyma.

Diagnosis and Classification of Chronic Pancreatitis

At present the diagnosis of chronic pancreatitis rests primarily on the clinical features and imaging modalities with support from function studies. In future refinements in terms of types or distributions of lesions may be available from percutaneous needle biopsy samples and statements as to the aetiology, grading and anatomy may be possible from these and other sources. Attempts have been made to apply an hypothesis which is aetiologically inclusive, with the notion that there is one basic lesion causing chronic pancreatitis, although this lesion may be produced by various causes. This is attractive and although this hypothesis needs confirmation, it seems reasonable to postulate that the basic lesion in chronic pancreatitis is the sequence of protein plug/stone formation consequent on changes in the juice, particularly related to pancreatic stone protein (lithostathine), and that these juice changes have varying causes including alcoholism and duct hypertension. Nevertheless, it is important always to include aetiology in the classification, since, at least for alcohol induced pancreatitis, this has important implications for the prognosis of pain, preservation of function and calcification.

Various imaging modalities are helpful in the classification of chronic pancreatitis. Ultrasound is non-invasive and in experienced hands gives much information. It can define duct and parenchymal morphology and will allow percutaneous biopsy and percutaneous pancreatography with duct pressure measurements. There is good correlation with ERCP findings (Jones et al. 1988). ERCP is useful, particularly for diagnosis of duct obstruction in the region of the sphincter of Oddi (Venu et al. 1989). Pancreatography is used as the basis for classification of severity (Axon 1989).

CT is generally less useful in the diagnosis and classification of chronic pancreatitis, although it may help to exclude other conditions such as carcinoma, and may be helpful to research and planning an operation.

Pancreatic function testing is rarely helpful in diagnosis or classification. Correlation with imaging techniques is only good in the later stages of the disease (Malfertheiner and Buchler 1989). Correlation is also poor with morphologically derived classifications of severity.

With these constraints in mind, the following classification is proposed, based on the morphological and aetiological information currently available.

Chronic Calcifying Pancreatitis

This is the commonest form of chronic pancreatitis although not all patients have overt calcification. Various aetiologies of this group are described but alcohol is by far the commonest known cause, particularly in Europe, the United States and Japan. Pathologically there is an irregular distribution of lesions of varying intensity throughout the parenchyma. The crucial lesion is the intraduct protein precipitate plug which subsequently calcifies with the formation of stones (calculi). Associated with this plug there is atrophy of the duct lining cells and duct stenosis occurs, and cysts of various size or areas of acute pancreatitis may be present. It is postulated that a combination of the stimulatory effect of alcohol, which produces a viscid juice, with a reduction in citrate and bicarbonate output and a defect in secretion of the stone protein (lithostathine) lead to the production of a protein plug. This plug obstructs the flow of juice with patchy effects. Not all alcoholics develop chronic pancreatitis and it may be that a genetic susceptibility, mediated through abnormalities of production of lithostathine is the underlying factor. Epidemiological data have implicated an associated high fat and high protein diet in the development of this disease (Durbec and Sarles 1978). The changes, both morphological and functional, are said to be progressive even if the primary cause is eliminated, but this has not been convincingly demonstrated.

Tropical Pancreatitis

The lesions in this condition are very similar to those found in chronic calcifying pancreatitis and the differential diagnosis rests on the history and the geographical location of the patient. The patients are usually young, of either sex, and come from a region where the diet is very low in protein and very low in fat (Kerala in South India, Zaire and Nigeria), both for children and adults, particularly mothers. Neonatal or prenatal subnutrition may be an important factor here, but further studies, particularly in respect of secretion of the stone protein (lithostathine) are required.

Hereditary Pancreatitis

In this rare condition, it is postulated that a congenital lack of the protein stabiliser lithostathine allows the formation of calcifying plugs. This is a hypothesis that awaits confirmation. The condition affects either sex and may run in families.

Hypercalcaemic Pancreatitis

Supersaturation of pancreatic juice with calcite presumably leads to swamping of the stabilising mechanism which maintains calcium in solution. This can occur in any condition of hypercalcaemia but is most uncommon.

Obstructive Pancreatitis

This results from obstruction of the main pancreatic duct prior to the development of the lesions. There is a uniform upstream dilatation of the main pancreatic duct, and intraductal protein plugs and calcium-containing stones are not usually found. The duct epithelium is preserved. The reversibility of this intrapancreatic change is uncertain if the obstruction is overcome (is it really chronic pancreatitis?). Possible causes of this relatively rare form of chronic pancreatitis include trauma, stenosis of the ampulla, either due to a benign or malignant tumour, scars following acute pancreatitis, etc.

Pancreatic Fibrosis

Diffuse fibrosis with exocrine destruction is described (Martin and Bedossa 1989; Bedossa et al. 1989). There may be a mononuclear cell infiltrate and the lesion may be more frequent in old age. This condition may be asymptomatic (and therefore undiagnosable), but it is seen in patients with hyperlipoproteinaemia and may be ischaemic in origin. It is also seen in asymptomatic alcoholics.

Conclusions

A classification of chronic pancreatitis can now be based on aetiology, severity grading, and if possible, anatomy and histopathology, for example, marked chronic calcifying pancreatitis due to alcohol, or moderate obstructive chronic pancreatitis due to an ampullary tumour.

We are probably at the beginning of a classification which will include aetiological data on a molecular basis, but many questions remain. These include which patients will require surgery and which will become pain-free – indeed the relationships between pain, function and histopathological findings all need exploring. The dynamics of chronic pancreatitis are still to be studied – what is irreversible, why does inflammatory change persist or progress, and what are the dynamics of calcification? We still need more information concerning genetic predispositions. Agreed criteria for mild, moderate and marked disease are required and new techniques may give us insights into pancreatic function. If doctors can talk the same language we shall improve the prospects for the alleviation of this dreadful disease.

References

Axon ATR (1989) ERCP in chronic pancreatitis. Radiol Clin North Am 27:39–49

Bedossa P, Lemaigre G, Bacci J, Martin E (1989) Quantitative estimation of the collagen content in normal and pathological pancreas tissue. Digestion 44:7–13

Durbec JP, Sarles H (1978) Multicentre survey of the aetiology of pancreatic diseases. Relationship between the relative risk of developing chronic pancreatitis and alcohol, protein and lipid consumption. Digestion 18:337–350

Gyr KE, Singer MV, Sarles H (1984) Pancreatitis: concepts and classification. Excerpta Med Int Congr Ser 642, Amsterdam

Jones SN, Lees WR, Frost RA (1988) Diagnosis and grading of chronic pancreatitis by morphological criteria derived by ultrasound and pancreatography. Clin Radiol 39:43–48

Malfertheiner P, Buchler M (1989) Correlation of imaging and function in chronic pancreatitis. Radiol Clin North Am 27:51–64

Martin E, Bedossa P (1989) Diffuse fibrosis of the pancreas: a peculiar pattern of pancreatitis in alcoholic cirrhosis. Gastroenterol Clin Biol 13:579–584

Sarles H (1965) Pancreatitis symposium, Marseilles. Karger, Basel

Sarles H, Adler G, Dani R et al. (1989a) Classifications of pancreatitis and definition of pancreatic disease. Digestion. 43:234–236

Sarles H, Bernard JP, Johnson C (1989b) Pathogenesis and epidemiology of chronic pancreatitis. Ann Rev Med 40:453–468

Sarles H, Bernard JP, Gullo L (1990) Pathogenesis of chronic pancreatitis. Gut 31:629–632

Sarner M, Cotton PB (1984) Classification of pancreatitis. Gut 25:756–759

Venu RP, Geenen JE, Hogan W et al. (1989) Idiopathic recurrent pancreatitis. Dig Dis Sci 34:56–60

Chapter 16

The Geographical Distribution of Chronic Pancreatitis

H. Sarles

Introduction

There is some confusion in the literature between the different types of pancreatitis, even though these have different causes and geographical localisation in the world. Following the Marseille–Rome 1988 Classification (Sarles et al. 1989a,b) acute pancreatitis is defined not as a disease but as a series of lesions (oedema, fat necrosis, necrosis, haemorrhagic necrosis) which may be due to either extrapancreatic causes such as gall stones, hyperlipidaemia or may be a complication of chronic pancreatic lesions such as chronic pancreatitis or pancreatic cancer. Acute pancreatitis may recur when its cause persists. When it is not due to a chronic pancreatic lesion, it heals without sequelae if the patient survives. Though frequently confused with chronic pancreatitis when it recurs, acute pancreatitis will not be studied here. There are very few studies on the geographical distribution of acute pancreatitis.

As shown previously, chronic pancreatitis is a group of different diseases with different features and causes (Payan et al. 1972; Sahel et al. 1986; Sarles et al. 1989a, b). The less frequent form of chronic pancreatitis is obstructive pancreatitis, which is due to obstruction of pancreatic ducts prior to the development of chronic pancreatitis. The obstruction may be caused by tumours or scars. This type of lesion is not often reported. It is mostly diagnosed by endoscopic retrograde pancreatography, mainly in developed countries, but this does not mean that its real frequency is greater in these countries (Sarles et al. 1988).

It has been shown that the majority of cases of chronic pancreatitis present with particular lesions, which differ from those of obstructive pancreatitis (Payan et al. 1972; Sahel et al. 1986). These patients develop calcified pancreatic calculi, visible on abdominal radiographs after a number of years of evolution (Bernades et al. 1983; Ammann et al. 1986). Therefore, we proposed the name "chronic calcifying pancreatitis" with calcified and precalcified stages for this form of chronic pancreatitis. This disease is a pancreatic lithiasis (Sarles et al. 1989c).

A recent paper has shown that there are at least two different and common types of pancreatic lithiasis. The most frequent one is characterised by regularly calcified calculi and is strongly associated with alcoholism or malnutrition. It is the only type to deserve the name "chronic calcifying pancreatitis". The second type is much less frequent. In these cases pancreatic calculi consist of small insoluble, degraded proteins without affinity for calcium. They are radiolucent but with time their core may be covered by a shell of calcium carbonate which gives the appearance of a target. These radiolucent or target calculi are not related to alcoholism, tobacco or nutritional disorders but are frequently hereditary (Sarles et al. 1991). There are no data on the geographical distribution of this type of pancreatic calculi. Our personal cases came from France, Italy and Algeria.

This chapter will therefore deal with the geographical distribution of chronic calcifying pancreatitis or pancreatic lithiasis with regularly calcified calculi which is the best known form of chronic pancreatitis because it is by far the most frequent and also because it is easily diagnosed by simple radiographs of the abdomen.

White (1966) was probably the first author to study the geographical distribution of chronic pancreatitis. Later, different multicentre studies organised by our group tried to correlate the frequency and the type of chronic pancreatitis in different countries to local dietary conditions (Sarles 1973; Sarles et al. 1979) in order to define the aetiology of the disease. One difficulty is that there are no good data on the prevalence of the disease either in autopsy material or in the general population. In the autopsy material, it varies from 0 to 4 per 1000. In Marseille, USA and Brazil, it is approximately 4 per 1000 (Sarles 1973; Sarles et al. 1979).

It has been shown that there are two different areas of chronic calcifying pancreatitis: in the Western world and also in some tropical countries, the disease is associated with heavy alcohol consumption and generally begins its clinical course in the third to fifth decade of life; males are usually affected. In some centres of tropical Asia and Africa, and rarely in Latin America, chronic calcifying pancreatitis begins during the first and second decades, almost as frequently in females as in males, and its frequency seems to be related to malnutrition lasting for some generations. This type of chronic pancreatitis is not related to alcohol consumption (Sarles et al. 1979).

Chronic Calcifying Pancreatitis in Temperate Countries

Europe

Some years after the disappearance of the starvation or simple nutritional restriction observed during the Second World War, the frequency of calcifying pancreatitis increased at different speeds in different European countries. This followed the increase of alcohol consumption and began probably in France:

in the hospitals of Marseille, only two cases were observed from 1943 to 1946 (unpublished data). The first large series was published in the 1950s (Société Française de Gastroenterologie 1965) but not only alcohol consumption but also fat and protein consumption increased during this period.

It was shown that there was a linear correlation between alcohol consumption and the relative risk of the disease (Durbec and Sarles 1978). This means that there is no statistical threshold of toxicity but a continuous spectrum of individual sensitivities to alcohol, starting with predisposed patients who will develop chronic pancreatitis even with such low intakes as 1–20 g alcohol per day. There is also a linear relationship between the logarithm of the risk and the daily intake of protein and a U-shaped curve for fat consumption with the lowest risk for 80–100 g fat per day (Durbec and Sarles 1978). The increased risk associated with tobacco smoking has been shown by different authors in the USA (Yen 1982; Lowenfels et al. 1987). Among our patients, 94% are both smokers and drinkers compared with 80% in liver cirrhosis. Smoking is significantly related to the risk of developing chronic pancreatitis but not liver cirrhosis. Moreover, the mean age of clinical onset of pancreatitis is lower among smokers (unpublished data). The risk associated with alcohol, fat, protein and tobacco are additive on the logarithm, that is, they multiply each other. This has very large effects on the risk due to a given quantity of alcohol.

Until recently, French patients with chronic calcifying pancreatitis had a higher intake of fat and protein than matched controls (Sarles et al. 1965). This difference disappeared recently (unpublished data), suggesting that during the period of dietary restrictions seen after the war, the risk associated with relatively high fat, high protein intake was significant. With a general increase of dietary intakes, there is now no difference between patients and controls, so there must be a maximum level of fat and protein intake beyond which the risk of chronic calcifying pancreatitis does not increase further.

After France, an increased frequency of chronic calcifying pancreatitis parallel to an increased alcohol consumption was found in Italy and Germany. In these countries the same increased consumption of alcohol, protein and fat was found in patients compared with controls (Gullo et al. 1977; Goebell et al. 1980).

In the 1970s a multicentre study of European cases defined two regions: Southern Europe (Portugal, Italy, Switzerland, France) where alcohol consumption increased earlier and Northern Europe where alcohol consumption was lower, and began to rise later. In this second area, the frequency of females, of non-alcoholic cases and of patients who did not (yet) present with radiographically visible calculi was higher (Sarles 1973; Sarles et al. 1979). The frequency of chronic calcifying pancreatitis increased progressively in Northern Europe as seen in Denmark (Andersen et al. 1982) and in Britain (Read et al. 1976; Johnson and Hosking 1991).

Asia

The only temperate Asian country where chronic calcifying pancreatitis is well documented is Japan (Nakamura and Nodo 1991). Alcohol consumption is the most frequent aetiological factor accounting for 58.7% of the cases (72.0% in males and 8.3% in females). The male to female ratio is 2.42:1 which is very

low compared to Europe and 58.9% of female cases are idiopathic. These
features are characteristic for countries where alcohol consumption is relatively
low as was the case in North Europe 15 years after the Second World War.

North America

Chronic calcifying pancreatitis has been the subject of many reports from the
USA (White 1966). The present position seems to be similar to Europe with
a large predominance of males and alcohol as the main aetiological factor.
Apparently there is no difference in the consumption of protein and fat between
patients and controls (Pitchumoni et al. 1980), which corresponds to the present
position in France.

South America

In Argentina and Chile which have a temperate climate, chronic calcifying
pancreatitis is similar to Europe and North America (Sarles 1973; Sarles et al.
1979).

Australia

The only study of the nutritional conditions of chronic pancreatitis patients
(Wilson et al. 1985) found a significant relation with alcohol consumption but
not with fat and protein. Nevertheless, the number of patients and controls
was very small and patients consumed more fat and protein than did controls,
although this was not statistically significant. This seems to correspond to the
present position in France and North America.

Chronic Calcifying Pancreatitis in the Tropics

Tropical Pancreatitis

This form was first reported in India by Kini (1937) and then by Zuidema
(1959) in Indonesia. The largest series was published by Geevarghese (1986)
in the South Indian state Kerala.

This form which is also called calcified pancreatic diabetes, is characterised
in the same way as alcoholic chronic calcifying pancreatitis by the formation
of pancreatic calculi after a certain time of evolution. The biochemical
composition of the calculi in alcoholic temperate and in tropical pancreatitis
is similar (Montalto et al. 1988). The clinical onset of tropical pancreatitis is
much younger than in the temperate disease: it is generally observed in the
two first decades of life. The male predominance is variable and in exceptional

series, there is a female predominance (Mohan et al. 1985; Balakrishnan 1986; Geevarghese 1986).

Chronic Calcifying Pancreatitis in Tropical Asia

The best-known area of tropical chronic pancreatitis is the South Indian state Kerala (Geevarghese 1986) but the disease exists in other Indian states such as Tamil Nadu, Orissa, Karnataka and Andhra Pradesh (Balakrishnan 1986). Indian studies have shown that in that country, the frequency of the disease is not correlated with consumption of cassava or with kwashiorkor although these two factors have been proposed by others as possible causes. A nutritional inquiry carried out in Kerala which compared the data from different tropical countries and from Europe showed that tropical chronic pancreatitis was apparently correlated with very low fat intakes (around 30 g per day) associated with low protein intakes (around 50 g) (Balakrishnan et al. 1988). The toxic effect of fat-poor diets on the pancreas has been shown by Durbec and Sarles (1978).

Tropical pancreatitis is only found in areas with poor nutritional conditions for some generations. For instance, it has never been described in areas such as Hungary where malnutrition was very severe during the Second World War, though at this time, kwashiorkor was a frequent disease in children (Veguelhi 1950). This suggests that the disease, the onset of which is generally in childhood, could be due to nutritional disorders in the children but might also be transmitted by malnourished parents. The fact that young rats born from undernourished mothers have increased pancreatic levels of secretory enzymes, particularly proteases, which persist into adulthood (Sarles et al. 1987) could support this hypothesis.

Tropical pancreatitis is also frequent in Thailand (Vannasaeng et al. 1988) where nutritional conditions are probably similar to those of India.

Tropical Pancreatitis in Africa

In tropical Africa, the tropical type of chronic pancreatitis is mostly found in Nigeria (Olurin and Olurin 1969; Osuntokun 1970) and in Zaire (Sonnet et al. 1960). In contrast, in countries with similar climates such as Senegal (Carayon et al. 1967), Ivory Coast (Sauniere et al. 1986), Uganda (Shaper 1964) and Natal (Moyshal 1973), pancreatitis is generally observed in alcoholics. As in India, there is no correlation in Africa between the frequency of tropical chronic pancreatitis and either the consumption of cassava or kwashiorkor (Sauniere et al. 1986).

In the two sub-tropical extremes of the African continent, chronic calcifying pancreatitis is frequent in Cape Town where it has has been extensively studied (Marks et al. 1973) and is related to alcoholism. In contrast, it is exceptional in the Moslem Magreb where alcohol is prohibited (Aubry et al. 1988). A recent paper has demonstrated some juvenile cases in Tunisia, not related to alcoholism and observed in poor populations (Chatti et al. 1990). If this is confirmed, it will show that tropical pancreatitis may occur in an area larger than was previously believed.

Chronic Calcifying Pancreatitis in Latin America

In the tropical part of Latin America, chronic pancreatitis has been extensively studied in Brazil (Mott et al. 1975; Dani et al. 1986) and in Mexico (Uscanga et al. 1985; Robles-Diaz et al. 1990). In these two countries where the average protein and fat intake are frequently low, chronic pancreatitis is mostly related to alcohol consumption, and the protein and fat intake of alcoholic patients, though low, is significantly higher than that of matched controls. Nevertheless some cases presenting with the juvenile tropical type have been reported in Brazil (Mott et al. 1975).

Conclusion

The most frequent type of chronic pancreatitis, pancreatic lithiasis with homogeneously calcified calculi is observed all around the world but with very different frequencies. The so-called occidental form is generally related to alcohol consumption. Its clinical onset is usually in the adult male aged 20–50 years. The disease is observed in the rich countries or in rich layers of developing countries. In certain European countries, after the dietary restrictions during the war and in developing countries, the fat and protein intake of patients was or is higher than those of matched controls from the same populations. This difference has disappeared in Europe but not in developing countries.

The tropical form or tropical calcific diabetes is in contrast found in very poor populations. Its clinical onset is generally in childhood. Epidemiological studies have ruled out the role of cassava or kwashiorkor. Our enquiries suggest the possible role of low fat, low protein intakes in the diet of the patient but possibly also of the parents.

Before ending, it is necessary to reiterate that chronic pancreatitis is not the sole cause of pancreatic insufficiency in tropical countries: compared to the pancreatic secretion of matched European controls, the enzyme secretion of apparently normal young Algerians is slightly decreased (Palasciano et al. 1979), the pancreatic secretion of children from Abidjan is much reduced and of children from Dakar very low indeed without pancreatic symptoms in any of these groups (Sauniere and Sarles 1988). In these countries, chronic pancreatitis is exceptional. The lesions responsible for this insufficiency are not well known but might be diffuse fibrosis.

References

Ammann RW, Buehler H, Bruehlmann W et al. (1986) Acute (nonprogressive) alcoholic pancreatitis: prospective longitudinal study of 114 patients with recurrent alcoholic pancreatitis. Pancreas 1:195–204

Andersen BN, Pedersen NT, Scheel J, Worning H (1982) Incidence of alcoholic chronic pancreatitis in Copenhagen. Scand J Gastroenterol 17:247–252

Aubry P, Attia Y, Barabe P et al. (1988) Geographical distribution and pathogenesis of chronic calcifying pancreatitis in tropical zones. Results of a multicentre survey in French-speaking black Africa. Gastroenterol Clin Biol 12:420–424

Balakrishnan V (1986) Chronic pancreatitis in India. Indian Society of Pancreatology, Trivandrum, India.

Balakrishnan V, Sauniere JF, Hariharan M, Sarles H (1988) Diet, pancreatic function and chronic pancreatitis in South India and in France. Pancreas 3:30–35

Bernades P, Belghiti J, Athouel M et al. (1983) Histoire naturelle de la pancréatite chronique. Etude de 120 cas. Gastroenterol Clin Biol 7:8–13

Carayon A, Onde M, Rousselet M (1967) Evolution de la pathologie pancréatique de L'Africain (à propos de 26 observations). Bull Soc Med Afr Noire Langue Fr 12:287–293

Chatti N, Chaieb L, Jemmi L et al. (1990) Juvenile idiopathic chronic calcifying pancreatitis: report of 10 cases from central Tunisia. Pancreas 5:354–357

Dani R, Penna FJ, Nogueira CED (1986) Etiology of chronic calcifying pancreatitis in Brazil: a report of 329 consecutive cases. Int J Pancreatol 1:399–406

Durbec JP, Sarles H (1978) Multicentre survey of the etiology of pancreatic diseases. Relationship between the relative risk of developing chronic pancreatitis and alcohol, protein and lipid consumption. Digestion 18:337–350

Geevarghese PJ (1986) Calcific pancreatitis. Causes and mechanisms in the tropics compared with those in the subtropics. Varghese Publishing House, Bombay

Goebell H, Hotz J, Hoffmeister H (1980) Hypercaloric nutrition as aetiological factor in chronic pancreatitis. Z Gastroenterol 18:94–97

Gullo L, Costa PL, Labo G (1977) Chronic pancreatitis in Italy. Aetiological clinical and histological observations based on 253 cases. Rendiconti Gastroenterol 9:97–104

Johnson CD, Hosking SW (1991) National statistics for diet, alcohol consumption and chronic pancreatitis in England and Wales 1960–1988. Gut 32:(in press)

Kini MG (1937) Multiple pancreatic calculi with chronic pancreatitis. Br J Surg 25:705

Lowenfels AB, Zwemer FL, Jhangiani S, Pitchumoni CS (1987) Pancreatitis in a native American Indian population. Pancreas 2:694–697

Marks IN, Banks S, Louw JH (1973) Chronic pancreatitis in the Western Cape. Digestion 9:447–453

Mohan V, Mohan R, Susheela L et al. (1985) Tropical pancreatic diabetes in South India: heterogeneity in clinical and biochemical profile. Diabetologia 28:229–232

Montalto G, Multigner L, Sarles H, De Caro A (1988) Organic matrix of pancreatic stones associated with nutritional pancreatitis. Pancreas 3:262–268

Mott C de B, Ohki Y, Barros MIB et al. (1975) Aspectos clinicos e laboratoriais das pancretives chronicas: observacao de 80 casos. Rev Assoc Med Minas Gerais 21:281–284

Moyshal MG (1973) A study of chronic pancreatitis in Natal. Digestion 9:438–446

Nakamura K, Nodo K (1991) Etiological aspects of chronic pancreatitis in Japan. In: Sarles H, Johnson CD, Sauniere JF (eds) Pancreatitis. Arnette Blackman, Paris

Olurin EO, Olurin O (1969) Pancreatic calcification: a report of 45 cases. Br Med J 4:534–539

Osuntokun BO (1970) The neurology of non-alcoholic pancreatic diabetes mellitus in Nigerians. J Neurol Sci 11:17–43

Palasciano G, Sauniere JF, Laugier R, Sarles H (1979) Pancreatic response to secretin-CCK-PZ in European and North African adults and children. Gut 20:1063–1065

Payan H, Sarles H, Demirdjian M et al. (1972) Study of the histological features of chronic pancreatitis by correspondance analysis. Identification of chronic calcifying pancreatitis as an entity. Biomedicine 18:663–670

Pitchumoni CS, Sonnenshein M, Candido FM, Panacharam P, Cooperman JM (1980) Nutrition in the pathogenesis of alcoholic pancreatitis. Am J Clin Nutr 33:631–636

Read G, Braganza JM, Howat HT (1976) Pancreatitis. A retrospective study. Gut 17:945–952

Robles-Diaz G, Vargas F, Uscanga L, Fernandes-Del Castillo C (1990) Chronic pancreatitis in Mexico City. Pancreas 5:479–483

Sahel J, Cros C, Durbec JP et al. (1986) Multicentre pathological study of chronic pancreatitis. Morphological regional variations and differences between chronic calcifying pancreatitis and obstructive pancreatitis. Pancreas 1:471–477

Sarles H (1973) An international survey on nutrition and pancreatitis. Digestion 9:389–403

Sarles H, Sarles JC, Camatte R et al. (1965) Observations on 205 confirmed cases of acute pancreatitis, recurring pancreatitis and chronic pancreatitis. Gut 6:545–559

Sarles H, Cros RC, Bidart JM and the International Group for the Study of Pancreatic Diseases (1979) A multicentre inquiry into the etiology of pancreatic diseases. Digestion 19:110–125

Sarles H, Lahaie R, Dollet JM et al. (1987) Effects of parental malnutrition on enzyme content of rat pancreas. Dig Dis Sci 32:520–528

Sarles H, Cambon P, Choux R et al. (1988) Chronic obstructive pancreatitis due to tiny (0.6 to 8 mm) benign tumours obstructing pancreatic ducts: report of three cases. Pancreas 3:232–237

Sarles H, Adler G, Dani R et al. (1989a) The pancreatitis classification of Marseilles Rome 1988. Scand J Gastroenterol 24:651–652

Sarles H, Adler G, Dani R et al. (1989b). Classifications of pancreatitis and definition of pancreatic diseases. Digestion 43:234–236

Sarles H, Bernard JP, Johnson CD (1989c) Pathogenesis and epidemiology of chronic pancreatitis. Ann Rev Med 40:453–468

Sarles H, Camarena J, Gomez-Santana G (1991) Radiolucent and calcified pancreatic lithiasis. Two different diseases. Role of alcohol and heredity. Scand J Gastroenterol (in press)

Sauniere JF, Sarles H (1988) Exocrine pancreatic function and protein-calorie malnutrition in Dakar and Abidjan (West Africa). Silent pancreatic insufficiency. Am J Clin Nutr 48:1233–1238

Sauniere JF, Sarles H, Attia Y et al. (1986) Exocrine pancreatic function of children from the Ivory Coast compared to French children. Effect of kwashiorkor. Dig Dis Sci 31:481–486

Shaper AG (1964) Aetiology of chronic pancreatic fibrosis with calcification seen in Uganda. Br Med J 1:1607–1609

Société Française de Gastroenterologie (1965) Les ulceres de l'oesophage. Les pancréatites chroniques. Rapport présenté aux Journées Françaises de Gastroenterologie. Masson et Cie Editeur, Paris

Sonnet J, Brisbois P, Bastin JP (1960) Chronic pancreatitis with calcification in Congolese bantus. Trop Geogr Med 18:97–113

Uscanga L, Robles-Diaz G, Sarles H (1985) Nutritional data and aetiology of chronic pancreatitis in Mexico. Dig Dis Sci 30:110–113

Vannasaeng S, Nitiyanant W, Vichayanrat A (1988) Case-control study on risk factors associated with fibrocalculous pancreatic diabetes. Diab Med 5:835–839

Veguelhi (1950) Nutritional oedema. Ann Pediatr 175:349–377

White TT (1966) Pancreatitis. Arnold, London

Wilson JS, Bernstein L, McDonald C et al. (1985) Diet and drinking habits in relation to the development of alcoholic pancreatitis. Gut 26:882–887

Yen S, Hsieh CC, MacMahon B (1982) Consumption of alcohol and tobacco and other risk factors for pancreatitis. Am J Epidemiol 116:407–414

Zuidema PJ (1959) Cirrhosis and disseminated calcification of the pancreas in patients with malnutrition. Trop Geogr Med 11:70–74

Chapter 17

The Pathogenesis of Chronic Pancreatitis

J. P. Bernard and R. Laugier

Introduction

In 1946, some authors proposed that chronic pancreatitis was the consequence of repeated attacks of acute pancreatitis because they found that acute lesions were often superimposed on chronic lesions (Comfort et al. 1946). But the converse could also be true, that acute lesions are a complication of chronic pancreatitis. If the assumption of these authors was correct, the age of onset of acute and chronic pancreatitis should be the same, and their aetiological data should be similar. In fact, the supposed cause, acute pancreatitis, is observed in patients 13 years older than those with chronic pancreatitis, the supposed consequence (Sarles et al. 1965). Moreover, aetiological data in patients presenting with acute or chronic pancreatitis are significantly different.

This has been the basis of the two Marseilles classifications which distinguish between acute and chronic pancreatitis (Sarles et al. 1965, 1989).

The recent Marseilles–Rome classification (Sarles et al. 1989) defined acute pancreatitis as "a spectrum of inflammatory lesions in the pancreas and also in peripancreatic tissues: oedema, necrosis, hemorrhagic necrosis, fat necrosis". Chronic pancreatitis was defined as "the presence of chronic inflammatory lesions characterised by the destruction of exocrine parenchyma and fibrosis and, at least, in the later stages, the endocrine parenchyma. It is frequently complicated in the early stages of its evolution by attacks of acute pancreatitis which are responsible for recurrent episodes of pain and which may represent the only clinical symptom. After some years, both exocrine (steatorrhoea) and endocrine (diabetes) insufficiency develops and acute attacks decrease in frequency and later on, disappear.

Two types of large computer-based studies of chronic pancreatitis (Payan et al. 1972; Sahel et al. 1986) and spatial reconstruction of extralobular and intralobular ducts from chronic pancreatitis patients and normal controls (Nakamura et al. 1972; Akao et al. 1986) led to similar conclusions: chronic pancreatitis is not one disease but a group of at least two different diseases which could be distinguished by their features and causes.

Obstructive Pancreatitis

Obstructive pancreatitis is due to the occlusion of the main pancreatic duct or of one of its collateral branches, by a lesion such as a slowly growing tumour, a fibrous scar after necrosis or a congenital anomaly. The lesions are regularly distributed in the occluded territories, the ductal epithelium is relatively well preserved, pancreatic calculi are not found and protein precipitates are rare.

Calcifying Chronic Pancreatitis (CCP)

CCP is the usual form of chronic pancreatitis, representing more than 95% of cases. Although CCP may be secondary to alcohol, hypercalcaemia or hereditary or idiopathic in subtropical countries and is probably nutritional in tropical countries, the pancreatic lesions are similar regardless of aetiology (Nakamura et al. 1972; Payan et al. 1972; Sahel et al. 1986). They are characterised by their patchy distribution: the intensity of the lesions of one lobule or group of lobules (and of the corresponding duct which drains them) is different from neighbouring lobules, which may vary from a completely normal appearance to complete destruction. Ductal lesions are important (atrophy of epithelium, stenosis, dilatation) and are often associated with perineural inflammatory infiltration with mononuclear cells and fibrosis.

A morphometric ultrastructural study of the acinar and ductal cells (Tasso et al. 1973) showed that the first lesion of CCP, which appears before lesions of the duct and acinar cells, was the formation in the ducts of eosinophilic protein plugs. All transitions exist between these precipitates and calcified calculi (Payan et al. 1972; Harada et al. 1982, 1983) which may be visible on X-ray films of the abdomen, after some years of evolution (Bernades et al. 1983; Ink et al. 1984).

CCP thus appears to be a lithiasis. As this disease has different causes with similar pathological lesions, there must be common mechanisms for the different aetiological forms.

Mechanisms Common to Different Forms of CCP

The protein precipitates that are the first step in the disease consist largely of a proteinaceous, fibrillar material. Morphological studies suggest that mature calculi derive from protein plugs when calcite is deposited on the network of fibrillar protein (Kern et al. 1984; Bockman et al. 1986). The biochemical composition of the calculi is identical in the alcoholic, idiopathic and tropical forms (Montalto et al. 1988): these calculi contain predominantly calcium salts, mostly calcium carbonate (calcite), associated with an organic matrix made up of a variable quantity of fibrillar protein (de Caro et al. 1984).

The proteinaceous material present in stones and in plugs is a low-molecular-weight protein (de Caro et al. 1979, Guy et al. 1983): pancreatic stone protein (PSP) which has recently been renamed lithostathine (Sarles et al. 1990). Nevertheless, in some exceptional cases in non-alcoholic patients, different types of calculi have been found: either large (2 cm diameter) stones which resembled marble and consisted only of calcite without lithostathine (Sarles et al. 1982) or else X-ray-transparent stones composed only of proteinaceous material without calcium salts (Multigner et al. 1987). The pathogenesis of CCP therefore revolves around two problems: precipitation of calcium and precipitation of protein.

Precipitation of Calcium

As pancreatic juice is supersaturated in calcium (Moore and Vérine 1987), it is surprising that so few people develop pancreatic calculi. It is necessary to assume the existence of one or more calcium stabilisers able to prevent the precipitation of calcium in normal pancreatic juice.

Lithostathine is probably one of these stabilisers. This molecule is present in normal pancreatic juice as a group of four glycoproteins (molecular weight 17000–22000) (de Caro et al. 1987). The molecule is synthesised as a 144 amino acid single chain in the endoplasmic reticulum of the acinar cell which contains a specific messenger RNA for lithostathine (Giorgi et al. 1985). Lithostathine is concentrated with enzymes in zymogen granules (Lechene de la Porte et al. 1986). The secretory forms of lithostathine are hydrolysed by trypsin and transformed into a smaller form of molecular weight 15000 (lithostathine H) which is insoluble at physiological pH and devoid of biological activity. A similar fibrillar protein named "pancreatic thread protein" (PTP) has been isolated in bovine and human pancreatic juice (Gross et al. 1985a, b). The partial amino acid sequence given by these authors strongly suggests that PTP is similar to lithostathine H, the trypsin-degraded fragment of lithostathine.

Lithostathine is present in the pancreatic juice of five mammalian species which have so far been studied (Bernard et al. 1991). The role of this protein is to inhibit nucleation and crystal growth of calcium carbonate in pancreatic juice (Multigner and de Caro 1987). Lithostathine acts by blocking specific growth sites on the crystal surface. The biological activity of lithostathine is carried by the N-terminal undecapeptide (unpublished observations). Similar molecules which prevent crystallisation of calcium salts are already known in saliva (Hay et al. 1979), urine (Nakagawa et al. 1983) and bile (Shimizu et al. 1989).

What is the role of lithostathine in the pathogenesis of chronic pancreatitis? Three separate series of experiments suggest reduced synthesis of lithostathine synthesis in chronic pancreatitis.

Firstly, the concentration of lithostathine measured by radial immunodiffusion or enzyme-linked immunosorbent assay with polyclonal antibodies and related to secretory proteins is significantly decreased in pancreatic juice of patients with CCP of different aetiologies. When lithostathine concentration is estimated by radioimmunoassay with a monoclonal antibody raised against lithostathine

H, there is no clear distinction between CCP patients and controls (Provansal-Cheylan et al. 1989; Schmiegel et al. 1990). This discrepancy could be because lithostathine estimation in pancreatic juice requires precise experimental conditions: activation of the juice or storage might induce hydrolysis of the molecule and release of the insoluble lithostathine H residue, which polymerises and precipitates.

Second, the messenger RNA levels of lithostathine, chymotrypsinogen, trypsinogen and colipase in CCP and control pancreas were compared: lithostathine mRNA was three times lower in CCP than in controls, whereas the other mRNA were not altered. This strongly suggests that lithostathine gene expression is specifically reduced in CCP patients (Giorgi et al. 1989).

Finally, immunolocalisation studies demonstrated smaller amounts of lithostathine in the rough endoplasmic reticulum and zymogen granules of acinar cells from CCP patients than in normal tissue (Lechene de la Porte et al. 1986). This suggests that there is a reduced rate of synthesis and secretion of lithostathine.

Precipitation of Protein

The morphological and biochemical studies discussed above showed that the first visible lesion of CCP was the precipitation in a fibrillar form of the 133 C-terminal fragment of lithostathine (lithostathine H), associated with some other pancreatic proteins. Pancreatic calculi also consist of different degraded residues of lithostathine. The mechanism of hydrolysis is not understood. It is logical to assume that it could be due to enzymatic cleavage by trypsin, but the presence of active trypsin in the acinar lumen has not been demonstrated. Thus, the possibility of spontaneous autocatalytic cleavage of an abnormal lithostathine molecule is not ruled out.

Role of Local Factors

As soon as the ductal epithelium is in contact with plugs or stones, the basal membrane disappears (Kennedy et al. 1987) and thereafter ductal cells atrophy (Payan et al. 1972). This allows the transudation of interstitial fluid, which increases the concentration of serum proteins (Clemente et al. 1971) and calcium in pancreatic juice (Gullo et al. 1974). These changes increase in turn the risk of precipitation of proteins and calcium.

This increased concentration of calcium, which is secondary to the earliest lesions of the disease, could explain why calculi frequently appear after some years of clinical evolution and thereafter grow rapidly (Bernades et al. 1983; Ammann et al. 1984).

Mechanisms Particular to Different Forms of CCP

Alcoholic CCP

In Europe, Japan and temperate areas of America and Africa, CCP is most frequently associated with alcoholism (Sarles 1973; Sarles et al. 1979). The disease is mainly observed in alcoholic males having a high protein and fat consumption, although the risk is also increased by a low fat diet (Durbec and Sarles 1978).

Cytotoxic Effects of Alcohol on the Pancreas

In the rat subjected to chronic administration of alcohol, either orally or intravenously, several studies have shown accumulation of lipid droplets in both acinar and ductal cells (Singh et al. 1982; Wilson et al. 1982). This probably results from ethanol metabolism in the acinar cell where both ethanol and acetaldehyde stimulate lipid biosynthesis and inhibit fatty acid oxidation (Durand et al. 1982).

The same results were observed on pancreatic specimens obtained at surgery from alcoholics. It appears that alcohol consumption is responsible for an increased fat content in the pancreas and perhaps for some fibrosis, as these are also found in asymptomatic alcoholic patients (Noronha et al. 1981). The increased fat content of acinar cells cannot explain all the biochemical modifications found in the pancreatic juice in CCP.

Modifications of Pancreatic Juice Due to Alcohol

In man as well as in dogs, chronic ethanol consumption increases the total concentration of protein in pancreatic juice, and decreases pH, bicarbonate and citrate secretion, as well as the concentration of the secretory trypsin inhibitor, and the ratio of cationic to anionic trypsinogen (Tiscornia et al. 1973; Sarles et al. 1983; Noel-Jorand and Sarles 1983; Rinderknecht et al. 1985; Sahel et al. 1986; Sarles 1986). The increased concentration (and output) of secretory proteins is probably due, at least partly, to an increased biosynthesis by the acinar cells (Boyd et al. 1985). The mechanism of this increased secretion is neural, cholinergic and vagally mediated (Noel-Jorand and Sarles 1983). These modifications of pancreatic juice induced by alcohol probably play a role in the formation of protein plugs which are more frequently found in the pure pancreatic juice of alcoholic dogs or men than in controls. Precipitation of calcium may be facilitated by a decrease in citrate secretion (Boustière et al. 1985) and perhaps also, by a direct effect of alcohol which decreases lithostathine secretion (Provansal-Cheylan et al. 1989). The mechanism of this last effect is unknown.

Hypercalcaemic Chronic Calcifying Pancreatitis

Hypercalcaemia is also a cause of chronic calcifying pancreatitis, which may be secondary to hyperparathyroidism. The modifications of pancreatic juice induced by chronic hypercalcaemia have been described in the dog and the cat. In the dog, chronic hypercalcaemia induces a decrease of bicarbonate secretion associated with an increased protein secretion and formation of protein plugs (Noel-Jorand et al. 1981). The same changes were observed in man (Goebell 1976). In the cat, hypercalcaemia decreases bicarbonate secretion without modification of protein concentration, but significantly increases the ductal permeability for calcium ions (Layer et al. 1985).

The mechanism of these changes induced by hypercalcaemia has been shown to involve an increased release of cholecystokinin in the cat (Layer et al. 1985), and in the dog, a decreased sensitivity of ductal cells to secretin with an increased sensitivity of acinar cells to acetylcholine and CCK analogues (Noel-Jorand et al. 1981). During hypercalcaemia, pancreatic lithogenesis could be related to an increased concentration of proteins in association with an increased concentration of calcium in pancreatic juice (Layer et al. 1985).

Tropical Pancreatitis

The mechanisms involved in tropical pancreatitis are not known. The disease is observed in non-alcoholic children and young adults of both sexes living in South India, Indonesia and some parts of Africa such as Nigeria and Zaire (Mohan et al. 1985; Sarles 1986). Kwashiorkor and cassava consumption have been implicated (Pitchumoni and Thomas 1973; Clain et al. 1981), but other studies conducted in different areas to compare the type of diet and the incidence of tropical pancreatitis have shown that neither of these factors plays a part (Mohan et al. 1985; Saunière and Sarles 1988), although tropical pancreatitis is never encountered in countries in which protein malnutrition does not exist. At present two factors seem to play a role in the development of tropical pancreatitis (Balakrishnan et al. 1988): very low fat diets (less than 30 g per day) and probably low protein intake (less than 50 g per day).

Malnutrition of the mother during pregnancy may also play a role in the disease of the child: in young rats born from animals submitted to a moderately restricted protein diet, the pancreas showed an increase of protein content, especially proteases. This modification persisted for several months after weaning (Sarles et al. 1987). As in CCP in subtropical countries, pathophysiology of tropical pancreatitis appears to involve nutritional and also possibly other predisposing factors.

Predisposing Factors

Not all alcoholics nor all subjects submitted to hypercalcaemia or living in tropical areas develop pancreatitis. There is a hereditary autosomal dominant form of CCP with variable penetrance, as observed in two reports (Comfort and Steinberg 1952; Stafford and Grand 1982). One case of total lack of lithostathine was observed in a non-alcoholic woman presenting with giant calculi (Sarles et al. 1982).

These cases represent the extremes of genetic influence on CCP. In other cases it is possible that there might be a genetically programmed predisposition. The risk of finding another case in the family of a patient presenting with CCP is greater than in the general population (Sarles and Camatte 1966). A higher risk of developing CCP is also associated with blood group O (Marks et al. 1973; Gullo et al. 1977); however, data on the HLA groups are contradictory (Sarles 1986). Our current working hypothesis is that decreased or abnormal biosynthesis and secretion of lithostathine, which may be congenital or acquired, could explain the predisposition to the noxious action of alcohol and different diets but could also be the cause of hereditary and idiopathic pancreatitis. Further genetic studies using molecular biology techniques will be needed to confirm this.

References

Akao S, Bockman DE, Lechene de la Porte P, Sarles H (1986) Three-dimensional pattern of ductuloacinar associations in normal and pathological human pancreas. Gastroenterology 90:661–668

Ammann RW, Akovbiantz A, Lagiarder F, Schueler G (1984) Course and outcome of chronic pancreatitis. Longitudinal study of a mixed medical–surgical series of 245 patients. Gastroenterology 86:820–828

Balakrishnan V, Sauniere JF, Hariharan M, Sarles H (1988) Diet, pancreatic function and chronic pancreatitis in South India and in France. Pancreas 3:30–35

Bernard JP, Adrich Z, Montalto G, Sarles H, Dagorn JC, de Caro A (1991) Inhibition of nucleation and crystal growth of calcium carbonate by human lithostathine. Pancreas (in press)

Bernardes P, Belghiti J, Athouel M, Mallardo N, Breil P, Fekete F (1983) Histoire naturelle de la pancréatite chronique. Etude de 120 cas. Gasteroenterol Clin Biol 7:8–13

Bockman, DE, Kennedy RH, Multigner L, de Caro A, Sarles H (1986) Fine structure of the organic matrix of human pancreatic stones. Pancreas 1:204–210

Boustiere C, Sarles H, Lohse J, Durbec JP, Sahel L (1985) Citrate and calcium secretion in the pure human pancreatic juice of alcoholic and nonalcoholic men and of chronic pancreatitis patients. Digestion 32:1–9

Clain JE, Barbezat GO, Marks IN (1981) Exocrine pancreatic enzyme and calcium secretion in health and pancreatitis. Gut 22:355–358

Clemente F, Ribeiro T, Figarella C, Sarles H (1971) Albumine IgG et IgG dans le suc pancréatique human normal chez l'adulte. Clin Chim Acta 33:317–324

Comfort MW, Steinberg AG (1952) Pedigree of a family with hereditary chronic relapsing pancreatitis. Gastroenterology 21:54–63

Comfort MW, Gambill EE, Baggenstoss AH (1946) Chronic relapsing pancreatitis – a study of 29 cases without associated disease of the biliary gastrointestinal tract. Gastroenterology 6:239–285

de Caro A, Lohse J, Sarles H (1979) Characterization of a protein isolated from pancreatic calculi of men suffering from chronic calcifying pancreatitis. Biochem Biophys Res Commun 87:1176–1182

de Caro A, Multigner L, Lafont H, Lombardo D, Sarles H (1984) The molecular characteristics of a human pancreatic acidic phosphoprotein that inhibits calcium carbonate crystal growth. Biochem J 222:669–677

de Caro A, Bonicel J, Rouimi P, de Caro J, Sarles H, Rovery M (1987) Complete amino acid sequence of an immunoreactive form of human pancreatic stone protein isolated from pancreatic juice. Eur J Biochem 168:201–207

Durand S, Estival A, Clemente F, Douste-Blazy L, Ribet A (1982) The decrease of the non-secretory phospholipase A in rat pancreas during a chronic alcohol intoxication. Biomedicine 36:254:256

Durbec JP, Sarles H (1978) Multicenter survey of the etiology of pancreatic diseases. Relationship between the relative risk of developing chronic pancreatitis and alcohol protein and lipid consumption. Digestion 18:337–350

Giorgi D, Bernard JP, de Caro A et al. (1985) Pancreatic stone protein. I. Evidence that it is encoded by a pancreatic messenger ribonucleic acid. Gastroenterology 89:381–386

Giorgi D, Bernard JP, Rouquier S, Iovanna J, Sarles H, Dagorn JC (1989) Secretory pancreatic stone protein messenger RNA. Nucleotide sequence and expression in chronic calcifying pancreatitis. J Clin Invest 84:100–106

Goebell H (1976) The role of calcium in pancreatic secretion and disease. Acta Hepatogastroenterol 32:151–161

Gross J, Brauer AW, Bringhurst RF, Corbett C, Margolies MN (1985a) An unusual bovine pancreatic protein exhibiting pH-dependent globule-fibril transformation and unique amino acid sequence. Proc Natl Acad Sci USA 82:5627–5631

Gross J, Carison RI, Brauer AW, Margolies MN, Warshaw AL, Wands JR (1985b) Isolation, characterization and distribution of an unusual pancreatic human secretory protein. J Clin Invest 76:2215–2216

Gullo L, Sarles H, Mott CB, Tiscornia OM, Pauli AM, Pastor J (1974) Pancreatic secretion of calcium in healthy subjects and various diseases of the pancreas. Rendiconti Gastroenterol 6:35–44

Gullo L, Costa PL, Labo G (1977) Chronic pancreatitis in Italy; aetiological, clinical and histological observations based on 253 cases. Rendiconti Gastroenterol 9:97–104

Guy O, Robles-Diaz G, Adrich Z, Sahel J, Sarles H (1983) Protein content of precipitates present in pancreatic juice of alcoholic subjects and patients with chronic calcifying pancreatitis. Gastroenterology 84:102–107

Harada H, Ueda O, Yasuoka M et al. (1982) Scanning electron microscopic studies on protein plugs obtained from patients with chronic pancreatitis. Gastroenterol Jpn 17:98–101

Harada H, Takeda M, Tanaka J, Miki H, Ochi K, Kimura I (1983) The fine structure of pancreatic stones as shown by scanning electron microscopy and X-ray probe microanalyser. Gastroenterol Jpn 18:530–537

Hay DI, Moreno E, Schlesinger TH (1979) Phosphoprotein inhibitors of calcium phosphate precipitation from salivary secretion. Inorg Perspect Biol Med 2:271–285

Ink O, Labayle D, Buffet C, Chaput JC, Etienne JP (1984) Pancréatite chronique alcoolique: relations de la douleur avec le severage et la chirurgie pancréatique. Gastroenterol Clin Biol 8:419–425

Kennedy RH, Bockman DE, Uscanga L, Choux R, Grimaud JA, Sarles H (1987) Pancreatic extracellular matrix alterations in chronic pancreatitis. Pancreas 2:61–72

Kern HF, Warshaw AL, Scheele GA (1984) Fine structure of protein precipitations in acinar lumina of the normal human pancreas and in chronic pancreatitis. In: Gyr KE, Singer MV, Sarles H (eds) Pancreatitis. Concepts and classification. Excerpta Medica, Amsterdam, pp 101–105

Layer P, Hotz J, Eysselein VE et al. (1985) Effects of acute hypercalcemia on exocrine pancreatic secretion in the cat. Gastroenterology 88:1168–1174

Lechene de la Porte P, de Caro A, Lafont H, Sarles H (1986) Immunocytochemical localization of pancreatic stone protein in the human digestive tract. Pancreas 1:301–308

Marks IN, Bank S, Louw JH (1973) Chronic pancreatitis in the Western Cape. Digestion 9:447–453

Mohan V, Mohan R, Susheela L et al. (1985) Tropical pancreatic diabetes in South India: heterogeneity in clinical and biochemical profile. Diabetologia 28:229–232

Montalto G, Multigner L, Sarles H, de Caro A (1988) Organic matrix of pancreatic stones associated with nutritional pancreatitis. Pancreas 3:262–268

Moore EW, Verine HJ (1987) Pancreatic calcification and stone formation: a thermodynamic model of calcium in pancreatic juice. Am J Physiol 252:707–718

Multigner L, de Caro A (1987) Kinetic studies on calcium carbonate crystal growth inhibition by human pancreatic stone protein. Digestion 38:43

Multigner L, Mariani A, Daudon M, Schmiegel WH, Sarles H, de Caro A (1987) Pancreatic stone protein and radiolucent pancreatic stones. Digestion 38:44

Nakagawa Y, Abram V, Kerby FJ, Kaiser ET, Coe SL (1983) Purification and characterization of the principal inhibitor of calcium oxalate monohydrate crystal growth in human urines. J Biol Chem 258:12594–12600

Nakamura K, Sarles H, Payan H (1972) Three-dimensional reconstruction of the pancreatic ducts in chronic pancreatitis. Gastroenterology 62:942–949

Noel-Jorand MC, Sarles H (1983) Simultaneous mechanisms on exocrine pancreatic secretion initiated by alcohol in the conscious dog. Dig Dis Sci 28:879–888

Noel-Jorand MC, Verine HJ, Sarles H (1981) Dose-dependent and long-lasting effects of repeated intravenous injections of calcium on the canine secretin-stimulated pancreatic juice secretion. Eur J Clin Invest 11:25–31

Noronha M, Salgadinho A, Ferrieira de Almedia MJ, Dreiling DA, Bordalo O (1981) Alcohol and the pancreas. I. Clinical associations and histopathology of minimal pancreatic inflammation. Am J Gastroenterol 76:114–119

Payan H, Sarles H, Demirdjian M, Gauthier AP, Cros RC, Durbec JP (1972) Study of the histological features of chronic pancreatitis by correspondence analysis. Identification of chronic calcifying pancreatitis as an entity. Biomedicine 18:663–670

Pitchumoni CS, Thomas E (1973) Chronic cassava toxicity. Possible relationship to chronic pancreatic disease in malnourished populations. Lancet ii:1397–1398

Provansal-Cheylan M, Mariani A, Bernard JP, Sarles H, Dupuy P (1989) Pancreatic stone protein: quantification in pancreatic juice by enzyme linked immunosorbent assay and comparison with other methods. Pancreas 4:680–689

Rinderknecht H, Stace NH, Renner IG (1985) Effects of chronic alcohol abuse on exocrine pancreatic secretion in man. Dig Dis Sci 30:65–71

Sahel J, Cros C, Durbec JP et al. (1986) Multicenter pathological study of chronic pancreatitis. Morphological regional variations and differences between chronic calcifying pancreatitis and obstructive pancreatitis. Pancreas 1:471–477

Sarles H (1973) An international survey on nutrition and pancreatitis. Digestion 9:389–403

Sarles H (1986) Etiopathogenesis and definition of chronic pancreatitis. Dig Dis Sci 31:91S–107S

Sarles H, Camatte R (1966) Etiopathogenesis of pancreas. In: Recent advances in gastroenterology, vol 4. Proceedings of the third World Conference of gastroenterology, Tokyo

Sarles H, Sarles JC, Camatte R et al. (1965) Observations on 205 confirmed cases of acute pancreatitis, recurring pancreatitis and chronic pancreatitis. Gut 6:545–559

Sarles H, Cros RC, Bidart JM, International Group for the Study of Pancreatic Diseases (1979) A multicenter inquiry into the etiology of pancreatic diseases. Digestion 19:110–125

Sarles H, de Caro A, Multigner L, Martin E (1982) Giant pancreatic stones in teetotal women due to absence of the "stone protein"? Lancet ii:714–715

Sarles H, Laugier R, Boustiere C (1983) Pancreatic lithiasis alcoholic pancreatic pathogenesis. Progr Gastroenterol 4:189–212

Sarles H, Lahaie R, Dollet JM, Beck B, Michel R, Debry G (1987) Effect of parental malnutrition on enzyme content of rat pancreas. Dig Dis Sci 32:520–528

Sarles H, Adler G, Dani R et al. (1989) The pancreatitis classification of Marseilles Rome 1988. Scand J Gastroenterol 24:651–652

Sarles H, Dagorn JC, Giorgi D, Bernard JP (1990) Renaming pancreatic stone protein as lithostathine. Gastroenterology 99:900–901

Sauniere JF, Sarles H (1988) Exocrine pancreatic function and protein-calorie malnutrition in Dakar and Abidjan (West Africa). Silent pancreatic insufficiency. Am J Clin Nutr 48:1233–1238

Schmiegel W, Burchert M, Kalthoff H et al. (1990) Immunochemical characterization and quantitative distribution of pancreatic stone protein in sera and pancreatic secretions in pancreatic disorders. Gastroenterology 99:1421–1430

Shimizu S, Sabsay B, Veis A, Ostrow JD, Rege RV, Dawes LG (1989) Isolation of an acidic protein from cholesterol gallstones, which inhibits the precipitation of calcium carbonate in vitro. J Clin Invest 84:1990–1996

Singh M, La Sure MM, Bockman DE (1982) Pancreatic acinar cell function and morphology in rats chronically fed an ethanol diet. Gastroenterology 82:425–434

Stafford RJ, Grand RJ (1982) Hereditary disease of the exocrine pancreas. Clin Gastroenterol 11:141–170

Tasso F, Stemmelin N, Sarles H, Clop J (1973) Comparative morphometric study of the human pancreas in its normal state. Biomedicine 18:134–144

Tiscornia OM, Gullo L, de Barros Mott C et al. (1973) The effect of intragastric ethanol administration upon canine exocrine pancreatic secretion. Digestion 9:490–501

Wilson JS, Colley PW, Sornia L, Pirola RC, Chapman BA, Soner JB (1982) Alcohol causes a fatty pancreas. A rat model of ethanol-induced pancreatic stenosis. Alcoholism (NY) 6:117–121

Chapter 18

The Molecular Biology of Lithostathine (Pancreatic Stone Protein)

D. Giorgi and J. C. Dagorn

Introduction

Pancreatic secretion of mammals contains about 20 principal protein species (Rinderknecht 1986). Most of these secretory proteins are directly implicated in the digestive process. Our laboratory has reported the presence in human pancreas of a protein apparently devoid of enzyme activity (Montalto et al. 1986) and named secretory pancreatic stone protein (PSP-S) because of its immunological identity with the pancreatic stone protein, the major component of the protein matrix present in calculi of patients suffering from chronic calcifying pancreatitis (CCP). In human pancreatic juice collected over an appropriate mixture of protease inhibitors, PSP-S comprised four species with apparent M_r between 16 and 20 kDa, named PSP-S2 to PSP-S5 (de Caro et al. 1988). However, immunoprecipitation of in vitro translation products of pancreatic RNAs showed that PSP-S was synthesised as a single polypeptide (Giorgi et al. 1985a). Hence, PSP-S is a protein entity with a molecular weight heterogeneity probably due to posttranslational processing. An additional PSP-S form (PSP-S1) appears in pancreatic juice upon activation. PSP-S1 with a M_r of 15 kDa derives from PSP-S2-5 by trypsin-like cleavage of an Arg–Ile bond in the NH_2-terminal part of the protein (Rouimi et al. 1987).

PSP-S1 and the form present in the calculi have the same amino acid sequence, which derives from that of PSP-S2-5 (de Caro et al. 1989): their pI are, however, different. The amino acid sequence of PSP-S2-5 comprises 144 amino acids. Trypsin-like cleavage of an Arg–Ile bond in position 11 generates an NH_2-terminal undecapeptide and the 133 amino acid polypeptide of PSP-S1. The abundance of PSP-S in juice (10%–14% of total protein) suggests that it plays an important role in pancreatic function. Experiments in vitro have shown that PSP-S inhibited calcium carbonate crystal growth (Multigner and de Caro 1987). Evidence that normal pancreatic secretion is supersaturated in calcium carbonate (Moore and Verine 1985) prompted us to suggest that the physiological role of PSP-S could be related to its inhibitory properties.

Demonstration that PSP-S concentration was diminished in the juice of patients presenting with CCP supported that hypothesis (Multigner et al. 1985). Other biological fluids like saliva or urine are supersaturated in calcium salts. The presence of proteins controlling calcium salt crystallisation has been demonstrated in these secretions (de Caro et al. 1988). We chose to rename PSP as lithostathine to clarify the PSP-S nomenclature and to account for its physiological role (Sarles et al. 1990). Lithostathines S2 to S5 (S for secretory) are the 144 amino acid secretory forms present in pancreatic juice. Lithostathine H1 and H2 (H for hydrolysed) are respectively the undecapeptide generated by trypsin-like cleavage of lithostathine S2-5 in juice and the remaining 133 amino acid form. Lithostathine C (C for calculi) is the 133 amino acid form present in calculi. Recently we have shown that the purified amino terminal undecapeptide (lithostathine H1) was able to inhibit calcite crystal growth with an efficacy similar to that of lithostathine S whereas lithostathine H2 had no effect (J. P. Bernard, 1990, personal communication). Characterisation of lithostathine by our group resulted from studies on the physiopathology of CCP. The protein was described by others, in different circumstances: Scheele et al. (1981) observed, by double-dimension gel analysis of human pancreatic proteins, the presence of several spots in the 16–19 kDa region with acidic isoelectric points which were eventually attributed to the secretory form of lithostathine. The presence of a 15 kDa protein forming fibrillar aggregates has been reported in bovine (Gross et al. 1985a) and human (Gross et al. 1985b) pancreatic tissues. This protein was named PTP for pancreatic thread protein. Sequence comparison between PTP and lithostathine S revealed that PTP was identical to lithostathine H2 (133 amino acid form). Finally, Terazono et al. (1988) described in the rat a transcript named *reg* expressed in regenerating pancreatic islets but not in mature islets. The encoded protein was proposed to play a specific role in islet regeneration. The human counterpart of the rat *reg* transcript was also isolated.

A complete sequence identity was observed between human lithostathine S and *reg* (Stewart 1989) and between rat lithostathine and *reg* mRNAs (Rouquier et al. 1991). It is now clearly established that lithostathine, PTP and *reg* are the product of the same gene (Watanabe et al. 1990; Rouquier et al. 1991).

Human Lithostathine

Human Lithostathine mRNA Sequence

A human pancreatic cDNA library was constructed in λ gt10. It was screened with a synthetic 23-mer oligonucleotide (Giorgi et al. 1989) whose sequence was derived from preliminary lithostathine protein sequence data. EcoR1-generated inserts purified from positive clones were subcloned into M13 vectors and sequenced.

The complete sequence of prelithostathine mRNA and the deduced sequence of the encoded protein are shown in Fig. 1. The size of that mRNA, estimated by Northern blot analysis of total pancreatic RNA is around 900 nucleotides.

```
agagattgttgatttgcctcttaagcaagagattcattgcagctcagc ATG GCT CAG ACC AGC    63
                                                  Met Ala Gln Thr Ser     5

TCA TAC TTC ATG CTG ATC TCC TGC CTG ATG TTT CTG TCT CAG AGC CAA GGC   114
Ser Tyr Phe Met Leu Ile Ser Cys Leu Met Phe Leu Ser Gln Ser Gln Gly    22

CAA GAG GCC CAG ACA GAG TTG CCC CAG GCC CGG ATC AGC TGC CCA GAA GGC   165
Gln Glu Ala Gln Thr Glu Leu Pro Gln Ala Arg Ile Ser Cys Pro Glu Gly    39
                                           ↑
ACC AAT GCC TAT CGC TCC TAC TGC TAC TAC TTT AAT GAA GAC CGT GAG ACC   216
Thr Asn Ala Tyr Arg Ser Tyr Cys Tyr Tyr Phe Asn Glu Asp Arg Glu Thr    56

TGG GTT GAT GCA GAT CTC TAT TGC CAG AAC ATG AAT TCG GGC AAC CTG GTG   267
Trp Val Asp Ala Asp Leu Tyr Cys Gln Asn Met Asn Ser Gly Asn Leu Val    73

TCT GTG CTC ACC CAG GCC GAG GGT GCC TTT GTG GCC TCA CTG ATT AAG GAG   318
Ser Val Leu Thr Gln Ala Glu Gly Ala Phe Val Ala Ser Leu Ile Lys Glu    90

AGT GGC ACT GAT GAC TTC AAT GTC TGG ATT GGC CTC CAT GAC CCC AAA AAG   369
Ser Gly Thr Asp Asp Phe Asn Val Trp Ile Gly Leu His Asp Pro Lys Lys   107

AAC CGC CGC TGG CAC TGG AGC AGT GGG TCC CTG GTC TCC TAC AAG TCC TGG   420
Asn Arg Arg Trp His Trp Ser Ser Gly Ser Leu Val Ser Tyr Lys Ser Trp   124

GGC ATT GGA GCC CCA AGC AGT GTT AAT CCT GGC TAC TGT GTG AGC CTG ACC   471
Gly Ile Gly Ala Pro Ser Ser Val Asn Pro Gly Tyr Cys Val Ser Leu Thr   141

TCA AGC ACA GGA TTC CAG AAA TGG AAG GAT GTG CCT TGT GAA GAC AAG TTC   522
Ser Ser Thr Gly Phe Gln Lys Trp Lys Asp Val Pro Cys Glu Asp Lys Phe   158

TCC TTT GTA TGC AAG TTC AAA AAC  tagaggcagctggaaaatacatgtctagaactgat   581
Ser Phe Val Cys Lys Phe Lys Asn                                       166

ccagcaattacaacggagtcaaaaattaaaccggaccatctctccaactcaactcaacctggacactc   649

tcttctctgctgagtttgccttgttaatcttcaatagttttacctaccccagtctttggaaccctaaa   717

taataaaaataaacatgttttccactaaaa                                        747
```

Fig. 1. Complete sequence of prelithostathine mRNA and deduced sequence of the encoded protein. The sequence was obtained from the cloned cDNA. Non-coding sequences are in lowercase letters and the two polyadenylation sites are underlined. In the protein sequence of prelithostathine S, the prepeptide is underlined and the Arg–Ile bond whose hydrolysis generates the lithostathine H forms is marked by an *arrow*. (From Giorgi et al. 1989, with permission.)

The size of the cDNA clone is 743 nucleotides excluding the poly(A) tail. This 3′ poly(A) end attached to mature lithostathine S mRNA is about 125 nucleotides long. The 3′ non-translated region comprises 197 nucleotides. Two canonical polyadenylation signals (AATAAA) are present in tandem in positions 719 and 725. The 5′ non-translated sequence comprises 74 nucleotides before the translation initiation ATG codon.

Analysis of Encoded Prelithostathine S

A single open reading frame was present in the mRNA sequence, corresponding to a preprotein of 166 amino acids with a M_r of 18690 (Fig. 1). The amino acid sequence was found to be identical to that established by de Caro et al. (1989) for lithostathine S. Prelithostathine S comprises a 22 amino acid prepeptide presenting with typical structural features of signal peptides. Mature lithostathine S is a 144 amino acid polypeptide.

Similarities Between Lithostathine and Other Proteins

A computer search for overall sequence homology confirmed that lithostathine S was distinct from other pancreatic proteins described to date and demonstrated that no identity could be found between lithostathine H2 and trypsinogen which had been suggested by Amouric et al. (1987).

Searches conducted by Petersen (1988) and Patthy (1988) for partial homologies between lithostathine S and sequences from the NBRF database pointed to an interesting similarity (up to 31% homology) between lithostathine S, thrombomodulin and several lectins. Positions of disulphide bridges were remarkably conserved. Such homology raises the question of whether lithostathine shares with those proteins carbohydrate-binding or protein-binding properties. Searching the same database with a different window, we found a significant homology in the COOH-terminal region of lithostathine S and several serine proteases (Fig. 2). The homologous region surrounded a tripeptide involved in the specificity pocket of pancreatic serine proteases (Stroud et al. 1975).

These findings raise the possibility that the lithostathine gene arose from ancestor serine and lectin genes by the shuffling of exons encoding structural or functional domains from both protein families.

Structure of the Lithostathine/*reg* Gene

During the study of the *reg* protein, Watanabe et al. (1990) have isolated from a genomic DNA library a DNA fragment containing the sequence of the lithostathine/*reg* gene. They purified from a human genomic clone a 4,2 kb EcoR1 fragment containing the entire lithostathine/*reg* gene sequence (Fig. 3). The *reg* gene is composed of six exons and five introns and contains canonical TATA boxes and CCAAT box-like sequences localised at −27 and −100 base pairs upstream from the transcriptional initiation site. Genomic DNA analysis from normal human pancreas indicated that *reg* gene is represented as a single copy per haploid genome. During this study, at least two *reg*-related sequences were demonstrated.

Lithostathine S	S	G	S	L	V	S	Y	K	S	W	G	I	G	A	P	S	S	V	N	P	G
Bov. TgI	S	G	K	L	Q	G	I	V	S	W	G	S	G	C	A	Q	K	N	K	P	G
Hum. TgI	N	G	Q	L	Q	G	V	V	S	W	G	N	G	C	A	Q	K	N	K	P	G
Hum. Plasm. Kal.	M	W	R	L	V	G	I	T	S	W	G	E	G	C	A	R	R	E	Q	P	G
Bov. ChTgA	A	W	T	L	V	G	I	V	S	W	G	S	S	T	C	S	T	S	T	P	G

Fig. 2. Sequence homology in the COOH-terminal ends of human lithostathine S and serine proteases. Sequence comparison was obtained by searching the National Biomedical Research Fund database with the FASTP program (Lipman and Parson 1985). Sequence alignment was possible without introducing deletions. Bov. TgI, bovine trypsinogen I; Hum. TgI, human trypsinogen I; Hum. Plasm. Kal., human plasmatic kallikrein; Bov. ChTgA, bovine chymotrypsinogen A. (From Giorgi et al. (1989), with permission.)

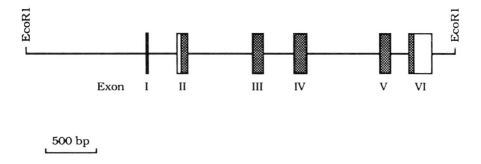

500 bp

Fig. 3. Structure of the lithostathine/*reg* gene. The six exons are indicated as boxes; filled boxes and open boxes indicate protein coding regions and untranslated regions, respectively. (From Watanabe et al. (1990), with permission.)

Expression of the Lithostathine Gene in CCP

Previous studies in our laboratory (Multigner et al. 1985; Provansal-Cheylan et al. 1989) have shown that lithostathine concentration is lowered in the pancreatic juice of patients presenting with CCP, suggesting that expression of its gene might be decreased in the disease. To test that hypothesis we quantified lithostathine mRNA concentration in the pancreas of CCP patients and in controls by dot-blot hybridisation measurements using a human lithostathine cDNA probe.

Fig. 4 represents the mRNA concentrations of lithostathine S and other secretory pancreatic proteins in the pancreas of CCP patients and controls. Lithostathine S mRNA was three times lower in CCP than in controls whereas trypsinogen, chymotrypsinogen and colipase mRNA concentrations showed no significant differences between the two groups. Thus, a decrease in tissue lithostathine S mRNA seems to be specifically associated with CCP and could account for the decreased lithostathine concentration observed in the pancreatic juice of CCP patients. In addition, decreased lithostathine gene expression seems to be a primary event in the disease since lithostathine mRNA levels of patients with lesions similar to those of CCP (e.g. in obstructive pancreatitis) are not altered, whereas in a patient with very mild lesions of CCP and no pancreatic insufficiency lithostathine mRNA was lower than in controls.

Rat Lithostathine

Animal Model for Lithostathine Gene Expression Studies

Epidemiological studies have shown that alcohol intake and a lipid-rich diet increased the risk of developing CCP (Sarles 1973). An animal model was needed to test these factors on lithostathine gene expression. Proteins immunologically related to human lithostathine and of similar size could be detected in the pancreatic juice of all mammals tested (cow, dog, monkey, pig

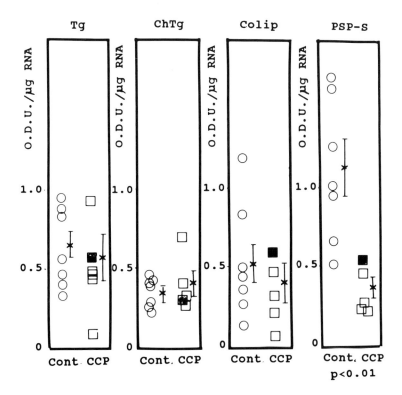

Fig. 4. mRNA concentrations of trypsinogen, chymotrypsinogen, colipase, and lithostathine S in the pancreas of CCP patients and in controls. mRNA concentrations were measured by dot-blot hybridisation of equal amounts of RNA from controls (Cont.) or CCP tissues (CCP) to ^{32}P-labelled cDNA probes. They were expressed as arbitrary OD_{492} U/µg RNA obtained after scanning the autoradiograms of the blots. O, individual data controls; □, individual data CCP patients; X, mean values (±SE) for each group. ■ in the CCP groups, the patient presenting with a mild form of the disease. The significance of the difference in lithostathine S mRNA concentration between controls and CCP patients was estimated by the Wilcoxon test. (From Giorgi et al. (1989), with permission.)

and rat) (J. P. Bernard, 1990, personal communication). Inhibition of calcium carbonate crystal growth by these proteins was demonstrated in dog and rat. More extensive studies conducted in the rat showed that a single immunoreactive form was present (M_r 17000) which bound to calcium carbonate crystals with a K_d similar to human lithostathine (J. P. Bernard, 1990, personal communication). Using a human cDNA probe, we have cloned and sequenced rat lithostathine mRNA (Rouquier et al. 1991). The rat lithostathine mRNA is 783 nucleotides long and encodes a preprotein of 165 amino acids including a prepeptide of 21 amino acids; rat and human lithostathine S show 70% identity and the mature proteins have the same length (144 amino acids). Given this high degree of similarity, rat lithostathine also presents sequence homologies with pancreatic serine proteases and lectins, as already described for the human protein (Giorgi et al. 1989).

Effect of Ethanol Consumption on Lithostathine Gene Expression

Epidemiological studies have shown that in Western countries, CCP is almost always linked to chronic alcohol consumption (Sarles 1973). However, most alcoholics never show clinical symptoms of the disease. Previous studies indicated that chronic ethanol intoxication (20% ethanol) in the rat could induce pancreatic lesions similar to those of human chronic pancreatitis (Sarles et al. 1971). Lithostathine gene expression was, therefore, studied in rats submitted to 20% ethanol intoxication for 4 months. No difference could be found in lithostathine mRNA concentration between alcohol-drinking and control rats. In this protocol, ethanol had no direct effect on lithostathine gene expression. Hence, alcohol might facilitate stone formation by interacting with parameters other than lithostathine, or by altering lithostathine gene expression only in individuals with a genetic predisposition.

Regulation of Lithostathine Gene Expression by Food Content

Epidemiological studies have also pointed out the role of nutritional status in the risk of developing CCP (Sarles 1973). We compared lithostathine mRNA concentrations using dot-blot techniques in the pancreas of rats adapted to different diets to determine whether lithostathine gene expression was influenced by food composition. Results and details of the dietary composition are given in Table 1. Three groups of rats (I, II, III) were adapted to diets containing 15%, 25% or 70% protein respectively. Data shown in Table 1 indicate that lithostathine mRNA concentration was 3.2 and 12.3 times higher in groups II and III (high protein) than in group I (low protein), whereas chymotrypsinogen B (ChTgB) and trypsinogen I (TgI) mRNA concentrations increased only four times in group III. On the other hand, amylase mRNA concentrations were related to diet carbohydrate content, as described by Giorgi et al. (1984). It is very intriguing that concentration of a mRNA encoding a protein devoid of proteolytic activity should be 12 times higher with a high protein diet than

Table 1. Quantification of lithostathine S, amylase, trypsinogen I (TgI), and chymotrypsinogen B (ChTgB) mRNAs in total pancreatic RNA from animals adapted to different diets

mRNA	Diets		
	I	II	III
Lithostathine S	65.1 ± 6.6	207.7 ± 19.7	802.4 ± 79.7
Amylase	751.3 ± 78.2	83.6 ± 9.4	385.8 ± 39.8
Tg I	78.7 ± 7.7	151.5 ± 16.2	277.8 ± 28.5
ChTgB	103.4 ± 11.2	270.2 ± 26.6	407.1 ± 46.4

Results (in arbitrary scanner units/microgram of RNA) are expressed as arithmetical means ±SE ($n=4$) of the dot-blot experiments.
Composition (% w/w) of the diets in protein, lipid, and carbohydrate: I, 15, 4, 75; II, 25, 58, 11; III, 70, 4, 20, respectively.
From Rouquier et al. (1991), with permission.

with a low protein diet when protease (TgI, ChTgB) mRNA concentrations were only four times greater in the same conditions (Giorgi et al. 1985b). This can be related to the similarity reported above between lithostathine and serine proteases, suggesting that the two molecules could derive from a common ancestor gene. The lithostathine gene could have retained during evolution part of the promoter region of the protease gene family.

Lithostathine and Pancreatic Regeneration

Claims were made (Terazono et al. 1988) that lithostathine/*reg* was expressed in regenerating islets but not in mature islets, and was therefore involved in the regeneration process. This was surprising because of the high level of lithostathine/*reg* gene expression in mature exocrine tissue and also because lithostathine is a secretory crystal growth inhibitor. To get further insight into that problem, we studied the expression of the gene in exocrine and endocrine tissue during regeneration following subtotal pancreatectomy. Important expression was confirmed in regenerating islets. However, it remained negligible compared to expression in exocrine tissue. This was later confirmed by Miyaura et al. (1991). A transient 3–4-fold increase in expression was also observed in exocrine tissue in the early hours of regeneration. A similar observation was made during taurocholate-induced acute pancreatitis in the rat: lithostathine/*reg* mRNA concentration increased threefold during the day following induction and then returned to control levels, whereas regeneration proceeded. It was concluded that increased expression of the gene was temporally correlated to tissue inflammation rather than to regeneration. Expression during islet cell regeneration suggests that lithostathine/*reg* mRNA is synthesised at an early stage of pancreatic cell differentiation. Acinar and islet cells being of the same embryological origin (Pictet et al. 1972), dedifferentiated cells expressing the gene might be present during acute pancreatic inflammation and in regenerating islets as well.

Other Roles for Lithostathine?

Previous studies (Gross et al. 1985a,b) showed that the hydrolysed form of lithostathine (H2 form) (PTP), was detected as a fibrillar protein forming filaments in bovine and human pancreas. More recently, accumulation of lithostathine/PTP was detected in several areas of brain from patients presenting with Alzheimer's disease (Ozturk et al. 1989) and in the human developing brain (de la Monte 1990). Other studies (Watanabe et al. 1990) reported that lithostathine/*reg*/PTP was detected in several gastrointestinal tumors (stomach, colon, rectum). These data suggest that the lithostathine/*reg* gene is expressed during the development or dedifferentiation of other tissues than pancreas. Whether its function in those tissues is related to its properties of binding calcium salt crystals or to its lectin-like structure remains unknown.

Conclusion

Lithostathine is an inhibitor of calcium carbonate crystal growth synthesised by the exocrine pancreas and presenting structural homology with lectins. Expression of the lithostathine gene is regulated by food composition and increases with dietary protein content. Chronic calcifying pancreatitis is associated with decreased lithostathine gene expression which seems primary to the disease. Structural or functional alterations in the promoter region of the lithostathine gene are therefore expected in CCP patients, but remain to be characterised.

Exocrine pancreas is the only mature tissue where lithostathine expression has been demonstrated. The gene is, however, activated during differentiation of several other tissues, suggesting that lithostathine might be more than a crystal growth inhibitor.

References

Amouric M, Barthe C, Kopeyan C, Figarella C, Guy-Crotte O (1987) Protein X, a proteolysis product of human pancreatic juice. Immunological relationship to trypsinogen I. Biol Chem Hoppe Seyler 368:1525–1532

de Caro A, Multigner AL, Dagorn JC, Sarles H (1988) The human pancreatic stone protein. Biochimie (Paris) 70:1209–1214

de Caro A, Adrich Z, Fournet B et al. (1989) N-terminal sequence extension in the glycosylated forms of human pancreatic stone protein. The 5-oxoproline N-terminal chain is O-glycosylated on the 5th amino acid residue. Biochim Biophys Acta 994:281–284

de la Monte SM, Ozturk M, Wands JR (1990) Enhanced expression of an exocrine pancreatic protein in Alzheimer's disease and the developing human brain. J Clin Invest 86:1004–1013

Giorgi D, Bernard JP, Lapointe R, Dagorn JC (1984) Regulation of amylase messenger RNA concentration in rat pancreas by food content. EMBO J 3:1521–1524

Giorgi D, Bernard JP, De Caro A et al. (1985a) Pancreatic stone protein. I Evidence that it is encoded by a pancreatic messenger ribonucleic acid. Gastroenterology 89:381–386

Giorgi D, Renaud W, Bernard JP, Dagorn JC (1985b) Regulation of proteolytic enzyme activities and mRNA concentrations in rat pancreas by food content. Biochem Biophys Res Commun 127:937–942

Giorgi D, Bernard JP, Rouquier S, Iovanna J, Sarles H, Dagorn JC (1989) Secretory pancreatic stone protein messenger RNA. Nucleotide sequence and its expression in chronic calcifying pancreatitis. J Clin Invest 84:100–106

Gross J, Brauer AW, Bringhurst RF, Corbett C, Margolies MN (1985a) An unusual bovine pancreatic protein exhibiting pH-dependent globule-fibril transformation and unique amino acid sequence. Proc Natl Acad Sci USA 82:5627–5631

Gross J, Carlson RI, Brauer AW, Margolies MN, Warshaw AL, Wands JR (1985b) Isolation, characterization and distribution of an unusual pancreatic human secretory protein. J Clin Invest 76:2115–2126

Lipman DJ, Parson WR (1985) Rapid and sensitive protein similarity searches. Science 227:1435–1441

Miyaura C, Chen L, Appel M, et al. (1991) Expression of reg/PSP, a pancreatic exocrine gene: Relationship to changes in islet β-cell mass. Mol Endocrinol (in press)

Montalto G, Bonicel J, Multigner L, Rovery M, Sarles H, de Caro A (1986) Partial amino acid sequence of human pancreatic stone protein, a novel pancreatic secretory protein. Biochem J 238:227–232

Moore EW, Verine HJ (1985) Pathogenesis of pancreatic and biliary $CaCO_3$ lithiasis: the solubility product (K'sp) of calcite determined with the Ca^{++} electrode. J Lab Clin Med 106:611–618

Multigner L, de Caro A (1987) Pancreatic stone protein. Kinetic studies on calcium carbonate crystal growth inhibition by human pancreatic stone protein. Digestion 38:43–44

Multigner L, Sarles H, Lombardo D, De Caro A (1985) Pancreatic stone protein. II Implication in stone formation during the course of chronic calcifying pancreatitis. Gastroenterology 89:387–391

Ozturk M, de la Monte SM, Gross J, Wands J (1989) Elevated levels of an exocrine pancreatic secretory protein in Alzheimer disease brain. Proc Natl Acad Sci USA 86:419–423

Patthy L (1988) Homology of human pancreatic stone protein with animal lectins. Biochem J 253:309–311

Petersen TE (1988) The amino-terminal domain of thrombomodulin and pancreatic stone protein are homologous with lectins. FEBS Lett 231:51–53

Pictet RL, Clark WR, Williams RH, Rutter WJ (1972) An ultrastructural analysis of the developing embryonic pancreas. Dev Biol 29:436–467

Provansal-Cheylan M, Mariani A, Bernard JP, Sarles H, Dupuy P (1989) Pancreatic stone protein: quantification in pancreatic juice by enzyme-linked immunosorbent assay and comparison with others methods. Pancreas 4:680–689

Rinderknecht H (1986) Pancreatic secretory enzymes. In: Go VLW, Gardner JD, Brooks FP, Lebenthal E, DiMagno EP, Scheele JA (eds) The exocrine pancreas: biology, pathology and diseases, Raven Press, New York, pp163–183

Rouimi P, Bonicel J, Rovery M, De Caro A (1987) Cleavage of the Arg-Ile bond in the native polypeptide chain of the human pancreatic stone protein. FEBS Lett 216:195–199

Rouqier S, Verdier JM, Iovanna J, Dagorn JC, Giorgi D (1991) Rat pancreatic stone protein messenger RNA. Abundant expression in mature exocrine cells, regulation by food content, and sequence identity with the endocrine reg transcript. J Biol Chem 266:786–787

Sarles H (1973) An international survey on nutrition and pancreatitis. Digestion 9:389–403

Sarles H, Lebreuil G, Tasso F et al. (1971) A comparison of alcoholic pancreatitis in rat and man. Gut 12:377–388

Sarles H, Dagorn JC, Giorgi D, Bernard JP (1990) Renaming pancreatic stone protein as 'lithostathine'. Gastroenterology 99:900–905

Scheele G, Bartelt D, Bieger W (1981) Characterization of human exocrine pancreatic proteins by two-dimensional isoelectric focusing/sodium dodecylsulphate gel electrophoresis. Gastroenterology 80:461–473

Stewart TA (1989) The human reg gene encodes pancreatic stone protein. Biochem J 260:622–623

Stroud RM, Krieger M, Koeppe RE, Kossiakoff AA, Chambers JL (1975) Structure–function relationships in the serine proteases. In: Reich E, Rifkin DB, Shaw E (eds) Proteases and biological control. Cold Spring Harbor Laboratory, New York, pp13–32

Terazono K, Yamamoto H, Takasawa S et al. (1988) A novel gene activated in regenerating islets. J Biol Chem 263:2111–2114

Watanabe T, Yonekura H, Terazono K, Yamamoto H, Okamoto H (1990) Complete nucleotide sequence of human reg gene and its expression in normal and tumoral tissues. The reg protein, pancreatic stone protein, and pancreatic thread protein are one and the same product of the gene. J Biol Chem 265:7432–7439

Chapter 19

Endoscopic Therapy in Chronic Pancreatitis

A. R. W. Hatfield

Over the last few years, the role of endoscopic sphincterotomy and gallstone removal in severe acute pancreatitis has been well established. However, the role of a variety of endoscopic manoeuvres in chronic pancreatitis is far less well established. There are indeed many endoscopic techniques which could be used in the non-surgical management of this condition. These include sphincterotomy, dilatation, stent insertion, drainage tube insertion and pancreatic stone removal or lithotripsy. Although these techniques are technically possible and represent enormous challenges for the endoscopist, the clinician must question whether they are actually helpful for the patient.

One of the earlier procedures was the use of endoscopic sphincterotomy to divide either the biliary or the pancreatic sphincter to improve drainage in patients with chronic pancreatitis. This would seem to have no relevance in the majority of patients with chronic pancreatitis, unless there is clear evidence of a discrete and localised stenosis of the papilla of Vater. A few such patients are seen following iatrogenic damage to the papilla sustained during previous endoscopic attempts at therapy.

Duct Occlusion

About ten years ago there was a vogue for instilling tissue glue into the pancreatic duct system at the time of endoscopic retrograde cholangiopancreatography (ERCP) in patients with severe painful chronic pancreatitis, in the hope that this might obliterate the pancreatic duct system and cause atrophy of the gland and so reduce the pain. This technique caused horrendous post-procedure pancreatitis and produced no lasting benefit to the patient, so the technique has been abandoned.

Pancreas Divisum (Isolated Dorsal Pancreas)

Endoscopic therapy has been used in patients with pancreatitis secondary to pancreas divisum, in an attempt to improve drainage from the dorsal pancreatic system at the level of the accessory papilla. Initial attempts to improve pancreatic drainage via endoscopic sphincterotomy of the accessory papilla produced very little sustained benefit, and such sphincterotomies were associated with complications and often would close up rapidly. In retrospect, such attempts were unwise and very careful surgery with a sphincteroplasty at the level of the accessory papilla with a mucosa to mucosa anastomosis is more appropriate.

In patients with pancreas divisum it is logical to attempt a trial period of endoscopic drainage of the dorsal pancreas to see whether pain can be improved. This is best achieved by temporary endoscopic stenting. After a small accessory papilla sphincterotomy, an 8, 10 or 12 FG prosthesis can be inserted into the pancreatic duct system to provide drainage. There is debate as to whether the stent should be extremely short just to straddle the area of the accessory papilla, or whether it should be longer with a series of side holes. It is also uncertain as to whether these stents should be left in for a short period of time – 1–2 months – or whether they can be left in for up to 6 months. In patients in whom pain has been improved by a period of endoscopic drainage it is logical to attempt a more permanent surgical drainage procedure to the pancreas, providing the dorsal duct is dilated.

There is an argument that it would be better to perform a pancreaticojejunostomy without a previous endoscopic intervention in order to have a dilated duct for anastomosis. This follows from the observation that prior endoscopic stenting of the obstructive biliary tree makes it far more difficult to perform an adequate biliary anastomosis at a later date, due to the duct being decompressed and somewhat inflamed and thickened, which makes any anastomosis technically difficult. The same problems would undoubtedly apply to the pancreatic duct system, but might be even more problematical for the surgeon.

Failure to relieve symptoms after a trial of endoscopic stenting of the dorsal duct system in pancreas divisum suggests that the patient might be better treated with a resection rather than a drainage procedure.

Pseudocysts

Reports of technical success of pseudocyst drainage using endoscopically placed drainage tubes demonstrate that the technique works to a degree. Using the gastric route or the medial wall of the second part of the duodenum, a pseudocyst can be punctured using a sheathed needle passed down the endoscope. A guide wire is inserted over which a pigtail drainage catheter can be passed and left in situ. The size of the drainage tube is limited by the diameter of the channel of the endoscope and the other disadvantage is the length of the drainage tube, which is then rerouted through the nose in the same way as a nasobiliary drainage catheter. In the vast majority of cases, when non-surgical management of pseudocysts is indicated, this is best achieved by direct percutaneous puncture under ultrasound guidance, using shorter and larger diameter drainage catheters.

Pancreatic Duct Drainage

In European endoscopic literature, one often sees extremely attractive pictures of stents in main pancreatic ducts across neoplastic strictures to "improve drainage". This sort of manoeuvre is treating a radiograph and not the patient. Marked steatorrhoea due to carcinoma of the pancreas is not common, and when it does occur can be treated adequately with pancreatic replacement therapy. In patients with chronic pancreatitis with obstruction due to stones or strictures and associated exocrine insufficiency and steatorrhoea, endoscopic stenting is equally irrelevant, as the loss of function is probably mainly due to destruction of the gland itself and not just to the apparent obstruction.

Endoscopic procedures such as dilatation and stent insertion performed to relieve pain in chronic pancreatitis in patients with stricture or pancreatic duct stones are certainly possible, but in my own experience such manoeuvres are often disappointing. It is well known that the incidence of obstructing lesions such as stones or strictures is similar in patients with and without pain, and very often strictures and stone formation are secondary to the chronic pancreatitis process, rather than a primary cause for pain. There is certainly a small group of patients in whom proximal obstruction due to stricture or pancreatic stone formation appears to be a major cause of recurrent attacks, particularly if the remainder of the pancreas looks relatively normal. Theoretically, an attempt to improve the drainage from the pancreas in these patients might not only relieve pain, but might also preserve what exocrine and endocrine function remains and stop further deterioration. The evidence to support this approach is sparse.

Fig. 1(a) shows a pancreatogram of a 40-year-old woman who had 5 years of severe painful chronic pancreatitis following previous endoscopic sphincterotomy for gallstones, complicated by pancreatitis. The patient probably developed a proximal pancreatic stricture as a result. In this patient the stricture was dilated using a 6 mm Olbert catheter passed over a guide wire that had been inserted into the pancreatic duct system (Fig. 1b). Successful dilatation was obtained on radiological grounds and although this benefited the patient in the short term, she eventually needed a subtotal pancreatectomy for recurrent severe attacks of pancreatitis.

Lithotripsy

Occasionally, one sees patients with a solitary pancreatic calculus obstructing the pancreatic duct adjacent to the papilla, and it is tempting to remove such

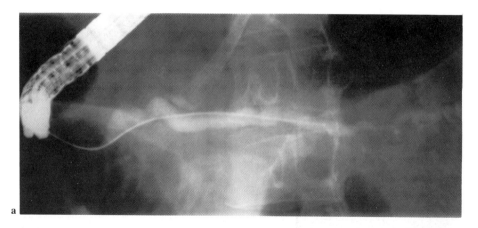

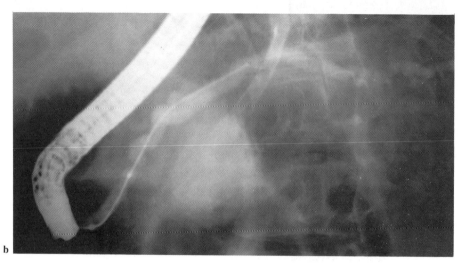

Fig. 1. a This pancreatogram shows a stricture in the proximal pancreatic duct adjacent to a stenosed sphincterotomy site. **b** The pancreatic duct has been cannulated with a guide wire, over which has been passed an Olbert dilatation catheter which has been fully inflated with successful dilatation of the stricture.

a calculus on the grounds that it may be cause for symptoms. Unfortunately, many of these calculi are encased in an area of fibrosis and cannot be removed even following pancreatic sphincterotomy. In such cases, the use of extracorporeal shock-wave lithotripsy (ESWL) can be extremely successful in fragmenting the calculus so that the fragments can then pass out of the pancreatic duct via the sphincterotomy. This sequence of events is shown in Fig. 2. In a 38-year-old man with severe painful chronic pancreatitis a single calculus was demonstrated at ERCP. Following sphincterotomy it proved impossible to extract the stone from the pancreatic duct system. ESWL successfully fragmented the calculus, and at the follow-up ERCP the pancreatic duct system was completely clear and draining well. In this particular patient, dramatic resolution of his pancreatic pain was achieved.

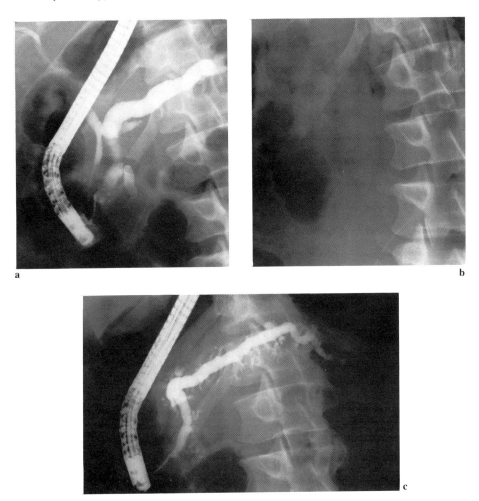

Fig. 2. a This pancreatogram shows a large calcified stone impacted in the proximal pancreatic duct adjacent to the papilla. b This abdominal radiograph, taken 24 h after extracorporeal lithotripsy, shows the pancreatic calculus fragmented with a much reduced size. c This pancreatogram, performed two weeks after shock-wave lithotripsy, shows that there is no residual calculus and the pancreatic duct is draining freely through the pancreatic sphincterotomy.

Conclusion

In conclusion, although many endoscopic techniques are available that may be used in patients with chronic pancreatitis, there are relatively few patients in whom they may actually be appropriate. These techniques are of importance. First, in the temporary drainage of the dorsal pancreatic duct system in pancreas divisum to see whether pain can be relieved, prior to a permanent surgical procedure. Second, proximal pancreatic obstruction due to solitary calculus may be the single most important indication for endoscopic therapy. In uncommon cases, a combination of endoscopic sphincterotomy and ESWL offers an effective alternative management to surgery.

Chapter 20

Pathophysiology of Acute Pancreatitis

K. Ohlsson and S. Genell

Introduction

It is generally agreed that the main aetiological factors of pancreatitis are bile tract disease and alcoholism. Despite much experimental work the mechanism by which these factors induce pancreatitis is still obscure. The time-honoured concept is that the fundamental cause of the pathological changes in acute pancreatitis is autodigestion of the organ, mediated by the pancreatic enzymes (Chiari 1886). Though this proposal is still generally accepted, our knowledge of acute pancreatitis is today still far from complete and no unanimity has been achieved concerning the enzymatic processes leading to the typical anatomical and pathophysiological alterations. Nor has agreement been attained on the mechanism of the intrapancreatic activation of enzymes.

According to one recent theory, which has met with considerable interest, the intra-acinar activation of digestive enzymes results from their intracellular co-localisation with lysosomal hydrolases such as cathepsin B. The data supporting the theory were obtained from two experimental models of acute pancreatitis; one induced by feeding young female mice a choline-deficient, ethionine-supplemented diet (Koike et al. 1982) and another induced by infusing rats with a dose of the secretagogue caerulein in excess of that which stimulates a maximal rate of pancreatic protein secretion (Saluja et al. 1987).

However, these observations cannot be extrapolated to the situation in human pancreatitis, as the clinical disease obviously does not result from ethionine injections and is unlikely to be the result of supramaximal secretagogue stimulation. However, duct obstruction in rabbits has also been shown to cause co-localisation of digestive enzyme zymogens and lysosomal hydrolases within acinar cells (Saluja et al. 1989).

Although the critical initial process leading to the activation of enzymes is still obscure a large body of data supports the assumption that the intrapancreatic activation of digestive enzymes as well as injury to the gland by activated proteolytic and lipolytic enzymes are important early events in the pathogenesis of acute pancreatitis. This chapter summarises current knowledge about the endogenous turnover of pancreatic and leucocyte proteases and the relevant inhibitors, focusing on trypsin(ogen) and pancreatic secretory trypsin inhibitor (PSTI) in normal conditions and in acute pancreatitis.

Evidence is presented for the existence of a local protease–antiprotease imbalance; initially caused mainly by pancreatic proteases and then with an increasing contribution from leucocyte proteases which finally results in the activation of the cascade systems and severe pathophysiological changes.

Trypsin in Acute Pancreatitis

The trypsin concept recently gained extensive support from two studies of experimental pancreatitis showing that recombinant human PSTI (rhPSTI) effectively blocked the protease cascade and drastically improved survival rate. Acute haemorrhagic pancreatitis was induced in rats by intraductal injection of sodium taurocholate. In one group of rats the injection of taurocholate was preceded by the intraductal injection of rhPSTI. In a second group of rats rhPSTI was given intraperitoneally starting 15 min after the induction of acute pancreatitis. The survival rate in a control group of rats was 13%. In contrast, the survival rate in groups receiving rhPSTI intraductally or intraperitoneally was 80% and 63%, respectively (Ohlsson et al. 1989).

In a second study, haemorrhagic pancreatitis was induced in dogs by intraductal injection of bile. The survival rate in a control group of dogs was 40% after 24 h and 0 after 48 h. In contrast all the dogs which received a single intraductal dose of rhPSTI, either immediately before the bile injection or mixed with the bile, recovered from the disease. Detailed biochemical and immunohistological studies in the dog indicate that, whereas rhPSTI cannot prevent the initial detergent-induced tissue injury, it does completely prevent major trypsinogen activation and the trypsin-induced protease cascade. The animals can evidently cope with the non-specific tissue damage caused by the intraductal bile/bile acids (Ohlsson et al. 1989).

Between 0.01% and 0.1% of the total trypsinogen production in the pancreas is normally distributed to the extracellular tissue fluids surrounding the gland and eventually reaches the general circulation, resulting in a physiological serum concentration of trypsinogen of about 25–50 µg/l (Borgström and Ohlsson 1976, 1978a; Geokas et al. 1979). This endogenous trypsinogen is eliminated from the circulation without activation, most probably by glomerular filtration and variable tubular absorption in the kidney.

There is no consumption of or interaction with protease inhibitors during the normal endogenous turnover of trypsinogen, whereas after activation of trypsin as in acute pancreatitis, complexes between trypsin and plasma and local protease inhibitors have been demonstrated (Balldin and Ohlsson 1979). In recent studies, interest has been focused on the leakage of pancreatic enzymes through basolateral membranes of the acinar cell. One hypothesis is that this might be of significant importance in pancreatitis. The secretion products are blocked within the pancreas and cannot enter the duct in the normal way and are instead discharged through the basolateral membrane, thereby increasing the interstitial concentration of proenzymes (Andersson et al. 1990). Alpha-1 protease inhibitor (α_1PI) and alpha-2 macroglobulin (α_2M) are quantitatively the dominating trypsin inhibitors in serum (Table 1).

Pancreatic juice contains only trace amounts of these inhibitors, but it does contain a specific trypsin inhibitor, PSTI, at a concentration corresponding to about 2% of the total potential content of trypsin (Kazal et al. 1948; Eddeland and Ohlsson 1978a,b; Eddeland and Wehlin 1978). PSTI was originally thought to be produced only in the pancreatic gland but later results indicate that PSTI is also produced in various other secretory cells in the gastrointestinal tract, including the Paneth cells (Fukayama et al. 1986; Bohe et al. 1986, 1987).

Trypsin, initially bound by PSTI, is rapidly taken over by the protease inhibitors, mainly α_2M present in plasma and tissue fluids (Eddeland and Ohlsson 1978a–c). Thus trypsin–PSTI complexes are not found in plasma in acute pancreatitis. Trypsin is also preferentially bound by α_2M following the addition of small amounts of the enzyme to normal serum (Ohlsson et al. 1971; Balldin et al. 1981) (Fig. 1). The ratio between the amount of trypsin bound to α_2M and to α_1PI in vitro for man is about 70/30. Trypsin–α_2M complexes given intravenously to man are rapidly eliminated from the circulation, having a half-life in the circulation of 10 min (Ohlsson 1971b,c; Ohlsson and Laurell 1976). Pronounced complex formation thus leads to decreased plasma levels of α_2M, which is a finding in severe pancreatitis. The complexes are mainly phagocytosed and degraded in the liver by the Kupffer cells (Ohlsson 1971b,c) and the hepatocytes (Gliemann et al. 1983). A major part of the protease–α_2M complexes formed in the interstitial tissue is probably phagocytosed by local macrophages in the tissue and regional lymph nodes (Ekerot and Ohlsson 1982). The elimination of trypsin α_1PI complexes is less rapid, having a half-life in the circulation of 2–3 h.

High levels of trypsin-like immunoreactivity can be demonstrated in serum and peritoneal fluid during acute pancreatitis. The immunoreactive (ir) material is contained in two fractions with different molecular weights, free trypsinogen, and trypsin i complexed with protease inhibitors, mainly α_1PI (Borgström and Ohlsson 1978b; Geokas et al. 1979; Borgström and Lasson 1984). Likewise α_1PI-bound trypsin is present in serum and peritoneal exudates of dogs with experimental pancreatitis (Ohlsson 1971a; Ohlsson and Eddeland 1975). It should be added that trypsin bound by α_2M is not detectable by radioimmunoassay (Fig. 1). Thus the immunoreactive α_1PI-bound trypsin represents only a minor part of the active trypsin released. The presence of trypsin complexed with protease inhibitors indicates the formation of active trypsin during acute pancreatitis. Furthermore, active trypsin as well as elastase and chymotrypsin have been demonstrated in exudates collected directly from the pancreatic

Table 1. Main endogenous trypsin inhibitors

	Molecular mass (kDa)	Concentration in	
		Serum	Pancreatic juice
α_1PI	55	1.35 g/l	trace amounts
α_2M	725	1.8 g/l	trace amounts
PSTI	6.5	10–15 µg/l	50–100 mg/l

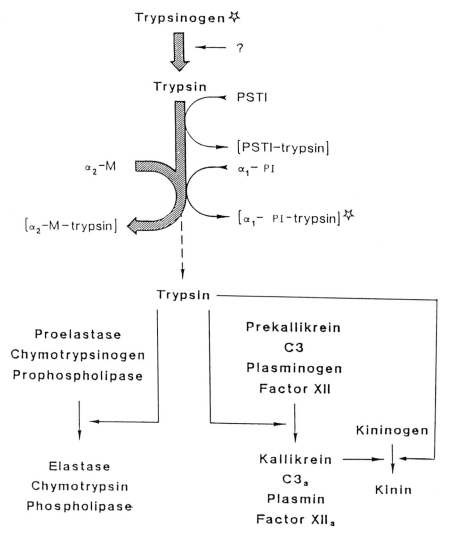

Fig. 1. Some interactions between proteases, inhibitors and the cascade systems during acute pancreatitis. ☆ immunoreactive trypsin.

surface in bile-induced pancreatitis in dogs (Ohlsson and Eddeland 1975). The release of active trypsin is a very early event in experimental pancreatitis (Ohlsson and Eddeland 1975; Ohlsson et al. 1989). This also appears to be true for human pancreatitis since the highest plasma levels of ir α_1PI-bound trypsin are often found within 24 h of the onset of symptoms of pancreatitis. (Borgström and Lasson 1984).

Early release of active trypsin is also supported by data from studies of ir trypsin in plasma after endoscopic retrograde cholangiopancreatography (ERCP) and papillotomy. Severe acute pancreatitis with a mortality of 70%–100% has been reported in 1%–2% of these procedures (Bilbao et al.

1976; Hamilton et al. 1983). A rise in serum amylase is in fact a regular finding after ERCP and transient abdominal pain is not uncommon but this has not been considered to constitute true pancreatitis (Raphael 1987). In a group of 50 patients undergoing ERCP, 12 had transient (24–48 h) abdominal pain compatible with mild pancreatitis. All of these patients had high amylase and high ir trypsinogen levels in their plasma within a few hours of ERCP. Furthermore, a simultaneous rise in plasma levels of ir α_1PI-bound trypsin was seen (unpublished). Active trypsin is probably of major pathogenetic significance since trypsin is able to activate all cascade systems as well as all the proenzymes in the pancreatic secretion (Fig. 1).

Peritoneal exudates from patients with severe acute pancreatitis contain a much higher concentration of α_1PI-bound trypsin than serum. Chymotrypsin and elastase are also found complexed with this inhibitor and with α_2M (Geokas et al. 1978; Balldin and Ohlsson 1979). In one study, about 15% of the α_1PI of the peritoneal exudate was found in a complexed form, while about 65% of the α_2M was enzyme-bound (Balldin and Ohlsson 1979). A further strong indication of pronounced α_2M consumption in pancreatitis is the low plasma levels found in severe cases (Lasson and Ohlsson 1984a; McMahon et al. 1984). The appearance of large amounts of inhibitor-bound elastase and chymotrypsin (Balldin and Ohlsson 1979; Satake et al. 1982) together with active phospholipase (PLA_2) (Schröder et al. 1980; Nevalainen 1988) in plasma and in the peritoneal exudates provides strong evidence of the release of active trypsin in areas with insufficient inhibitor protection, resulting in proenzyme activation. The different active enzymes may then contribute to the tissue damage.

Leucocyte Proteases

Recent data indicate that leucocyte proteases may be of pathophysiological significance in severe acute pancreatitis (Fritz et al. 1986; Balldin et al. 1989; Axelsson et al. 1990). Bile-induced canine pancreatitis was thus characterised by a pronounced release of leucocyte elastase during the later stage of the disease with very high levels, especially in the peritoneal exudate. This pattern parallels earlier observations of frequently seen heavy infiltration of polymorphonuclear (PMN) leucocytes into the necrotic areas of the gland in the same model (Bergenfeldt et al. 1989). These leucocytes are recruited as a part of the cascade events of the acute phase response. The clearly demonstrable but much less pronounced increase in the plasma level of leucocyte elastase is explained by the time taken for the complexes to reach the plasma and the probable elimination of large amounts of the complexes in the phagocytosing cells of the reticuloendothelial system (Ekerot and Ohlsson 1982).

Human PMN neutrophils contain large amounts of several serine proteases, which are active at neutral pH (Table 2). They have the capacity to degrade, or in some cases, activate a major part of the proteins within the cascade systems. Likewise all components of the connective tissue are potential substrates. Elastase is the most studied of these proteases and in several studies of sepsis (Fritz et al. 1986) it has been held responsible as an important

Table 2. Natural protease inhibitors of PMN leucocyte neutral proteases

	Azurophil granules			Collagenase specific granules[d]
	Elastase[a]	Cathepsin G[b]	NP4[c]	
Leucocyte content (μg/10^6 PMN)	3	1.5	3	0.07
Alpha$_1$-PI	90*	2*	60*	
Alpha$_2$-M	10*	86*	40*	+ +
Alpha$_1$-ACHY	0*	12*	0*	
β_1-anticollagenase				+ +
SLPI[e]		+ +	+	
UTI[f]	+			

* Percentage binding on addition of the protease to plasma in an amount corresponding to 1% of the total inhibiting capacity.
SLPI, secretory leucocyte protease inhibitor; UTI, urinary trypsin inhibitor.
[a] Ohlsson and Olsson (1974), Baugh and Travis (1976), Salvesen et al. (1987)
[b] Odeberg et al. (1975), Sinha et al. (1987)
[c] Ohlsson et al. (1990)
[d] MacCartney and Tschesche (1983)
[e] Ohlsson et al. (1988)
[f] Jönsson et al. (1982)

pathogenetic factor. The normal daily turnover of neutral leucocyte proteases has been estimated at about 1 g (Ohlsson and Olsson 1977). This normal turnover involves at least to some extent the plasma protease inhibitors, as judged by the finding that the immunoreactive elastase in plasma is present as elastase–α_1PI complexes. The major leucocyte protease inhibitors are shown in Table 2. SLPI is a low-molecular-weight (12 kDa) inhibitor, stable at acid pH, which has been isolated from parotid saliva and characterised (Thompson and Ohlsson 1986; Ohlsson et al. 1988). It is the dominating inhibitor in the respiratory tract mucosa and secretions and it is also found in the male and female genital tract. In addition to leucocyte proteases it also inhibits chymotrypsin very strongly and it is a relatively potent inhibitor of trypsin and human pancreatic elastase. We found that SLPI offers good protection in vitro against degradation of plasma proteins induced by leucocyte elastase (Axelsson et al. 1988; Björk et al. 1988). Its capacity to block trypsin-induced cleavage of C3 and kininogen in vitro in plasma was, however, much less than that for aprotinin (Balldin et al. 1980) and PSTI (Ohlsson 1986). In inflammatory pulmonary processes also, like those complicating acute pancreatitis, SLPI may help to protect the lung against tissue digestion by leucocyte proteases, besides its role in protecting the ciliated epithelium. High plasma levels of SLPI have been demonstrated in pneumonia (Fryksmark et al. 1984). Interestingly, we demonstrated recently that high levels of leucocyte elastase–α_1PI complexes in the peritoneal exudate in clinical pancreatitis was an early indication of local abscess formation which was evident several days prior to the clinical diagnosis of the abscess. Besides probable pathophysiological significance this observation has diagnostic potential as abscess formation is a severe complication to acute pancreatitis with a high mortality (Balldin et al. 1989).

PLA_2 is found not only in pancreatic juice, but also in various cellular materials. Neutrophils contain soluble Ca^{2+}-dependent secretory PLA_2 with an acidic pH optimum that is activated on phagocytosis. They also contain a membrane-bound, Ca^{2+}-dependent PLA_2 with a neutral pH optimum which is probably released into inflammatory exudates in acute pancreatitis and peritonitis. Biological inhibitors, like lipocortin, have been purified from stimulated macrophages and from inflammatory exudates. The relevance of lipocortins as PLA_2 inhibitors is, however, debatable at present, partly because of their tendency to bind to phospholipids rather than to PLA_2 (Davidsson and Dennis 1989).

The Cascade Systems

Complement

Trypsin-like enzymes play an important role in the normal function of the cascade systems. Thus activated trypsin can, if uninhibited, cause severe disturbances by irregular activation of these systems. The release of large amounts of vasoactive substances is then the natural consequence as evidenced by many studies (Balldin et al. 1980).

Low plasma levels of C3 are a frequent finding in acute pancreatitis, indicating consumption, as C3 is an acute phase reactant and other acute phase reactants such as α_1-antichymotrypsin, α_1PI and CRP show very high plasma levels in this disease. A strong indication of complement activation is also the regular finding of C3 degradation products in plasma. In peritoneal exudates C3 is frequently completely cleaved in severe pancreatitis (Balldin et al. 1981; Lasson et al. 1985). The release of C5a from C5 can cause the aggregation of leucocytes and these aggregates may be trapped in the lung and lead to tissue damage and impaired function. C3a and C5a may participate in the inflammatory response by affecting smooth muscle contraction in the arterioli and in the airway passages (Jacob and Hammerschmidt 1982; Roxvall et al. 1989). By inducing increased vascular permeability, they promote the formation of oedema. It has been shown that anaphylotoxins stimulate the biosynthesis of the arachidonate products, leukotrienes and prostaglandins, which may affect pulmonary haemodynamics and respiration (Stimler et al. 1982).

A detailed study of the complement system in acute pancreatitis showed evidence for activation via both the classical and the alternative pathway. Besides evidence of C3 degradation, C1Q and C4 showed low plasma levels early in the disease and C1r-1s-C1–inactivator complexes were present in particular after a few days of illness. Furthermore, properdin was often low and factor B was within the normal range although it is an acute phase reactant. Factor B products (Bb) were also present. Interestingly enough there was a discrepancy between functional and immunochemical levels for the C1 inhibitor, with low functional values explained by the presence of C1 inhibitor complexes with C1r-C1s. Again the most dramatic finding is in the peritoneal exudate, where the C1 inhibitor is completely consumed (Lasson et al. 1985).

Kallikrein–Kinin

The kallikrein–kinin system shows similar patterns to complement in severe pancreatitis with low plasma levels of prekallikrein and kininogen. Simultaneously complete degradation of kininogen and low levels of prekallikrein are found in the peritoneal cavity. The observation of low levels of low-molecular-weight kininogen, which is a poor substrate for plasma kallikrein, indicates the activity of other proteases, for example; glandular kallikrein and trypsin (Lasson and Ohlsson 1984b). It should be observed that only α_2M offers good protection against trypsin-induced C3 and kininogen cleavage, whereas α_1PI is without significant effect (Balldin et al. 1981; Lasson et al. 1983; Lasson and Ohlsson 1984b). In severe acute pancreatitis α_2M is frequently consumed in the peritoneal exudate concomitant with complete cleavage of C3 and kininogen which in both cases may be trypsin-induced, although massive amounts of free α_1PI are present (Balldin et al. 1981).

The Clotting System

Consumptive coagulopathy in severe attacks of acute pancreatitis is indicated by decreased values for prothrombin, platelets and fibrinogen (Walker et al. 1981; Agarwal et al. 1982). Antithrombin III (ATIII), the main inhibitor of thrombin, also inhibits factors IX, X, XI, XII, plasmin, tissue factor, kallikrein, trypsin and chymotrypsin. Low ATIII levels are a regular finding in severe pancreatitis, similar to the findings in sepsis. Often a marked discrepancy is found between the electroimmunoassay and the functional plasma levels. This denotes protease–ATIII complex formation. This was also seen directly on crossed immunoelectrophoretic analyses (Lasson and Ohlsson 1986). In severe attacks of acute pancreatitis fibrinolysis is indicated by the low plasminogen levels together with fibrinogen degradation products in most patients. We found that a low plasminogen level persisted for eight days, in contrast to the rapid return to normal of plasminogen in less than 48 h after low levels caused by intravenous streptokinase infusion (Nihlén and Ganrot 1967). This difference is compatible with continued plasminogen activation for several days in severe pancreatitis. Low levels have been found in septicaemia and in experimentally induced pulmonary insufficiency (Aasen et al. 1980). The plasma levels of alpha-2 antiplasmin (α_2AP), the main inhibitor of plasmin, are often high, but with a discrepancy between the electroimmunoassay and the functional values indicating complex formation or degradation. Such a discrepancy has also been seen in sepsis (Velasco et al. 1982). Crossed immunoelectrophoretic analysis of peritoneal exudates consistently showed complex formation, thus partly explaining the difference between immunochemical and functional levels. A further explanation of the difference may be limited proteolysis of α_2AP caused by leucocyte elastase (Gramse et al. 1984), which also has the capacity to degrade ATIII (Jochum et al. 1981). High levels of α_2AP seen in these pancreatitis patients after a few days of illness have previously been implicated as a cause of delayed fibrin elimination from the lungs with resultant disseminated intravascular coagulation and pulmonary insufficiency (Carlin et al. 1981; Berry et al. 1981).

Haemodynamic Effects of Acute Pancreatitis

Measurements of pancreatic blood flow in acute pancreatitis have given varying results. However, most authors report hypoperfusion in severe pancreatitis. Ischaemia probably precedes pancreatic necrosis but the degree of protease–antiprotease imbalance is related to pancreatic hypoperfusion in experimental as well as in clinical pancreatitis (Hjelmqvist et al. 1986). Vascular damage occurs both in capillary vessels and in larger vessels, probably partly caused by pancreatic and leucocyte elastase (Geokas 1977; Geokas et al. 1978; Stroud et al. 1981). Arterial thrombosis in pancreatitis has been reported to cause infarction and limited necrosis in the pancreas. The decreased perfusion in severe pancreatitis could lead to diminished wash-out of enzymes and an impaired inflow of plasma protease inhibitors.

The systemic circulation is under severe stress in acute pancreatitis. Oedema formation results in loss of plasma to the "third space", haemoconcentration and finally circulatory collapse. In experimental pancreatitis this is usually characterised by reduction in cardiac output and increased systemic vascular resistance, redistribution of blood flow with splanchnic hypoperfusion, preservation of cerebral and myocardial blood flows and finally a drop in blood pressure (Hjelmqvist 1990).

Clinically, hyperdynamic states with elevated cardiac index and low systemic resistance have been reported. Thus certain circulatory changes in pancreatitis resemble hyperdynamic septic shock while others resemble hypovolaemic shock. Pleural and pericardial effusions, ascites as well as inflammatory intraperitoneal and retroperitoneal exudates are frequent complications and side effects of acute pancreatitis, with a deleterious influence on organ function (Hjelmqvist 1990).

Remote Systemic Effects

The systemic effects of the released active enzymes can directly or indirectly cause complications in the lungs, kidneys, liver, the heart and brain, in blood coagulation and in electrolyte, carbohydrate and lipid metabolism.

Pulmonary dysfunction is seen in more than 50% of the patients with acute pancreatitis. It is usually reversible and is manifest as tachypnoea and mild hypoxaemia (Ranson et al. 1973). In severe cases of acute pancreatitis, however, the lung injury is frequently progressive and may be associated with acute respiratory failure and adult respiratory distress syndrome (Hayes et al. 1974; Imrie et al. 1977). Data have been presented which indicate that the lung injury may be dependent on complement activation with C5a release causing leucocyte accumulation, attachment and activation in the lung capillaries. The release of oxygen-derived free radicals would then cause endothelial cell injury and increased capillary leak, resulting in acute lung injury (Guice et al. 1989). The leucocyte proteases may then also contribute to the tissue injury.

The hypocalcaemia observed in severe cases is probably due to several causes. Besides calcium deposits in the necrotic adipose tissues, the low calcium level may be due to reduced parathormone levels due to cleavage of the pancreatic proteases (Brodrick et al. 1981), release of calcitonin by glucagon, decrease of protein-bound calcium and a shift in the extracellular and intracellular calcium concentrations (Imrie et al. 1976).

Hypophosphataemia associated with increased phosphate excretion has been reported in acute pancreatitis and is ascribed to reduced tubular reabsorption. Such reduced serum phosphate levels may contribute to the cerebral states of disorientation frequently seen in severe acute pancreatitis (Jacobsson et al. 1982). The hyperglycaemia which accompanies acute pancreatitis may be caused by the destruction of islet cells, changes in the control variables with absolute or relative increase of glucagon levels, stress-induced increases of cortisol and catecholamines, or by pre-existing diabetes (Klose et al. 1982).

It is known that familial hyperlipoproteinaemia can cause acute pancreatitis, but acute pancreatitis itself can give an increase of the serum lipid concentration through increased lipolysis. Alcohol abuse can provoke pancreatitis as well as secondary hyperlipoproteinaemia (Löffler et al. 1976).

It should be realised that probably only the initial pathophysiological changes and tissue damage are the result exclusively of the intrapancreatic activation of the different digestive pancreatic enzymes. This process then triggers and is complicated by the cascade events leading to the general acute inflammatory response with stimulation of macrophages, fibroblasts and endothelial cells. This primary cellular reaction leads to the production and release of acute phase cytokines like interleukin 1, interleukin 6, tumour necrosis factor and interferon. The secondary systemic reaction includes leucocytosis, complement activation, increased serum glucocorticoids, decreased serum iron and zinc, enhanced uptake of amino acids and increased synthesis of acute phase proteins. The end result of this chain of events in severe acute pancreatitis is pancreatitic shock with multi-organ failure and a high mortality.

Acknowledgements. Supported by the Swedish Medical Research Council (projects no. B91-17X-03910-19A, B91-17K-08715-03C), the Swedish Cancer Society (project no. 1300-B91-06X), the Medical Faculty, University of Lund, Sweden, the Foundation of Malmö General Hospital for Cancer, the Albert Påhlsson Foundation and the Torsten and Ragnar Söderberg Foundations.

References

Aasen AO, Saugstad OD, Lium B (1980) Plasma antiplasmin activities in experimental lung insufficiency. Acta Chir Scand suppl. 499:113–121

Agarwal MB, Kamdar MS, Bapat RD, Mehta BC, Suryaprabha R, Rao PN (1982) Consumptive coagulopathy and fibrinolysis in experimental acute pancreatitis. J Postgrad Med 28:214–217

Andersson RJL, Braganza M, Case RM (1990) Routes of protein secretion in the isolated perfused cat pancreas. Pancreas 5:394–400

Axelsson L, Bergenfeldt M, Björk P, Olsson R, Ohlsson K (1990) Release of immunoreactive canine leucocyte elastase normally and in endotoxin and pancreatic shock. Scand J Clin Lab Invest 50:35–42

Axelsson L, Linder C, Ohlsson K, Rosengren M (1988) The effect of the secretory leukocyte protease inhibitor on leukocyte proteases released during phagocytosis. Biol Chem Hoppe-Seyler Suppl. 369:89–93

Balldin G, Ohlsson K (1979) Demonstration of pancreatic protease–antiprotease complexes in the peritoneal fluid of patients with acute pancreatitis. Surgery 85:451–456

Balldin G, Gustavsson E-L, Ohlsson K (1980) Influence of plasma protease inhibitors and Trasylol on trypsin-induced bradykinin-release in vitro and in vivo. Eur Surg Res 12:1–10

Balldin G, Eddeland A, Ohlsson K (1981) Studies on the role of the plasma protease inhibitors on in vitro C3-activation and in acute pancreatitis. Scand J Gastroenterol 16:603–609

Balldin G, Genell S, Ohlsson K (1989) Pancreatic abscess: formation, diagnostic procedures and treatment. Dig Dis 7:104–112

Baugh RJ, Travis JJ (1976) Human leukocyte granule elastase: rapid isolation and characterization. J Biochem 15:836–841

Bergenfeldt M, Axelsson L, Björk P, Olsson R, Ohlsson K (1989) Release of leukocyte elastase in severe acute pancreatitis in the dog. In: Thorsgaard N, Ebbehøj N (eds) Pankreas i Fokus V, MEDA AS, Copenhagen, pp 215–219

Berry AR, Taylor TV, Davies GC (1981) Pulmonary function and fibrinogen metabolism in acute pancreatitis. Br J Surg 68:870–873

Bilbao MK, Dotter CT, Lee TG, Katon RM (1976) Complications of endoscopic retrograde cholangiopancreatography (ERCP). Gastroenterology 70:314–320

Björk P, Axelsson L, Bergenfeldt M, Ohlsson K (1988) Influence of plasma protease inhibitors and the secretory leukocyte protease inhibitor on leukocyte elastase-induced consumption of selected plasma proteins in vitro in man. Scand J Clin Lab Invest 48:205–211

Bohe M, Borgström A, Lindström C, Ohlsson K (1986) Pancreatic endoproteases and pancreatic secretory trypsin inhibitor immunoreactivity in human Paneth cells. J Clin Pathol 39:786–793

Bohe M, Lindström CG, Ohlsson K (1987) Varying occurrence of gastroduodenal immunoreactive pancreatic secretory trypsin inhibitor. J. Clin Pathol 40:1345–1348

Borgström A, Lasson Å (1984) Trypsin–alpha1-protease inhibitor complexes in serum and clinical course of acute pancreatitis. Scand J Gastroenterol 19:1119–1122

Borgström A, Ohlsson K (1976) Radioimmunological determination and characterization of cathodal trypsin-like immunoreactivity in normal human plasma. Scand J Clin Lab Invest 36:809–814

Borgström A, Ohlsson K (1978a) Studies on the turnover of endogenous cathodal trypsinogen in man. Eur J Clin Invest 8:379–382

Borgström A, Ohlsson K (1978b) Immunoreactive trypsin in serum and peritoneal fluid in acute pancreatitis. Hoppe-Seyler's Z Physiol Chem 359:677–681

Brodrick JW, Largman C, Ray SB, Geokas MC (1981) Proteolysis of parathyroid hormone in vitro by sera from acute pancreatitis patients. Proc Soc Exp Biol Med 167:588–592

Carlin G, Einarsson M, Saldeen T (1981) Delayed elimination of fibrin from the lungs in rats given alpha2-antiplasmin. Thromb Haemost 46:757–758

Chiari H (1886) Ueber selbstverdaung des mensclichen pancreas. 17:69–96

Davidsson FF, Dennis EA (1989) Biological relevance of lipocortins and related proteins as inhibitors of phospholipase A2. Biochem Pharmacol 38:3645–3651

Eddeland A, Ohlsson K (1978a) Studies on the pancreatic secretory trypsin inhibitor in plasma and its complex with trypsin in vivo and in vitro. Scand J Clin Lab Invest 38:507–515

Eddeland A, Ohlsson K (1978b) A radioimmunoassay for measurement of human pancreatic secretory trypsin inhibitor in different body fluids. Hoppe-Seyler's Z Physiol Chem 359:671–675

Eddeland A, Ohlsson K (1978c) Purification and immunochemical quantitation of human pancreatic secretory trypsin inhibitor. Scand J Clin Lab Invest 38:261–267

Eddeland A, Wehlin L (1978) Secretin/cholecystokinin-stimulated secretion of trypsinogen and trypsin inhibitor in pure human pancreatic juice collected by endoscopic retrograde catheterization. Hoppe-Seyler's Z Physiol Chem 359:1653–1658

Ekerot L, Ohlsson K (1982) The elimination of alfa2-macroglobulin complexes from the arthritic joint. An experimental study in dogs. Scand J Plast Reconstr Surg 16:107–115

Fritz H, Jochum M, Dusvald et al. (1986) Granulocyte proteinases as mediators of unspecific proteolysis in inflammation. In: Tschesche H (ed) Proteinases in inflammation and tumor invasion. Walter de Gruter, Berlin, pp 1–23

Fryksmark U, Prellner T, Tegner H, Ohlsson K (1984) Studies on the role of antileukoprotease in respiratory tract disease. Eur J Resp Dis 65:201–209

Fukayama M, Hayashi Y, Koike M, Ogawa M, Kosaki G (1986) Immunohistochemical localization of pancreatic secretory trypsin inhibitor in fetal and adult pancreatic and extrapancreatic tissues. J Histochem Cytochem 227–235

Geokas MC (1977) Pancreatic elastase in human serum. Determination by radioimmunoassay. J Biol Chem 252:61–67

Geokas MC, Rinderknecht H, Brodrick JW, Largman C (1978) Studies on the ascites fluid of acute pancreatitis in man. Dig Dis 23:182–188

Geokas MC, Largman C, Brodrick JW, Johnson JH (1979) Determination of human pancreatic cationic trypsinogen in serum by radioimmunoassay. Am J Physiol 236:E77–E83

Gliemann J, Larsen TR, Sothrup-Jensen L (1983) Cell association and degradation of alpha2-macroblubulin–trypsin complexes in hepatocytes and adipocytes. Biochim Biophys Acta 756:230–237

Gramse M, Havemann K, Egbring RF (1984) Alpha2-plasmin inhibitor inactivation by human granulocyte elastase. Adv Exp Med Biol 167:253–261

Guice KS, Oldham KT, Caty MG, Johnson KJ, Ward PA (1989) Neutrophil dependent, oxygen-radical mediated lung injury associated with acute pancreatitis. Ann Surg 210:740–747

Hamilton I, Lintott DJ, Rothwell J, Axon ATR (1983) Acute pancreatitis following endoscopic retrograde cholangiopancreatography. Clin Radiol 34:543–546

Hayes ME, Rosenbaum RW, Zibelman M, Matsumoto T (1974) Adult respiratory distress syndrome in association with acute pancreatitis. Evaluation of positive end-expiratory pressure ventilation and pharmacologic doses of steroids. Am J Surg 127:314–319

Hjelmqvist B (1990) Experimental and clinical acute pancreatitis. A study with special reference to general hemodynamics, regional blood flow, protease–antiprotease imbalance and to the use of computed tomography. MD thesis, University of Lund, Sweden

Hjelmqvist B, Ohlsson K, Aronsen KF (1986) Protease–antiprotease imbalance, hemodynamic and regional blood flow changes in experimental pancreatitis. Scand J Gastroenterol Suppl 126:8–11

Imrie CW, Allam BF, Ferguson JC (1976) Hypocalcemia of acute pancreatitis: the effect of hypoalbuminaemia. Curr Med Res Opin 4:101–116

Imrie CW, Ferguson JC, Murphy D, Blumgart LH (1977) Arterial hypoxia in acute pancreatitis. Br J Surg 64:185–188

Jacob HS, Hammerschmidt DH (1982) Tissue damage caused by activated complement and granulocytes in shock lung, post perfusion lung, and after amniotic fluid embolism: ramifications for therapy. Ann Chir Gynaecol 71: Supplement 196:3–9

Jacobsson G, Hedstrand U, Nilsson B (1982) The cause of hypophosphatemia in acute pancreatitis. In: Hollender LF (ed) Controversies in acute pancreatitis. Springer, Berlin, Heidelberg, New York, pp 45–47

Jochum M, Lander S, Heimburger M, Fritz H (1981) Effect of human granulocyte elastase in isolated human antitrombin III. Hoppe-Seyler's Z Physiol Chem 362:103–109

Jönsson BM, Loeffler L, Ohlsson K (1982) Human granulocyte elastase is inhibited by the urinary trypsin inhibitor. Hoppe-Seyler's Z Phys Chem 363:1167–1175

Kazal LA, Spicer DS, Brahinsky RA (1948) Isolation of a crystalline trypsin inhibitor–anticoagulant protein from pancreas. J Am Chem Soc 70:3034–3040

Klose G, Klapdor R, Greten H (1982) Akute pancreatitis: Stoffwechselveränderungen sind diagnostische und prognostische Parameter. Klinikarzt 11:616–625

Koike HM, Steer ML, Meldolesi J (1982) Pancreatic effects of ethionine blockade of exocytosis and appearance of crinophagy and autophagy precede cellular necrosis. Am J Physiol 242:G297–G307

Lasson Å, Ohlsson K (1984a) Protease inhibitors in acute human pancreatitis. Correlation between biochemical changes and clinical course. Scand J Gastroenterol 19:779–786

Lasson Å, Ohlsson K (1984b) Changes in the kallikrein kinin system during acute pancreatitis in man. Thromb Res 35:27–41

Lasson Å, Ohlsson K (1986) Consumptive coagulopathy, fibrinolysis and protease–antiprotease interactions during acute pancreatitis. Thromb Res 41:167–183

Lasson Å, Dittmann B, Ohlsson K (1983) Influence of plasma protease inhibitors and aprotinin on trypsin-induced bradykinin release in vitro in man. Hoppe-Seyler's Z Physiol Chem 364:1315–1322

Lasson Å, Laurell A-B, Ohlsson K (1985) Correlation among complement activation, protease inhibitors and clinical course in acute pancreatitis in man. Scand J Gastroenterol 20:335–345

Löffler A, Löffler-Bock AH, Friedrich U (1976) Hyperlipoproteiämie und Pankreatitis. Leber Magen Darm 6:249–256

MacCartney HW, Tschesche H (1983) Latent and active human polymorphonuclear leucocyte collagenase.Isolation, purification and characterization. Eur J Biochem 130:171–178

McMahon MJ, Bowen M, Mayer AD, Cooper EH (1984) Relation of alfa2-macroglobulin and other antiproteases to the clinical features of acute pancreatitis. Am J Surg 147:164–170

Nevalainen TJ (1988). Review, phospolipase α_2 in acute pancreatitis. Scand J Gastroenterol 23:897–904

Nihlén JE, Ganrot P-O (1967) Plasmin, plasmin inhibitors and degradation products of fibrinogen in human serum during and after intravenous infusion of streptokinase. Scand J Clin Lab Invest 20:113–121

Odeberg H, Olsson I, Venge P (1975) Cationic proteins of human granulocytes, IV, esterase activity. Lab Invest 32:86–90

Ohlsson (1971a) Experimental pancreatitis in the dog. Appearance of complexes between proteases and trypsin inhibitors in ascitic fluid, lymph and plasma. Scand J Gastroenterol 6:645–652

Ohlsson K (1971b) Interactions in vitro and in vivo between dog trypsin and dog plasma protease inhibitors. Scand J Clin Lab Invest 28:219–223

Ohlsson K (1971c) Elimination of ^{125}I-trypsin alpha-macroglobulin complexes from blood by reticuloendothelial cells in dog. Acta Physiol Scand 81:269–272

Ohlsson K (1986) Influence of the human pancreatic secretory trypsin inhibitor on trypsin induced C3 and kininogen cleavage: an in vitro study. Scand J Gastroenterol 21:suppl 126:18–20

Ohlsson K, Eddeland A (1975) Release of proteolytic enzymes in bile-induced pancreatitis in dogs. Gastroenterology 69:668–675

Ohlsson K, Laurell C-B (1976) The disappearance of enzyme-inhibitor complexes from the circulation of man. Clin Sci Mol Med 51:87–92

Ohlsson K, Olsson I (1974) The neutral proteinases of human granulocytes. Isolation and partial characterization of granulocyte elastase. Eur J Biochem 42:519–527

Ohlsson K, Olsson I (1977) The extracellular release of granulocyte collagenase and elastase during phagocytosis and inflammatory processes. Scand J Haematol 19: 145–152

Ohlsson K, Ganrot P-O, Laurell C-B (1971) In vivo interaction between trypsin and some plasma proteins in relation to tolerance to intravenous infusion of trypsin in dog. Acta Chir Scand 137:113–121

Ohlsson K, Rosengren M, Stetler G et al. (1988). Structure, genomic organization and tissue distribution of human secretory leucocyte protease inhibitor (SLPI). A potent inhibitor of neutrophil elastase. In: Taylor JC, Mittman C (eds) Pulmonary emphysema and proteolysis. Academic Press, London, pp 307–324

Ohlsson K, Olsson R, Björk P et al. (1989) Local administration of human pancreatic secretory trypsin inhibitor prevents the development of experimental acute pancreatitis in rats and dogs. Scand J Gastroenterol 24:693–704

Ohlsson K, Linder C, Rosengren M (1990) Monoclonal antibodies specific for neutrophil proteinase 4. Biol Chem Hoppe-Seyler 371:549–555

Ranson JHC, Roses DF, Fink SD (1973) Early respiratory insufficiency in acute pancreatitis. Ann Surg 178:75–79

Raphael SC (1987) Endoscopic sphincterotomy: nonsurgical treatment of common bile duct stones. In: Muino J (ed) Therapeutic endoscopy in gastrointestinal surgery. Churchill Livingstone, New York, pp 271–277

Roxvall L, Bengtson A, Heideman M (1989) Anaphylatoxin generation in acute pancreatitis. J Surg Res 47:138–143

Saluja AKS, Hashimoto M, Saluja RE et al. (1987) Subcellular redistribution of lysosomal enzymes during caerulein-induced pancreatitis. Am J Physiol 251:G508–G516

Saluja A, Saluja M, Villa A et al. (1989) Pancreatic duct obstruction in rabbits causes digestive zymogen and lysosomal enzyme colocalization. J Clin Invest 84:1260–1266

Salvessen G, Farley D, Schuman J et al. (1987) Molecular cloning of human cathepsin G: structural similarity to mast cell and cytotoxic T lymphocyte proteinase. Biochemistry 26:2289–2293

Satake K, Chung Y-S, Umeyama K (1982) Serum elastase I levels in pancreatic disease. Am J Surg 144:239–244

Schröder T, Kivilaakso E, Kinnunen PKJ, Lempinen M (1980) Serum phospholipase A2 in human acute pancreatitis. Scand J Gastroenterol 15:633–638

Sinha S, Watorek W, Karr S et al. (1987) Primary structure of human neutrophil elastase. Proc Natl Acad Sci USA 84:2228–2232

Stimler NP, Bach MK, Bloor CM, Hugli TE (1982) Release of leukotrienes from guinea pig lung stimulated by C5a desArg anaphylatoxin. J Immunol 128:2247–2253

Stroud WH, Cullom JW, Andersson MC (1981) Hemorrhagic complications of severe pancreatitis. Surgery 90:657–665

Thompson RC, Ohlsson K (1986) Isolation, properties, and complete amino acid sequence of human secretory leucocyte protease inhibitor, a potent inhibitor of leucocyte elastase. Proc Natl Acad Sci USA 83:6692–6696

Velasco F, Torres A, Andres P, Duran MI (1982) Functional activities and concentrations of plasmin inhibitors in normal subjects and D.I.C. patients. Thromb Haemost 47:275–277

Walker ID, Gallimore MJ, Imrie CW, Davidson JF (1981) The coagulation, fibrinolytic and plasma kallikrein systems in acute pancreatitis. In: Davidson JF, Nilsson J, Åstedt B (eds) Progress in fibrinolysis. Vol. V. Churchill Livingstone, New York, pp 112–123

Chapter 21

Experimental Models of Acute Pancreatitis

C. Wilson and C. W. Imrie

Pancreatitis was first induced experimentally in dogs as early as the mid-19th century by the intraductal injection of bile and other substances (Bernard 1855). Since then numerous experimental models have been described which have furthered our understanding of the pathogenesis and pathophysiology of acute pancreatitis, both at a glandular and cellular level. Experimental models have also permitted study of the treatment of acute pancreatitis and its many complications. Various models of experimental pancreatitis are summarised in Table 1.

In the initiation of acute pancreatitis it has been assumed that pancreatic enzyme activation occurs outside the acinar cell, within the ducts or interstitial tissues, perhaps following duct rupture or leakage of pancreatic enzymes from the ducts. The activated pancreatic enzymes, or products of enzymatic activity such as lysolecithin (Schmidt and Creutzfeldt 1969), may then attack the acinar cells and cause autodigestion and pancreatic necrosis.

Theories supported by evidence from animal experiments which have sought to explain the pathogenesis of acute pancreatitis have included the bile reflux theory, pancreatic ductal obstruction/hypersecretion and duodenal reflux. All these are considered possible sequelae of gallstone migration with transient ampullary obstruction. These will be termed the "ductal" models of acute pancreatitis and each is examined in turn.

Table 1. Models of experimental pancreatitis

Ductal	Retrograde ductal infusion
	Ductal obstruction/hypersecretion
	Closed duodenal loop
	Ductal perfusion
Cellular	Diet-induced pancreatitis
	Caerulein hyperstimulation
Miscellaneous	Isolated, ex vivo perfused pancreas
	Immune pancreatitis

The other major group of experimental pancreatitis models may be termed the "cellular" models, as in these cases pancreatic enzyme activation appears to originate from within the acinar cell itself.

A final group of experimental models to be discussed includes the isolated, perfused, ex vivo pancreas preparation as popularised by Cameron and co-workers. Immune pancreatitis is also discussed but the relevance of these models to the human disease appears tenuous.

Ductal Models of Experimental Pancreatitis

Retrograde Ductal Infusion

Reflux of bile into the pancreatic duct was observed to have occurred at the post mortem of a patient with acute haemorrhagic pancreatitis, due to a gallstone impacted at the ampulla of Vater (Opie 1901). Numerous experimental studies have since confirmed that bile or bile salts injected retrogradely into the pancreatic duct can cause acute pancreatitis. As experience of the model has grown it has become clear that the presence of bile alone within the pancreatic duct appears to cause no deleterious effect (White and Magee 1960; Emslie et al. 1966; Konok and Thompson 1969). However, if bile is injected under pressure then acute pancreatitis results (Emslie et al. 1966). Other experiments have studied the retrograde infusion of bile mixed with trypsin or pancreatic juice and also of infected bile, all of which increased the severity of the resultant pancreatitis (Elliot et al. 1957; Konok and Thompson 1969).

The earliest studies used dogs as the experimental animal although all species appear susceptible to this method. Retrograde infusion of the bile salt sodium taurocholate in the rat has probably become the most widely studied model of this type. This method of inducing pancreatitis requires a general anaesthetic, laparotomy and cannulation of the pancreatic duct through the intact antimesenteric wall of the duodenum. Various volumes and concentrations of sodium taurocholate are then injected or slowly infused retrogradely into the bile–pancreatic duct with the bile duct temporarily clamped at the liver hilum above the pancreas (Fig. 1). Early macroscopic changes of pancreatic oedema and haemorrhage are usually apparent during the infusion. Subsequently a peritoneal exudate forms, and pancreatic necrosis and fat necrosis can be seen both macroscopically and microscopically, similar to the appearances of necrotising pancreatitis in man. The first histological change noted after taurocholate infusion was dissolution of the pancreatic ductal walls with destruction of the adjacent lobules (Aho et al. 1980). The blood vessels were engorged and had deformed walls. Aho et al. (1980) suggested that this may have been due to the detergent effect of the bile salts on the cell membranes of the ductal cells, proteolytic enzyme activation being a later feature, which produced the spreading acinar cell necrosis.

Taurocholate-induced pancreatitis tends to be a rapidly evolving disease, and death usually occurs within 24–48 h. The severity, and hence the mortality of the pancreatitis induced, can be varied by alteration of the rate and volume

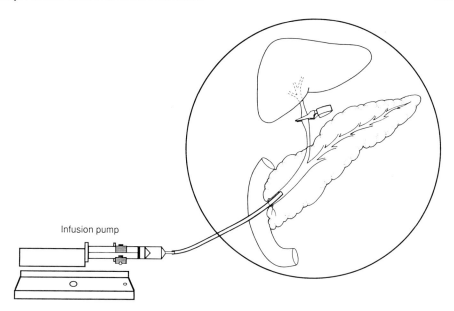

Fig. 1. Diagram of the induction of bile salt pancreatitis in the rat by retrograde ductal infusion. A manometer may be added to the infusion system to control the intraductal pressure.

infused (and hence the infusion pressure) and also by varying the bile salt concentration (Lankisch et al. 1979; Aho et al. 1980).

The earliest descriptions of this technique used a "freehand" injection of sodium taurocholate into the bile-pancreatic duct. Standardisation of the injection pressure is impossible by this method and would be expected to give rise to great variability in the severity of the initial pancreatic lesion. Injection volumes of 100μl or more produce gross ductal extravasation regardless of the pressure whereas at 50μl the amount of extravasation is closely related to the pressure generated (Armstrong et al. 1985a). If reflux of bile into the pancreatic duct is indeed the initial event in the pathogenesis of acute pancreatitis in man it is highly unlikely that the pressures developed within the duct would result in gross ductal rupture. In the investigation of this experimental model in the rat, small volumes of bile salt infused at physiological pressures should be used, to produce a standard, reproducible degree of injury.

This model tends to produce a severe, rapidly destructive pancreatitis with a high mortality. It has found its greatest application in the investigation of various therapies for the disease.

Ductal Obstruction/Hypersecretion

Simple ligation of the pancreatic duct produces atrophy of the pancreatic acinar tissue without pancreatitis (Radakovich et al. 1952) but extensive pancreatic oedema and also fat necrosis results from concurrently stimulating the gland with secretin (Popper and Necheles 1942; Radakovich et al. 1952). Ligation of the pancreatic duct with postoperative secretin stimulation results in increased intraductal pressure (Elliot et al. 1957) and the appearance of pancreatic enzymes in the lymphatics and blood vessels draining the pancreas (Papp 1976).

The addition of ischaemia, by temporary occlusion of the main pancreatic artery, was found to transform pancreatic oedema into necrosis (Popper et al. 1948; Menguy et al. 1957).

Obstruction of the pancreatic duct has been postulated to occur in man due to the (usually transient) impaction of a gallstone. Stimulation of pancreatic secretion would occur after eating a meal and indeed there is evidence in some cases that acute gallstone pancreatitis may come on within an hour or two of a large meal (Rich and Duff 1936; Menguy et al. 1957). This might be expected to produce pain and hyperamylasaemia and a mild, oedematous pancreatitis which is often found in association with gallstone disease.

Nowadays, this experimental model is rarely employed for research into acute pancreatitis. Ductal obstruction over a prolonged period of time leads to marked loss of acinar tissue and fibrosis and this model may well prove useful in the study of chronic obstructive pancreatitis.

Closed Duodenal Loop

The closed duodenal loop model of acute pancreatitis, first described by Seidel (1910), was popularised by Pfeffer et al. (1957). This technique was designed to minimise handling of the pancreas and to reduce the surgical trauma resulting from the retrograde ductal injection methods of inducing pancreatitis. In the initial studies on dogs the duodenum was divided just below the pylorus and again below the reflection of the pancreas onto the dorsal mesentery, thus creating a closed loop, 7–10 cm long. Bile was excluded by ligation of the common bile duct and gastric outflow was re-established by the construction of a gastroduodenostomy. Pancreatic oedema was the earliest change noted after 4 h. At 9 h small areas of haemorrhage had appeared in the head of the gland and two hours later the entire gland was haemorrhagic. Microscopically extravasated blood was noted prior to the development of focal parenchymal necrosis. Pfeffer et al. (1957) considered that the pancreatic lesion occurred as the result of the vascular injury. Others have suggested the involvement of a vasculitis (Rao et al. 1981). Many others consider that the pancreatitis in this model results from overdistension of the duodenal loop with the reflux of duodenal contents, which contain activated pancreatic enzymes, into the pancreatic duct. This would be supported by the finding that the pancreatitis can be prevented by either ductal ligation (McCutcheon 1968) or cannulation of the pancreatic duct (Paulino-Netto and Dreiling 1960).

Whether this mechanism applies in man is unknown, but it is likely that the sphincter of Oddi and the pressure gradient between the pancreatic duct and the duodenum act to prevent duodenopancreatic reflux. However, there is an increased incidence of pancreatitis following Polya (BII) as opposed to Bilroth I gastrectomy which has been attributed to afferent loop obstruction and duodenopancreatic reflux.

As originally described this model was complex to set up and expensive, given its use of the dog as the experimental animal. This model has since undergone modification and simplification and can now be applied to small animals such as the rat (Chetty et al. 1980) (Fig. 2). However, doubts remain

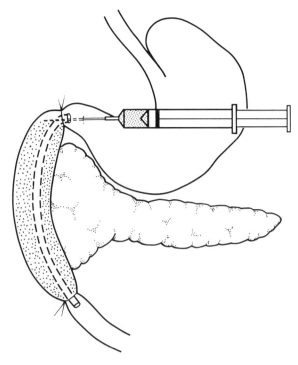

Fig. 2. Diagram of the induction of closed duodenal loop pancreatitis in the rat. A plastic tube has been inserted through the pylorus, via a gastrostomy, to re-establish gastrointestinal continuity. Bile, infected bile or other agents can be injected into the closed duodenal loop and speeds the development of the pancreatitis. Modified from Chetty et al. (1980).

concerning the validity of this experimental model and more recent work suggests that significant pathology occurs other than acute pancreatitis, namely duodenal wall necrosis, and pancreatic and peritoneal sepsis associated with bacteraemia (Dickson et al. 1986). The model appears to be associated with gross generalised sepsis, often with only mild degrees of pancreatitis. This is not typical of the disease in man, particularly in its early stages, and presently this model is rarely used for the study of acute pancreatitis.

Ductal Perfusion

A more controlled means of examining factors which lead to the initiation of acute pancreatitis may be provided by the ductal perfusion model as originally described by Reber et al. (1979). The pancreatic duct mucosal barrier normally acts to prevent diffusion of HCO_3^- from the pancreatic juice back into the bloodstream. This model was initially described in the cat and necessitated cannulation of the pancreatic duct at both the head and tail of the gland. (Fig. 3). The duct was then perfused in a cephalad direction with a standard solution of known pH and electrolyte composition. The flux of HCO_3^- and Cl^- anions could be determined before and after perfusion with the test solution.

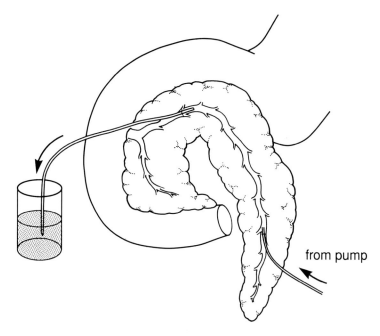

from pump

Fig. 3. Diagram showing the experimental set-up for in vivo perfusion of the pancreatic duct of the cat. (Modified from Reber and Mosley (1980).

The perfusion of the duct with sterile bile was not deleterious; however, perfusion with infected bile increased the anion flux (Reber and Mosley 1980). The pancreatic duct mucosal barrier was also damaged by ethanol, aspirin, hydrochloric acid and secondary bile acids (Reber et al. 1979). More recent work has shown that this technique can also be applied to a small animal model such as the rat (Olazabal 1983; Armstrong et al. 1985b). This model appears to be most valuable for examining agents implicated in the pathogenesis of acute pancreatitis.

Cellular Models of Experimental Pancreatitis

Diet-induced Pancreatitis

Young female mice fed a diet which is choline deficient and supplemented with DL-ethionine develop acute haemorrhagic pancreatitis within 5 days (Lombardi et al. 1975). Pancreatic necrosis was associated with increased amylase and lipase activity in the serum and the intraparenchymal activation of zymogens (Rao et al. 1976). In this model normal exocytosis was blocked, leading to the accumulation of zymogen granules within the acinar cells. Thereafter, lysosomes fuse with the zymogen granules (crinophagy). This results in the formation of large vacuoles which contain both pancreatic digestive zymogens and lysosomal hydrolases. These latter appear to be capable of activating trypsinogen (Fig. 4) (Rao et al. 1980; Steer et al. 1984). Thus it appears possible that in this model intracellular zymogen activation may occur. The release of activated pancreatic enzymes then follows as a result of pancreatic acinar cell necrosis rather than being the cause of it, as is thought in other models.

The severity (and lethality) of this model can be reduced by limiting the

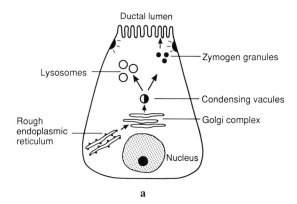

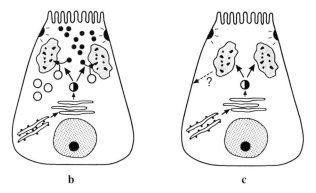

Fig. 4. a Pancreatic digestive and lysosomal enzymes are synthesised on ribosomes in the rough endoplasmic reticulum from where they are transported to the Golgi complex. Molecular sorting occurs in the Golgi complex and condensing vacuoles are formed which mature into zymogen granules that are ultimately discharged at the apical surface of the cell in response to secretagogue stimulation. Lysosomal enzymes are separated from digestive enzymes during condensing vacuole maturation, forming lysosomes. Modified from Steer et al. (1984). **b** In diet-induced pancreatitis the discharge of zymogen granules is blocked leading to their accumulation within the acinar cell. Subsequently they fuse with lysosomes producing large vacuoles containing both pancreatic digestive and lysosomal enzymes, which are capable of activating trypsinogen. Digestive enzyme activation leads to acinar cell necrosis and pancreatitis. Modified from Steer et al. (1984). **c** In hyperstimulation pancreatitis there is interference with the process of condensing vacuole maturation leading to the formation of large vacuoles containing both digestive and lysosomal enzymes. Alternatively zymogen granules and the large vacuoles may be discharged at the basolateral border of the cell giving rise to interstitial oedema and pancreatitis. Modified from Steer et al. (1984).

exposure to the diet, both in amount and in time (Gilliland and Steer 1980). This model has certain advantages in terms of its use of a small animal model and the ease of induction of the pancreatitis, without any operative intervention. However, the presence of oestrogens appears to be essential (Rao et al. 1982).

This model and the retrograde ductal infusion models have given conflicting results in the assessment of various treatments such as aprotinin (Manabe and Steer 1979; Imrie and Mackenzie 1981) and indomethacin (Lankisch et al. 1978; Coelle et al. 1983). While this may be due in part to factors such as the method and timing of administration of the therapeutic agent and interspecies variation, it also tends to suggest that this particular model is inherently different from the various retrograde ductal infusion models and, therefore, its relevance to the human disease is unclear.

Caerulein Hyperstimulation

In the rat, administration of supramaximal doses of the cholecystokinin (CCK)–pancreozymin analogue caerulein induces an acute interstitial pancreatitis (Lampel and Kern 1977). As in the diet-induced model discussed above, large vacuoles containing both pancreatic zymogens and lysosomal enzymes develop within the pancreatic acinar cells. Lampel and Kern (1977) believe that zymogen granules and the contents of these large vacuoles are discharged, not at the apical surface of the cell, but at the basolateral border of the cell and thus into the interstitial space. This gives rise to the interstitial oedema which particularly characterises this model.

Others dispute this theory of basolateral discharge and consider that secretagogue hyperstimulation interferes with the process of condensing vacuole maturation which normally separates the digestive zymogens from the lysosomal enzymes. As a result, both enzymes come into early contact leading to intravacuolar activation of the digestive enzymes and subsequently the development of pancreatitis (Watanabe et al. 1984).

The histological changes in this model include marked interstitial oedema, an acute inflammatory cell infiltrate and acinar cell necrosis. These changes appear within one hour of the onset of the caerulein infusion, are maximal at 12 h and have largely regressed by 24 h. Although originally described in the rat, this model is also applicable in the dog (Renner and Wisner 1983) and mouse (Niederau et al. 1984).

This model has, with the diet-induced model, been the centre of much recent interest, as they suggest an alternative pathogenesis of acute pancreatitis whereby trypsinogen is activated within large vacuoles by lysosomal hydrolases such as cathepsin B. The hyperstimulation model produces a mild, reversible pancreatitis and is perhaps most appropriate for investigations into the acinar cell function during and after the attack, rather than for studies of therapy.

In humans, two very rare forms of acute pancreatitis may be associated with supramaximal acinar cell stimulation: accidental ingestion of anticholinesterase insecticide (Dressel et al. 1979) and poisoning by the venom from the bite of the Trinidad scorpion (Bartholomew 1970).

Miscellaneous Models of Experimental Pancreatitis

Isolated, Ex Vivo Perfused Pancreas

The isolated, ex vivo, perfused dog pancreas was first described by Saharia et al. (1977) in Baltimore. The pancreas is isolated with a short cuff of duodenum. Perfusion catheters are placed in the splenic artery, superior mesenteric artery and portal vein and the pancreatic duct is cannulated. The preparation is then removed and connected to an oxygenated perfusion circuit in a humidity and temperature controlled chamber. Gallstone, alcoholic and ischaemic pancreatitis were reproduced by partial duct obstruction with secretin stimulation, infusion of free fatty acids and by two hours of warm ischaemia respectively (Sanfey et al. 1985).

On one level this experimental model is attractive, as it eliminates humoral and other influences which are an integral part of studies in vivo. However, it is an extremely complex model to set up, requires a large (and expensive) experimental animal and the preparations are not physiological, showing some functional deterioration even over the 4 hour period of study. Furthermore, the means of inducing the various types of pancreatitis are not generally accepted and other than the many studies reported from Cameron's group in Baltimore this model has not found widespread application.

Immune Pancreatitis Models

Acute pancreatitis can be induced in rabbits which have been sensitised to ovalbumin, by subsequent injection of ovalbumin into the pancreatic duct (Thal 1955). This form of experimental pancreatitis occurs as a result of the Arthus reaction and is associated with pronounced vascular lesions.

Induction of an intrapancreatic Schwartzmann reaction by the systemic and intraductal administration of bacterial endotoxin results in a haemorrhagic, necrotising pancreatitis (Thal and Brackney 1954). While these models highlight the role of the complement system in their pathogenesis (Seelig and Seelig 1975) their relevance to human acute pancreatitis is not clear and they have not found widespread application.

Relevance to Human Acute Pancreatitis

Histological Changes

The pancreas is an inaccessible organ and tissue for histological examination is rarely available, particularly in the early stages of an attack. Foulis (1980) has sought to investigate the initial lesion in human acute pancreatitis by examining the pancreas of patients who die with acute pancreatitis, including patients in whom the diagnosis was neither made nor suspected in life, some of whom had only mild or trivial degrees of necrosis. In nine patients there was only ductal inflammation and periductal necrosis, the pancreatitis being attributed to alcohol abuse in three patients, gallstones in two, metastatic tumour in one and of unknown aetiology in three. In another nine patients there was only perilobular necrosis without evidence of ductal inflammation, seven having suffered from shock due to visceral perforation or myocardial infarction. Foulis suggested that in alcohol- or gallstone-associated pancreatitis, as the initial site of necrosis was adjacent to the ducts, the initiating factors may be "duct-borne" which would fit with current concepts of the pathogenesis, at least of gallstone pancreatitis.

Ductal inflammation in acute pancreatitis has been noted by others. Blenkinsopp (1978) found this lesion in almost one-third of cases of acute pancreatitis, but also in 11 of 53 control patients. Other workers have found ductal inflammation only infrequently (Kloppel et al. 1984), which raises doubts about the validity of this hypothesis; the relevance of this finding remains uncertain.

The perilobular pattern of necrosis seen after shock is also observed in patients who develop pancreatitis following cardiac surgery (Feiner 1976) and can be explained on the basis of the lobular microcirculation. The majority of pancreatic lobules receive only one arterial branch and it is the peripheral portions of the lobule, particularly those opposite the entry of the lobular artery (furthest from the main arterial source) which are first to become ischaemic during hypotension or low-flow states (Foulis 1980). This pattern of necrosis was also seen in cases where pancreatitis was due to hypothermia; many of these patients had profound hypotension on admission to hospital (Foulis 1982).

Kloppel et al. (1984) in a review of 367 autopsy cases and three surgical specimens came to entirely different conclusions regarding the earliest lesion in human acute pancreatitis. In mild cases there was interstitial oedema, a mild inflammatory cell infiltrate and small foci of fat necrosis superficially and occasionally in the gland, but acinar cell necrosis was generally absent. In severe cases there were large areas of peripancreatic fat necrosis which extended deeply into the gland along the interstitial septa. These were invariably accompanied by necrosis of the adjacent acinar tissue. Using immunocytochemical techniques, the peripheral acinar cells within a lobule neighbouring an area of fat necrosis were found to be depleted of enzymes, whereas the more central acinar cells retained their enzyme content. No major differences were apparent between pancreatitis of varying aetiologies. Kloppel et al. interpreted this, and the fact that the ducts appeared intact, to indicate that the initial lesion was the discharge of enzymes by peripheral acinar cells (perhaps by basolateral release) into the surrounding interstitial tissue.

Cellular Events

The molecular events leading to the initiation of acute pancreatitis in man have not been fully elucidated. Many aetiological factors have been identified but it has not been possible to devise a unifying theory to account for the initiation of acute pancreatitis in all. It appears likely that the disease which we recognise clinically, biochemically and histologically as acute pancreatitis

Table 2. Characteristics of experimental models

Model	Animal	Surgery	Overall complexity	Relevance to man	Comments
Retrograde infusion	Any	+	+	+/-	Rapid onset. May be difficult to standardise. Can vary severity
Ductal obstruction/ hypersecretion	?Any	+	+ +	+/-	Only mild, non-lethal pancreatitis. Evolves slowly
Closed duodenal loop	Dogs, goats, rats	+ +	+ +	?	Sepsis predominates. Slowly evolving lethal pancreatitis
Duct perfusion	Cats, rats	+	+ +	+	Limited applications
Diet-induced pancreatitis	Mice	−	+	??	Small animal model. Can vary severity. No surgery
Caerulein-induced pancreatitis	Rats, mice, dogs	Vessel access	+	??	Slowly evolving, mild, non-lethal pancreatitis
Ex vivo perfused pancreas	Dogs	+ + +	+ + +	???	Artificial environment. Complex technology

may be the common response of the gland to a variety of different insults. In this review it can be seen that each experimental model results in a distinct type of pancreatitis with varying degrees of similarity to that seen in man.

Relevance of Experimental Models

Experimental models have been of immense value in furthering our understanding of the pathogenesis and pathophysiology of acute pancreatitis, particularly of events occurring at a cellular level. The characteristics of the various models described above are summarised in Table 2. However, it must be remembered that these models may not always be relevant to the human disease and any results and conclusions drawn from their study should be interpreted with great caution.

References

Aho HJ, Koskensalo SM-L, Nevalainen TJ (1980) Experimental pancreatitis in the rat. Sodium taurocholate-induced acute haemorrhagic pancreatitis. Scand J Gastroenterol 15:411–416
Armstrong CP, Taylor TV, Torrance HB (1985a) Pressure, volume and the pancreas. Gut 26:615–624
Armstrong CP, Taylor TV, Torrance HB (1985b) Effects of bile, infection and pressure on pancreatic duct integrity. Br J Surg 72:792–795
Bartholomew C (1970) Acute scorpion pancreatitis in Trinidad. Br Med J i:666–668
Bernard C (1855) Leçons de physiologie expérimentale appliquée à la médicine. J.B. Balliere, Paris. (Quoted by Frey CF (1986) Classification of pancreatitis: state of the art, 1986. Pancreas 1:62–68
Blenkinsopp WK (1978) The liver and pancreas in acute necrotising pancreatitis. J Clin Pathol 31:791–793

Chetty U, Gilmour HM, Taylor TV (1980) Experimental acute pancreatitis in the rat – a new model. Gut 21:115–117

Coelle EF, Adham N, Elashoff J, Lewin K, Taylor IL (1983) Effects of prostaglandin and indomethacin on diet-induced acute pancreatitis in mice. Gastroenterology 85:1307–1312

Dickson AP, Foulis AK, Imrie CW (1986) Histology and bacteriology of closed duodenal loop models of experimental acute pancreatitis in the rat. Digestion 34:15–21

Dressel TD, Goodale RL, Arneson MA, Borner JW (1979) Pancreatitis as a complication of anticholinesterase insecticide intoxication. Ann Surg 189:199–204

Elliot DW, Williams RD, Zollinger RM (1957) Alterations in the pancreatic resistance to bile in the pathogenesis of acute pancreatitis. Ann Surg 146:669–682

Emslie R, White TT, Magee DF (1966) The significance of reflux of trypsin and bile in the pathogenesis of human pancreatitis. Br J Surg 53:809–816

Feiner H (1976) Pancreatitis after cardiac surgery. A morphologic study. Am J Surg 131:684–688

Foulis AK (1980) Histological evidence of initiating factors in acute necrotising pancreatitis in man. J Clin Pathol 33:1125–1131

Foulis AK (1982) Morphological study of the relation between accidental hypothermia and acute pancreatitis. J Clin Pathol 35:1244–1248

Gilliland L, Steer ML (1980) Effects of ethionine on digestive enzyme synthesis and discharge by mouse pancreas. Am J Physiol 239:G418–G426

Imrie CW, Mackenzie M (1981) Effective aprotinin therapy in canine experimental bile-trypsin pancreatitis. Digestion 22:32–38

Kloppel G, von Gerkan R, Dreyer T (1984) Pathomorphology of acute pancreatitis. Analysis of 367 autopsy cases and 3 surgical specimens. In: Gyr KE, Singer MV, Sarles H (eds) Pancreatitis. Concepts and classification. Elsevier, Amsterdam, pp 29–35

Konok GP, Thompson AG (1969) Pancreatic ductal mucosa as a protective barrier in the pathogenesis of pancreatitis. Am J Surg 117:18–23

Lampel M, Kern HF (1977) Acute interstitial pancreatitis in the rat induced by excessive doses of a pancreatic secretagogue. Virchows Arch [A] 373:97–117

Lankisch PG, Koop H, Winckler K, Kunze H, Vogt W (1978) Indomethacin treatment of acute experimental pancreatitis in the rat. Scand J Gastroenterol 13:629–633

Lankisch PG, Koop H, Winckler K, Schmidt H (1979) Continuous peritoneal dialysis as treatment of acute experimental pancreatitis in the rat. I. Effect on length and rate of survival. Dig Dis Sci 24:111–116

Lombardi B, Estes LW, Longnecker DS (1975) Acute hemorrhagic pancreatitis (massive necrosis) with fat necrosis induced in mice by DL-ethionine fed with a choline-deficient diet. Am J Pathol 79:465–475

Manabe T, Steer ML (1979) Protease inhibitors and experimental acute hemorrhagic pancreatitis. Ann Surg 190:13–17

McCutcheon AD (1968) A fresh approach to the pathogenesis of acute pancreatitis. Gut 9:296–310

Menguy RB, Hallenbeck GA, Bollman JL, Grindlay JH (1957) Ductal and vascular factors in etiology of experimentally induced acute pancreatitis. Arch Surg 74:881–889

Niederau C, Ferell LD, Grendell JH (1984) Onset, course and regression of caerulin-induced acute necrotizing pancreatitis in mice. Dig Dis Sci 29:962

Olazabal A (1983) Effect of prostaglandins E_2 and I_2 and of indomethacin on deoxycholic acid-induced damage to the rat bile-pancreatic duct. Gastroenterology 84:928–934

Opie EL (1901) The aetiology of acute haemorrhagic pancreatitis. Bull Johns Hopkins Hosp 12:182–188

Papp M (1976) Pathogenesis of acute pancreatitis: pancreatic ductal-interstitial-vascular and lymphatic pathways. Acta Med Acad Sci Hung 33:191–206

Paulino-Netto A, Dreiling DA (1960) Chronic duodenal obstruction: a mechano-vascular etiology of pancreatitis. Am J Dig Dis 5:1006–1018

Pfeffer RB, Stasior O, Hinton JW (1957) The clinical picture of the sequential development of acute hemorrhagic pancreatitis in the dog. Surg Forum 8:248–251

Popper HL, Necheles H (1942) Edema of the pancreas. Surg Gynecol Obstet 74:123–124

Popper HL, Necheles H, Russell KC (1948) Transition of pancreatic edema into pancreatic necrosis. Surg Gynecol Obstet 87:79–82

Radakovich M, Pearse HE, Strain WH (1952) Study of etiology of acute pancreatitis. Surg Gynecol Obstet 94:749–754

Rao KN, Toma J, Lombardi B (1976) Acute hemorrhagic pancreatitis in mice: intraparenchymal activation of zymogens, and other enzyme changes in pancreas and serum. Gastroenterology 70:720–726

Rao KN, Zuretti MF, Baccino FM, Lombardi B (1980) Acute hemorrhagic pancreatic necrosis in mice. The activity of lysosomal enzymes in the pancreas and the liver. Am J Pathol 98:45–60

Rao KN, Eagon PK, Okamura K (1982) Acute hemorrhagic pancreatic necrosis in mice. Induction in male mice treated with estradiol. Am J Pathol 109:8–14

Rao SS, Watt IA, Donaldson LA, Crocket A, Joffe SN (1981) A serial histologic study of the development and progression of acute pancreatitis in the rat. Am J Pathol 103:39–46

Reber HA, Mosley JG (1980) The effect of bile salts on the pancreatic duct mucosal barrier. Br J Surg 67:59–62

Reber HA, Roberts C, Way LW (1979) The pancreatic duct mucosal barrier. Am J Surg 137:128–134

Renner IG, Wisner JR (1983) Exogenous secretin ameliorates ceruletide induced acute pancreatitis in the dog. Dig Dis Sci 28:946

Rich AR, Duff EL (1936) Experimental and pathological studies on the pathogenesis of acute haemorrhagic pancreatitis. Bull Johns Hopkins Hosp 58:212–259

Saharia P, Margolis S, Zuidema GD, Cameron JL (1977) Acute pancreatitis with hyperlipemia: studies with an isolated perfused canine pancreas. Surgery 82:60–67

Sanfey H, Bulkley GB, Cameron JL (1985) The pathogenesis of acute pancreatitis. The source and role of oxygen-derived free radicals in three different experimental models. Ann Surg 201:633–639

Schmidt H, Creutzfeldt W (1969) The possible role of phospholipase A in the pathogenesis of acute pancreatitis. Scand J Gastroenterol 4:39–48

Seelig R, Seelig HP (1975) The possible role of serum complement system in the formal pathogenesis of acute pancreatitis. Acta Hepatogastroenterol 22:263–268

Seidel H (1910) Bemerkungen zu meiner methode der experimentellen erzeugung der akuten haemorrhagischen pankreatitis. Zentralbl Chir 37:1601–1604

Steer ML, .Meldolesi J, Figarella C (1984) Pancreatitis. The role of lysosomes. Dig Dis Sci 29:934–938

Thal A (1955) Studies on pancreatitis. II. Acute pancreatic necrosis produced experimentally by the Arthus sensitization reaction. Surgery 37:911–917

Thal A, Brackney E (1954) Acute hemorrhagic pancreatic necrosis produced by local Schwartzman reaction. JAMA 155:569–574

Watanabe O, Baccino MF, Steer ML, Meldolesi J (1984) Supramaximal caerulin stimulation and ultrastructure of rat pancreatic acinar cell: early morphological changes during development of experimental pancreatitis. Am J Physiol 246:G457–G467

White TT, Magee DF (1960) Perfusion of the dog pancreas with bile without production of pancreatitis. Ann Surg 151:245–250

Chapter 22

Free Radicals and Antioxidants in Pancreatic Inflammation

Hilary Sanfey

While many clinical situations are known to initiate acute pancreatitis, our understanding of the pathogenesis of this disorder is still incomplete, despite the accumulation of a considerable amount of experimental data. Therefore, the treatment of acute pancreatitis is non-specific and often does not alter the course of the disease. Many recent studies have suggested that the local and systemic effects of this disease may be mediated by a common pathway, irrespective of the initiating stimulus. Previous experimental work has demonstrated that an increase in capillary permeability is an early step in the development of acute pancreatitis in experimental models of ischaemic (Sanfey et al. 1985a), alcoholic (Sanfey and Cameron 1984), gallstone (Broe and Cameron 1982) and caerulein-induced pancreatitis (McEntee et al. 1989). This capillary injury is thought to be mediated by the action of oxygen-derived free radicals.

Oxygen Free Radicals

Over the past ten years oxygen-derived free radicals have been identified as playing a role in the pathogenesis of many different diseases. Radiation-induced nucleic acid injury, oxygen toxicity in the pulmonary parenchyma (Fox 1984) and reperfusion injury in the small intestine (Parks et al. 1983), heart (Gardner et al. 1983), skin (Im et al. 1984, 1985) and kidney (Koyama et al. 1985) are but a few examples of cellular and subcellular injury induced by oxygen-derived free radicals. Oxygen free radicals are potent oxidising and reducing agents which contain an uneven number of electrons in their outer orbital. This renders them unstable and highly reactive, and therefore capable of participating in chain reactions which may be thousands of events long (Fridovich 1978; Del Maestro 1979; McCord 1983). Free radicals are capable of injuring tissues by degradation of hyaluronic acid and collagen in the extracellular matrix (Halliwell

1978) or by direct damage to cell membranes through the peroxidation of structural lipids which results in the formation of lipid peroxidative radicals and fragmentation products such as malondialdehyde, all of which are toxic and serve to amplify the ultimate destructive effect (Kellogg and Fridovich 1975; Goldstein and Weissman 1977). Experimental studies have also demonstrated that free radical flux can result in disruption of lysosomal membranes (Fong et al. 1973) and degradation of nucleic acids (Morgan et al. 1976).

Under normal conditions a small amount of oxygen undergoes univalent reduction during which several toxic intermediates are produced, including the superoxide radical (O_2^-), hydrogen peroxide (H_2O_2) and the hydroxyl radical ($OH^·$). These toxic species are generally rendered harmless by endogenous free radical scavengers such as superoxide dismutase (SOD) (McCord and Fridovich 1978) and by intracellular catalases and peroxidases (Del Maestro et al. 1980). However, in some pathological conditions oxygen free-radical production exceeds the scavenging capability of these enzymes (oxidative stress) and tissue injury results, often in the form of endothelial cell damage.

The enzyme xanthine oxidase, which is present in the tissues as the inactive xanthine dehydrogenase, is one of the most common sources of free radical generation. The irreversible activation of xanthine dehydrogenase to xanthine oxidase, a process termed D to O conversion, occurs in the presence of ischaemia (Parks and Granger 1983). Ischaemia also results in the accumulation of hypoxanthine following the breakdown of ATP. After reperfusion oxygen is delivered to the tissues, thereby providing xanthine oxidase with the two substrates necessary for free radical generation: hypoxanthine and oxygen. One of the primary manifestations of this type of injury, which is referred to as an ischaemia-reperfusion injury, is an increase in capillary permeability.

Acute Pancreatitis

Oedematous Pancreatitis

The possible role of oxygen free radicals in the pathogenesis of acute oedematous pancreatitis was evaluated about ten years ago by Sanfey et al. (1984) in isolated canine pancreas models which mimicked three common clinical situations. Alcoholic pancreatitis was simulated by free fatty acid infusion, gallstone pancreatitis by partial duct obstruction combined with secretin stimulation and ischaemic pancreatitis by subjecting the preparation to 2 h of total ischaemia. Pancreatitis was manifest in each model by the presence of pancreatic weight gain, oedema formation and hyperamylasaemia. Pretreatment with the free radical scavengers SOD and catalase brought about a significant decrease in all three parameters in each of these models. SOD alone was as effective in reducing the injury response in ischaemic pancreatitis as the combination of SOD and catalase suggesting that, as in other experimental models of ischaemia, the superoxide radical was the more important injurious agent. Since both SOD and catalase were required to reduce the injury produced by free fatty acid infusion and by partial duct obstruction/secretin stimulation it seems that both the superoxide and the hydroxyl radicals play an important role in the pathogenesis of these forms of acute pancreatitis.

The manifestations of acute pancreatitis in these three models were also significantly modified by pretreatment with the xanthine oxidase inhibitor allopurinol (Sanfey et al. 1985b), which is further evidence that oxygen free radicals mediate an early, common step in the pathogenesis of acute pancreatitis, no matter what is the nature of the initiating stimulus, and that xanthine oxidase is the common source of these free radicals. The same picture of acute pancreatitis was reproduced in the absence of ischaemia, by infusion of the enzyme xanthine oxidase and the substrate hypoxanthine (Sanfey 1986; Sanfey et al. 1986). Because allopurinol was equally protective against pancreatitis in all three models, activation of xanthine oxidase appears to be the common denominator, even in the absence of ischaemia. This has been confirmed by other investigators (Sarr et al. 1987a). Chymotrypsin is an active precursor of the process of proteolytic activation of xanthine oxidase from xanthine dehydrogenase in vitro (Batelli et al. 1973), and it is possible that gallstone obstruction or hyperlipidaemia might activate chymotrypsin from a chymotrypsin precursor, and so initiate the biochemical cascade which results in free radical production.

The role of oxygen free radicals has also been investigated in caerulein-induced acute oedematous pancreatitis. Guice et al. (1986) demonstrated that SOD and catalase administered 30 min after caerulein significantly reduced pancreatic weight and diminished the changes in pancreatic histopathology. These investigators suggested that caerulein induces oxidative stress within the acinar cells, which results in membrane damage with leakage of excess free radicals, pancreatic enzymes and cellular debris into the interstitium. This injury is further potentiated by activation of complement and leucocytes (Guice et al. 1987). Even when administered after the injury, exogenous scavengers appeared to be capable of providing protection to the pancreas. However, other investigators have found that in this model SOD reduces pancreatic weight gain but not hyperamylasaemia (Saluja et al. 1986). In contrast Wisner and Renner (1988) found that allopurinol reduced pancreatic weight gain by 45% and hyperamylasaemia by 60% in the caerulein-induced pancreatitis model.

Caerulein infusion has also been shown to be associated with a decrease in pancreatic tissue SOD activity corresponding with an increase in malondialdehyde, which is a byproduct of free radical-mediated peroxidation of unsaturated fatty acids. Gough et al. (1990) used chemiluminescence (a phenomenon based on the emission of light during chemical reactions which is dependent on free radical activity) to assess free radical activity in the caerulein-induced pancreatitis model. Chemiluminescence values were elevated compared with controls and appeared to peak at 20 min after induction of pancreatitis; thereafter the levels decreased to control values. The authors suggested that this short-lived burst of free radical activity might be the precipitating event which leads to microvascular injury. It appears therefore, from the available data, which are based on direct as well as indirect measurement of free radical activity, that the role of oxygen-derived free radicals is well established in models of acute oedematous pancreatitis.

Leucocytes and macrophages serve as important sources of free radical production in many free radical-mediated forms of tissue injury (McCord 1974;

Sacks et al. 1978). Sarr et al. (1987b) found that depletion of 98% of the circulating leucocytes had no effect on the manifestations of acute pancreatitis induced by free fatty acid infusion in the isolated canine pancreas model. These results were perhaps to be expected in view of the wealth of experimental data which suggest that xanthine oxidase is the source of oxygen free radicals in experimental pancreatitis. Xanthine oxidase is considered unimportant in leucocyte-mediated free radical generation, which is thought to be dependent on activation of membrane-bound NADPH oxidase (Kakinuma 1974; Badwey et al. 1981, 1984). At a cellular level, the probable source of free radicals in experimental pancreatitis is the endothelial cell, which has been shown to contain the essential components for superoxide production (Ratych et al. 1987).

Haemorrhagic Pancreatitis

Whereas the role of oxygen-derived free radicals appears to be well established in models of acute oedematous pancreatitis, their role in haemorrhagic pancreatitis is less well defined. The two most commonly studied models of acute haemorrhagic pancreatitis are choline-deficient dietary pancreatitis and taurocholate duct injection. A choline deficient diet prevents digestive enzyme secretion from the acinar cell. As a result, digestive enzyme levels and zymogen granule numbers increase within the pancreas. The accumulated zymogen granules are discharged into lysosomes by crinophagy, digestive enzymes are activated within the pancreas and fatal haemorrhagic pancreatic necrosis develops (Lombardi 1976). Rutledge et al. (1987) found that the degree of hyperamylasaemia and the high mortality rate usually associated with the choline deficient diet model were reduced by treatment with catalase but not by allopurinol or dimethylsulphoxide (DMSO). However the administration of heat-denatured catalase produced similar results which suggests that the apparent protective effect of catalase was not related to its antioxidant properties. Since both allopurinol and DMSO reduced peripancreatic oedema, Rutledge et al. postulated that the generation of oxygen free radicals may be responsible for the production of oedema but not the other features of acute haemorrhagic pancreatitis. However, other investigators have demonstrated that treatment with allopurinol (Degertekin et al. 1984) or with a combination of SOD and catalase (Bank et al. 1985) reduced the manifestations of acute pancreatitis in this model. An increase in xanthine oxidase and lipoperoxidase activity with a corresponding decrease in SOD activity have been demonstrated by Nonaka et al. (1989a,b), who measured free radical activity in this model directly using electron spin resonance. This technique detects molecules such as free radicals which have unpaired electrons. These investigators found increased hydroxyl radical activity in choline deficient diet pancreatitis, which suggests that oxygen-derived free radicals do play a role in the development of pancreatic lesions in this model.

Retrograde injection of sodium taurocholate into the pancreatic duct produces immediate interstitial oedema and sequential necrosis of duct and acinar cells. This is a readily reproducible model of acute haemorrhagic pancreatitis (Aho and Nevelainen 1980). Lankisch et al. (1989) studied the effect of allopurinol in both the choline deficient diet and the taurocholate models. They found no benefit in terms of changes in amylase levels or mortality rate. Similarly, MacGowan et al. (1987) found that pretreatment with allopurinol did not affect the mortality rate of rats with taurocholate-induced haemorrhagic pancreatitis. Other investigators have found that the beneficial effects of pretreatment with SOD and catalase were minimal and consisted of reduction in pancreatic weight gain only (Blind et al. 1988). Gough et al. (1990) evaluated free radical activity by chemiluminescence in the taurocholate model. Peak activity occurred at 15 min which is earlier than in the caerulein-induced pancreatitis model, suggesting that free radical activity parallels the onset of pancreatitis and is higher in the more aggressive model of haemorrhagic pancreatitis than in the oedematous pancreatitis model. SOD administered intraductally immediately after taurocholate infusion significantly reduced the chemiluminescence levels. This was associated with a corresponding decrease in amylase level. However, prophylaxis with allopurinol did not reduce chemiluminescence or serum amylase levels in these studies.

Braganza (1988) has not shown any benefit of antioxidant therapy in a ductal model of haemorrhagic pancreatitis. However, Koiwai et al. (1989) observed significant benefit from treatment with allopurinol, SOD and catalase in a rat model of reflux acute pancreatitis with necrosis but no evidence of haemorrhage. Since high concentrations of lipid peroxidation products have been found in bile from patients with pancreatitis (Braganza et al. 1983), Anderson et al. (1986) investigated the possibility that reflux of peroxidation products into the pancreatic duct might initiate attacks of pancreatitis. They found that intraductal administration of peroxidised linoleic acid caused a greater degree of pancreatic injury than either bile alone or non-peroxidised linoleic acid. Again, pancreatic haemorrhage was not a feature in this model of reflux pancreatitis. Therefore, the evidence is conflicting regarding the role played by oxygen free radicals in acute haemorrhagic pancreatitis. It is possible that free radicals initiate acute pancreatitis but play a minor role, if any, in the progression to acute haemorrhagic pancreatitis.

The earliest disturbance at a cellular level in acute pancreatitis is loss of secretory polarity so that an abnormally large fraction of secretions (zymogens not activated enzymes) is discharged from the basolateral membrane rather than into the duct lumen. Experimental hyperstimulation models of acute pancreatitis have demonstrated vacuoles containing digestive as well as lysosomal enzymes in the acinar cell cytoplasm which result from defective sieving in the Golgi apparatus (Braganza 1990). Fusion of the enzyme compartments merely represents the normal scavenging function of lysosomes in which oxygen free radicals are believed to play a part, since oxidative stress increases lysosomal fragility (Fig. 1). Recently, scanning and transmission electron microscopy have shown, as predicted, capillary distortion occurs within as little as 15 min and progresses within 2 h to vessel truncation and calibre variation secondary to disruption of endothelial cells (Kelly et al. 1989). Guyan et al. (1988) have suggested that the primary and secondary metabolites of oxygen do not directly activate the zymogens. It is still not clear what brings about the change to acute haemorrhagic pancreatitis. Lipid oxidation products are potent chemo-attractants and Braganza and Rinderknecht (1988) have suggested that haemorrhagic pancreatitis is initiated by the extracellular secretions from leucocytes which are drawn into the pancreatic interstitium. It is possible that leucocyte-activated plasmin and thrombin could activate

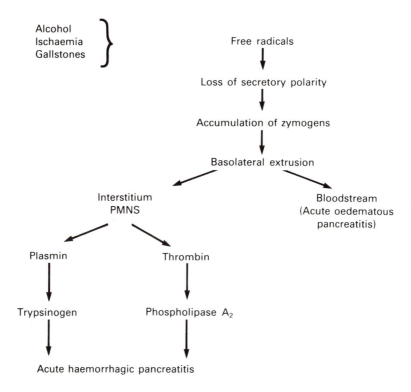

Fig. 1. Proposed mechanism for the role of oxygen free radicals in acute pancreatitis and the progression from oedematous to acute haemorrhagic pancreatitis. PMNS, polymorphonuclear leucocytes.

trypsinogen and pancreatic phospholipase A_2 respectively to produce haemorrhagic pancreatitis. While electron spin resonance and chemiluminescence studies have shown free radical activity in models of haemorrhagic pancreatitis, this activity appears to peak at an early stage in the disease in keeping with the theory that free radicals initiate acute pancreatitis but are less important in the progression to acute haemorrhagic pancreatitis.

Chronic Pancreatitis

In chronic pancreatitis, pancreatic structure remains irreversibly altered. These structural changes increase with each successive attack of pancreatitis. Free radicals may cause tissue injury in chronic pancreatitis by their ability to injure microtubules. The tissue extracellular spaces contain low concentrations of antioxidant enzymes, so free radicals liberated from cells can degrade cellular

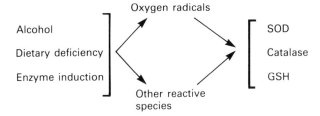

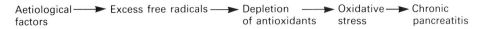

Fig. 2. Chronic pancreatitis: proposed mechanism for the role of oxidative stress.

supporting structures and provoke fibrosis. This mechanism is supported by the observation that administration of antioxidants to enzyme-induced hamsters over a 6-month period resulted in pancreatic lipoatrophy but without pancreatitis or fibrosis (Parker et al. 1986). Braganza (1988) has suggested that antioxidant stores are compromised in chronic pancreatitis (Fig. 2). There is indirect evidence of glutathione transferase B induction and these patients have large amounts of bilirubin in bile, changes which are similar to those seen in selenium-deficient animals exposed to enzyme inducers. Further support for the role of free radicals in chronic pancreatitis comes from the finding of increased levels of ferroxidase I activity with reduced levels of one or more antioxidants in serum (Martensson and Bolin 1986) and increased amounts of free radical markers including 9,11-linoleic acid in bile. An inadequate diet would appear to be the main reason why antioxidant supply runs out in patients with chronic pancreatitis (Braganza 1988) but excessive consumption of xenobiotics could be another important factor (Martensson and Bolin 1986). Malabsorbtion of antioxidants when pancreatic failure supervenes would compound these problems. In general the same pattern of antioxidant deficiency is found in patients with acute and chronic pancreatitis but the degree of antioxidant lack tends to be much higher in the latter. In a pilot study (Braganza et al. 1987) administration of an antioxidant cocktail prevented painful attacks of pancreatitis. It is possible, therefore, that chronic pancreatitis and idiopathic acute pancreatitis may be preventable by appropriate dietary advice and antioxidant supplementation in patients at risk.

References

Aho HJ, Nevelainen TJ (1980) Experimental pancreatitis in the rat. Ultrastructure of sodium taurocholate-induced pancreatic lesions. Scand J Gastroenterol 15:417–424

Anderson RL, Jeffrey IJ, Kay PM et al. (1986) Peroxidised linoleic acid and experimental pancreatitis. Int J Pancreatol 1:237–248

Badwey JA, Curnotte JT, Karnovsky ML (1981) Polyunsaturated fatty acids induce high levels of superoxide production by human neutrophils. J Biol Chem 256:640–653

Badwey JA, Curnotte JT, Robinson JM et al. (1984) Effects of free fatty acid on release of superoxide and on change of shape by human neutrophils. J Biol Chem 259:7870–7877

Bank S, Sandberg A, Aaron J et al. (1985) The effect of oxygen free radical scavengers on ethionine induced pancreatitis in mice. Dig Dis Sci 30:962 (abstract)

Batelli MG, Lorenzoni E, Stirpe F (1973) Milk xanthine oxidase type D (dehydrogenase) and type O (oxidase) purification, interconversion and some properties Biochem J 131:191–198

Blind JP, Marklund SL, Stenling R et al. (1988) Parenteral superoxide dismutase plus catalase diminish pancreatic oedema in sodium taurocholate-induced pancreatitis in the rat. Pancreas 3:563–567

Braganza JM (1988) Free radicals and pancreatitis. In: Rice-Evans C, Dormandy TL (eds) Free radicals chemistry, pathology and medicine. Richlieu Press, London, pp 357–381

Braganza JM (1990) Experimental acute pancreatitis. Curr Op Gastroenterol 6:763–768

Braganza JM, Rinderknecht H (1988) Free radicals and acute pancreatitis. Gastroenterology 94:1111–1112

Braganza JM, Wickens DG, Cawood P et al. (1983) Lipid peroxidation (free radical oxidation) products in bile from patients with pancreatic disease. Lancet ii:375–378

Braganza JM, Jeffrey IJM, Foster J et al. (1987) Recalcitrant pancreatitis: eventual control by antioxidants. Pancreas 4:489–494

Broe PJ, Cameron JL (1982) Experimental gallstone pancreatitis: pathogenesis and response to different treatment modalities. Ann Surg 195:566–573

Degertekin K, Van Meter A, Ertan K et al. (1984) Effect of hyperbaric oxygen therapy and a xanthine oxidase inhibitor on diet induced acute pancreatitis in mice. Gastroenterology 84:A1059 (abstract)

Del Maestro RF (1979) The influence of oxygen derived free radicals on in vitro and in vivo model systems. Acta Univ Upsal 340:32–40

Del Maestro RF, Thaw HH, Bjork J et al. (1980) Free radicals as mediators of tissue injury. Acta Physiol Scand 492:153–168 (suppl)

Fong KL, McKay PB, Poyer JL et al. (1973) Evidence that peroxidation of lysosomal membranes is initiated by hydroxyl free radicals produced during flavin enzyme activity. J Biol Chem 248:7792–7797

Fox RB (1984) Prevention of granulocyte mediated oxidant lung injury in rats by a hydroxyl radical scavenger, dimethylthiourea. J Clin Invest 74:1456–1464

Fridovich I (1978) The biology of oxygen radicals. Science 201:875–880

Gardner TJ, Stewart JR, Casale AS et al. (1983) Reduction of myocardial ischaemic injury with oxygen derived free radical scavengers. Surgery 94:423–432

Goldstein IM, Weissman G (1977) Effects of the generation of superoxide anion on permeability of liposomes. Biochem Biophys Res Commun 75:604–609

Gough D, Boyle B, Joyce WP et al. (1990) Free radical inhibition and serial chemiluminescence in evolving experimental pancreatitis. Br J Surg 77:1256–1259

Guice KS, Miller DE, Oldham KT et al. (1986) Superoxide dismutase and catalase. A possible role in established pancreatitis. Am J Surg 151:163–167

Guice KS, Oldham KT, Johnson KJ et al. (1987) Mechanisms of pancreatic capillary endothelial injury in acute pancreatitis. Surg Forum 34:144–146

Guyan PM, Braganza JM, Butler J (1988) The effect of oxygen metabolites on the zymogens of human pancreatic proteases. In: Rice-Evans C, Dormandy TL (eds) Free radicals, chemistry, pathology and medicine. Richlieu Press, London, pp 471–474

Halliwell B (1978) Biochemical mechanisms accounting for the toxic action of oxygen on living organisms. The key role of superoxide. Cell Biol Int Rep 2:113–128

Im MJ, Shen WH, Pak CJ et al. (1984) Effect of allopurinol on the survival of hyperemic island skin grafts. Plast Reconstr Surg 73:276–278

Im MJ, Manson PN, Bulkley GB et al. (1985) Effects of superoxide dismutase and allopurinol on the survival of acute island skin flaps. Ann Surg 201:357–359

Kakinuma K (1974) Effects of fatty acids on the oxidative metabolism of leukocytes. Biochim Biophys Acta 348:76–85

Kellogg EW, Fridovich I (1975) Superoxide, hydrogen peroxide and singlet oxygen in lipid peroxidation by a xanthine oxidase system. J Biol Chem 250:8812–8817

Kelly D, McEntee GP, McGeeney KF et al. (1989) Comparison of pathological changes in the local microvasculature in caerulein induced experimental haemorrhagic and oedematous pancreatitis. Digestion 43:152 (abstract)

Koiwai T, Oguchi H, Kawa S et al. (1989) The role of oxygen free radicals in experimental acute pancreatitis in the rat. Int J Pancreatol 5:135–143

Koyama I, Bulkley GB, Williams GM et al. (1985) The role of oxygen free radicals in mediating the reperfusion injury of cold preserved ischemic kidneys. Transplantation 40:590–595

Lankisch PG, Pohl U, Otto J et al. (1989) Xanthine oxidase inhibitor in acute experimental pancreatitis in rats and mice. Pancreas 4:436–440

Lombardi B (1976) Influence of dietary factors on the pancreatoxicity of ethionine. Am J Pathol 84:633–644

MacGowan S, Bouchier-Hayes DJ, Broe PJ (1987) Experimental pancreatitis: the effect of allopurinol. Gut 28:A368 (abstract)

Martensson J, Bolin T (1986) Sulfur amino acid metabolism in chronic relapsing pancreatitis. Am J Gastroenterol 81:1179–1184

McCord JM (1974) Free radicals in inflammation: Protection of synovial fluid by superoxide dismutase. Science 185:529–531

McCord JM (1983) The superoxide free radical: its biochemistry and pathophysiology. Surgery 94:412–414

McCord JM, Fridovich I (1978) The biology and pathology of oxygen radicals. Ann Intern Med 89:122–127

McEntee G, Leahy A, Cottell D et al. (1989) Three dimensional morphological study of the pancreatic microvasculature in caerulein induced experimental pancreatitis. Br J Surg 76:853–855

Morgan AR, Cone RL, Elgert TM (1976) The mechanism of DNA strand breakage by vitamin C and superoxide and the protective role of catalase and superoxide dismutase. Nucleic Acids Res 3:1139–1149

Nonaka A, Manabe T, Tamura K et al. (1989a) Changes of xanthine oxidase, lipid peroxide and superoxide dismutase in mouse acute pancreatitis. Digestion 43:41–46

Nonaka A, Manabe T, Asano N et al. (1989b) Direct ESR measurement of free radicals in mouse pancreatic lesions. Int J Pancreatol 5:203–211

Parker G, Branigan S, Houston JB et al. (1986) Potent induction of cytochromes P448 by corn oil in Syrian golden hamsters. Gut 27:A603 (abstract)

Parks DA, Granger DN (1983) Ischemia-induced microvascular changes. Role of xanthine oxidase and hydroxyl radical. Am J Physiol 245:G285–G289

Parks DA, Bulkley GB, Granger DN (1983) Role of oxygen derived free radicals in digestive tract diseases. Surgery 94:415–512

Ratych RE, Chuknyiska R, Bulkley GB (1987) The primary localisation of free radical generation after anoxia/reoxygenation in isolated endothelial cells. Surgery 102:122–131

Rutledge PL, Saluja AK, Powers RE et al. (1987) Role of oxygen derived free radicals in diet induced haemorrhagic pancreatitis in mice. Gastroenterology 93:41–47

Sacks T, Moldow CF, Craddock PR et al. (1978) Oxygen radicals mediate endothelial cell damage by complement stimulated granulocytes. J Clin Invest 61:1161–1167

Saluja A, Powers RE, Saluja M et al. (1986) The role of oxygen free radicals in caerulein-induced pancreatitis. Gastroenterology 90:1613 (abstract)

Sanfey H (1986) The pathogenesis of acute pancreatitis. MCh Thesis. Trinity College, Dublin

Sanfey H, Cameron JL (1984) Increased capillary permeability: an early lesion in acute pancreatitis. Surgery 96:485–491

Sanfey H, Bulkley GB, Cameron JL (1984) The role of oxygen derived free radicals in the pathogenesis of acute pancreatitis. Ann Surg 200:405–413

Sanfey H, Broe PJ, Cameron JL (1985a) Experimental ischemic pancreatitis: treatment with albumin. Am J Surg 150:297–300

Sanfey H, Bulkley GB, Cameron JL (1985b) The pathogenesis of acute pancreatitis: the source and role of oxygen derived free radicals in three different experimental models. Ann Surg 201:633–639

Sanfey H, Sarr MG, Bulkley GB et al. (1986) Oxygen derived free radicals and acute pancreatitis: a review. Acta Physiol Scand 548:109–118 (suppl)

Sarr MG, Bulkley GB, Cameron JL (1987a) Temporal efficacy of allopurinol during the induction of pancreatitis in the ex-vivo, perfused, canine pancreas. Surgery 101:342–345

Sarr MG, Bulkley GB, Cameron JL (1987b) The role of leukocytes in the production of oxygen derived free radicals in acute experimental pancreatitis. Surgery 101:292–296

Wisner JR, Renner IG (1988) Allopurinol attenuates caerulein induced acute pancreatitis in the rat. Gut 29:926–929

Chapter 23

The Microvasculature in Acute Pancreatitis

G. McEntee and D. Kelly

Introduction

Acute pancreatitis was first described in the late nineteenth century (Balser 1882) but the pathogenesis of this disease remains the subject of debate. Strategies for management of pancreatitis are non-specific and primarily supportive and reflect the current lack of understanding of the underlying disease process. However, there is considerable evidence to suggest that poor pancreatic perfusion is a major contributory factor in the development of pancreatitis and its associated complications. Clinical evidence is provided by the high incidence of pancreatitis following major surgery, such as cardiac (Warshaw and O'Hara 1978) and abdominal aortic surgery (Haas et al. 1985). Experimentally, local ischaemia may be used to induce pancreatitis by a variety of techniques ranging from simple occlusion of the major arterial supply (Popper et al. 1948) to Panum's classical experiment of local intra-arterial injection of wax particles (Panum 1862). In 1962 Pfeffer et al. produced pancreatitis of progressively increasing severity by injecting particles of decreasing size into the pancreatic circulation, suggesting that occlusion at a microvascular rather than an arterial or arteriolar level was the critical factor in determining the severity of disease. More recent experimental work has demonstrated a significant increase in capillary permeability at an early stage in the development of the disease process (Sanfey and Cameron 1984). All of these studies suggest that local pancreatic microcirculation plays an important role in the development of pancreatitis. This chapter reviews the changes seen in the pancreatic and systemic microvasculature, analyses their significance in the pathogenesis of the disease and discusses their clinical implications in terms of specific treatment of pancreatitis.

Alterations in Pancreatic and Systemic Microvasculature in Acute Pancreatitis

Distortion of the local vasculature in clinical pancreatitis was noted as early as 1936 by Rich and Duff. In an autopsy study of patients with haemorrhagic pancreatitis they observed several changes in the medium-sized vessels supplying the pancreas. These included adventitial condensation, swelling of the muscle fibres in the media and fraying of the internal elastic lamina. For obvious reasons the majority of attempts to investigate pancreatic microcirculation in pancreatitis have been experimental studies. Several techniques have been used including simple histological examination, intravital microscopy, angiography, intra-arterial injection of staining agents such as methylene blue, and electron microscopic imaging of microvascular casts. The majority of these studies have used the biliary pancreatitis model, in which a haemorrhagic form of pancreatitis is induced by retrograde injection of bile acids or trypsin into the pancreatic duct.

The microvascular changes described in the various studies are relatively consistent and differ only in time of onset after induction of pancreatitis. In 1954, Thal noted decreased capillary flow to the inflamed areas of the pancreas within 5 min of induction of pancreatitis, followed by capillary stasis and rupture with erythrocyte extravasation (Thal 1954). The findings were supported by Papp et al. (1966) using the technique of rubidium clearance. They demonstrated a reduction in pancreatic perfusion of the inflamed areas with redistribution of capillary blood flow to non-involved areas within 3 h (Papp et al. 1966). The same workers using polyvinyl chloride (PVC) and India ink gelatin casts subsequently provided further evidence for reduced capillary flow to involved areas by demonstrating occlusion of terminal arterioles with stump-like terminations of the gelatin cast, poor capillary filling and an increase in arteriovenous shunting (Papp et al. 1969). More recent studies using microvascular casting techniques and intravital microscopy report marked impairment of pancreatic microvasculature commencing 30 min after induction of pancreatitis (Schiller and Anderson 1975).

Using a combination of scanning electron microscopy (SEM) and microvascular casting, our laboratory has recently obtained a detailed three-dimensional view of the microcirculation not only in the retrograde bile injection model (Kelly et al. 1989a) but also in the reversible and relatively mild oedematous model induced by caerulein infusion (McEntee et al. 1989). In addition we have studied the changes seen in the microcirculation of the liver, lung and kidney, organs known to be impaired in acute pancreatitis, and have compared the changes seen in the two models (Delaney et al. 1990; Kelly et al. 1989b). Furthermore, we correlated the findings with transmission electron microscopy (TEM) studies of the microvasculature in cross section and with TEM changes seen in the acinar cell itself (Kelly et al. 1991b).

Using retrograde ductal injection of 0.2 ml 5% sodium taurocholate we induced haemorrhagic pancreatitis in the rat. SEM studies of casts of the local circulation demonstrated changes in the microvasculature as early as 15 min after induction of pancreatitis with variation in capillary diameter and blindly ending capillary cast buds. These changes progressed with time and at 12 h there was a dramatic reduction in the previously dense capillary network due to failure of the capillaries to fill. Furthermore, there was evidence of capillary disruption with leakage of cast material from the typically smooth capillary mould. Similar changes were noted in the caerulein model, and were detectable within 30 min of commencing the infusion. As in the haemorrhagic model these changes progressed with time but the degree of distortion was considerably less at all stages in the caerulein than in the haemorrhagic model (Fig. 1a,b). TEM studies provided evidence of intravascular thrombosis in the haemorrhagic model but only red cell congestion and stasis were noted in the caerulein model.

A further study of the caerulein model demonstrated changes in the acinar cell prior to any detectable changes in the microvasculature suggesting that the latter was a consequence rather than a cause of pancreatitis in this model.

The systemic microvasculature was assessed in the two experimental models by obtaining casts of the liver, lung and kidney at designated time intervals following induction of pancreatitis. Haemorrhagic pancreatitis was associated with demonstrable distortion of the hepatic (Fig. 2a,b) and pulmonary microvasculature (Fig. 3a,b) at the earliest period studied (15 and 60 min respectively); these changes progressed with time. No changes were noted in the renal microvasculature until 12 h when incomplete filling of the glomeruli was seen (Fig. 4a,b). Intravascular thrombosis was also demonstrated in TEM studies of the hepatic microcirculation but not in the pulmonary or renal vessels. Despite the fact that the caerulein model is associated with a reversible mild oedematous pancreatitis, microvascular changes were also seen in both the liver and the lung at the earliest period studied (30 and 60 min, respectively) but the kidney was spared. Once again the changes seen in the caerulein model were less than those seen in haemorrhagic pancreatitis and there was no evidence of intravascular thrombosis in any of the organs studied in the caerulein model.

Pathogenesis of Microvascular Changes in Acute Pancreatitis

It is clear that experimental pancreatitis at least is associated with gross distortion of the local and systemic microvasculature and our experience suggests that this occurs, albeit to varying degrees, regardless of the type of experimental model used. The retrograde bile injection model is thought to exert its effect on the pancreas by the interstitial route. Rupture of the ductoacinar junction releases pancreatic juices into the interstitial spaces resulting in vasospasm and gross microvascular disruption. The local ischaemia thus induced produces a typically severe haemorrhagic pancreatitis (Bockman et al. 1971). The caerulein hyperstimulation model on the other hand exerts its effect primarily within the acinar cell. Intracellular autophagic vacuoles develop which coalesce with the zymogen granules and subsequently release their contents laterally between cells and hence into the interstitial space at the base of the acinar cells (Lampel and Kern 1977). The presence of pancreatic

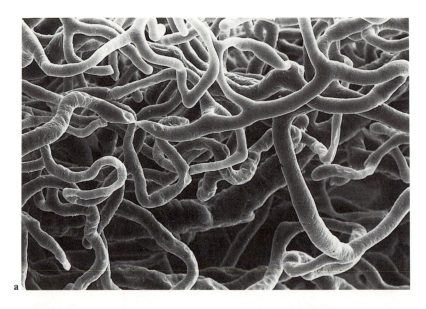

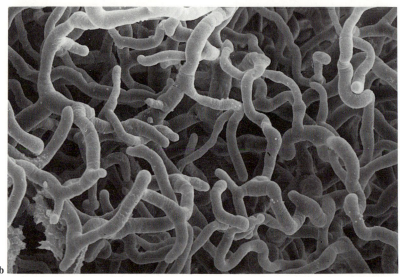

Fig. 1. a, SEM view of pancreatic vascular cast in control animal. The microvascular bed is characterised by a dense network of interlacing vessels. × 650. **b**, SEM view of a pancreatic vascular cast 4 h after induction of caerulein pancreatitis. Note the numerous blind ending capillary buds and blebs of cast material on the surface of the cast. × 600.

enzymes in the local interstitial spaces is the end result in both models. Presumably those factors present in the pancreatic juices which cause local microvascular distortion subsequently pass into the circulation and exert their effects systemically. It remains unclear why the retrograde bile injection model should produce such a severe and irreversible pancreatitis whereas the caerulein

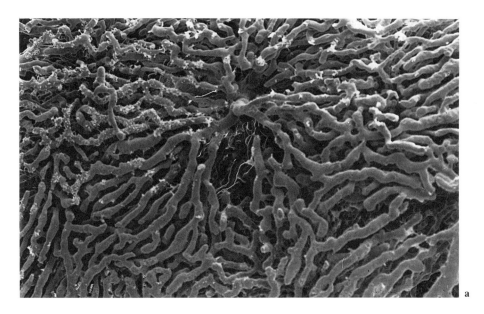

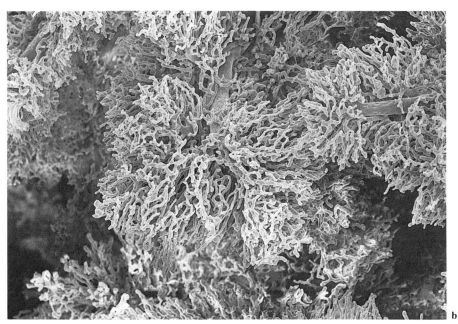

Fig. 2. a, SEM view of hepatic vascular cast in control animal. The central vein is visible in the centre of the micrograph, with sinusoids radiating to the periphery. × 110. **b**, 12 hours after induction of bile salt pancreatitis the normal anatomical arrangement has been severely disrupted. There is loss of normal vascular density and the vessels outlined are tortuous and terminate abruptly. × 100.

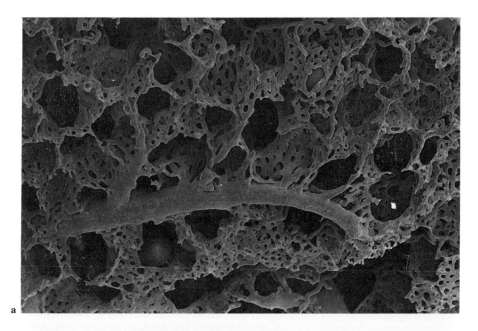

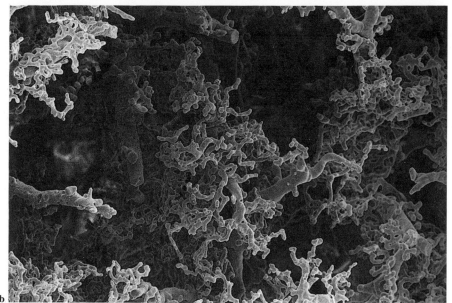

Fig. 3. a, SEM view of pulmonary microvasculature in the control animal. The capillaries form basket like structures around the alveoli. × 180. **b**, SEM view of pulmonary vasculature 12 h after induction of bile salt pancreatitis. The basket type arrangement is lost and the vessels are tortuous and end abruptly. Blebs of cast material are visible on the surface of the major vessel trunks. × 130.

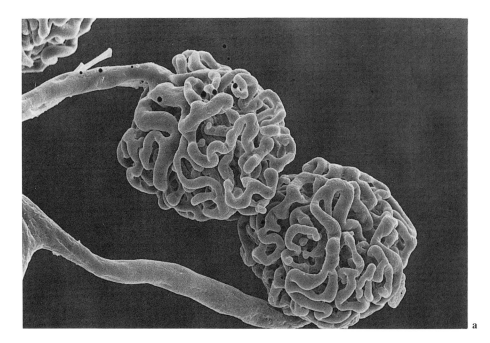

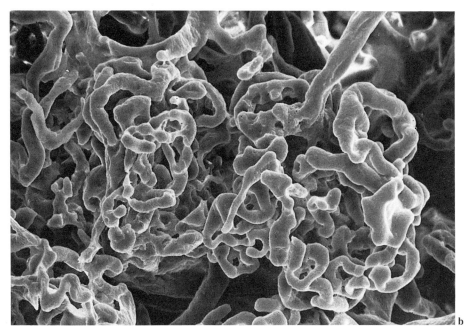

Fig. 4. a, SEM view of vascular cast of glomeruli in the control animal. × 390. **b**, Abnormal glomeruli found 12 h after induction of pancreatitis. The vessels are tortuous in outline and many terminate abruptly. × 430.

model produces a reversible oedematous form. The former is associated with TEM evidence of intravascular thrombosis and a greater degree of microvascular disruption – presumably both factors result in a greater degree of local ischaemia in the haemorrhagic model. Other factors known to decrease local tissue perfusion and increase local ischaemia include haemoconcentration due to loss of intravascular volume and increased interstitial pressure due to obstructed lymph drainage (Anderson and Schiller 1968). The increased microvascular disruption seen in the haemorrhagic model suggests that the degree of haemoconcentration and the degree of lymph drainage may be greater in the haemorrhagic rather than the oedematous model.

Oxygen free radicals have recently been implicated in the development of acute pancreatitis and are thought to be responsible for the early alteration in capillary permeability (Sanfey et al. 1986; Gough et al. 1990). Perhaps a comparison of oxygen free radical release in the two models may help to elucidate those factors responsible for determining the severity of pancreatitis and provide a rational basis for specific therapy.

Clinical Implications

Our experience and that of other workers suggests that distortion of the local and systemic microvasculature is a universal finding in acute pancreatitis regardless of the underlying aetiology. Moreover, the degree of distortion reflects the subsequent severity of the disease. The microvascular changes demonstrated experimentally have been used clinically in the evaluation of the severity of the disease. Failure clearly to outline the pancreas using contrast enhanced computed tomography is indicative of severe local microvascular disruption and is a reliable indicator of underlying pancreatic necrosis (Nuutinen et al. 1986).

Unfortunately, evidence of microvascular disruption has found little clinical application to date in terms of specific therapy. Restoration of intravascular volume remains the primary therapeutic goal and ideally should be introduced as early as possible to minimise intravascular fluid loss. However, patients typically present many hours following the onset of symptoms, by which time intravascular volume may already be significantly depleted, which will further aggravate local pancreatic ischaemia and increase the likelihood of haemorrhagic rather than oedematous pancreatitis. Several solutions, both crystalloid and colloid, have been used successfully to restore intravascular volume but few have any beneficial effect on local pancreatic perfusion. Some encouraging results have been obtained recently using high molecular weight dextran (60 or 70) which has known antithrombotic properties (Klar et al. 1990). Experimentally, dextran not only improves cardiac output but also increases pancreatic perfusion (Lehtola et al. 1986). This experimental work has been supported by some preliminary clinical experience in which red blood cells were withdrawn from the patient in exchange for similar volumes of dextran 70, in order to reduce the haematocrit to 30% (Klar et al., unpublished data).

An alternative approach to management is to introduce treatment aimed at the prevention or reduction of microvascular distortion at a molecular level. It has been suggested that oxygen free radicals are implicated in the alteration of capillary permeability which occurs early in the pathogenesis of the disease. If this is so, perhaps treatment with oxygen free radical scavengers might be beneficial. However, the greatest obstacle to developing successful specific forms of therapy for acute pancreatitis remains the almost inevitable delay in presentation for treatment. In the absence of detailed clinical data, the weight of experimental evidence suggests that a sequence of pathological events occurs early in the development of pancreatitis which if not corrected or minimised will produce a severe and sometimes irreversible haemorrhagic pancreatitis in a significant proportion of patients. If any specific forms of therapy are to be identified and evaluated they should be introduced at an early stage in the disease process where they are likely to exert their influence on those factors which determine the subsequent severity of the disease.

References

Anderson NC, Schiller WR (1968) Microcirculatory dynamics in the normal and inflamed pancreas. Am J Surg 115:118–127

Balser W (1882) First foreign description of pancreatitis on clinical level. Virchows Arch [A] 90:52–54

Bockman DE, Schiller WR, Anderson MC (1971) Route of retrograde flow in the exocrine pancreas during ductal hypertension. Arch Surg 103:321–329

Delaney C, McEntee G, Cottell D, McGeeney K, Fitzpatrick J (1990) The effect of caerulein induced pancreatitis on the hepatic microvasculature. Br J Surg 77:294–296

Gough D, Boyle B, Joyce W et al. (1990) Free radical inhibition and serial chemiluminescence in evolving experimental pancreatitis. Br J Surg 77:1256–1260

Haas GS, Warshaw AL, Daggett WM, Aretz HT (1985) Acute pancreatitis after cardiopulmonary bypass. Am J Surg 149:508–515

Kelly D, McEntee G, Cottell D, McGeeney K, Fitzpatrick JM (1989a) Diffuse vascular injury is a critical factor in the extrapancreatic organ impairment of acute haemorrhagic pancreatitis. Digestion 43:152

Kelly D, McEntee G, Delaney C, McGeeney K, Fitzpatrick JM (1989b) Correlation of ultrastructural acinar cell changes with changes in the local microvasculature in caerulein induced pancreatitis. Gut 30:A742

Klar E, Messmer K, Warshaw AL, Herfarth C (1990) Pancreatic ischaemia in experimental acute pancreatitis: mechanism, significance and therapy. Br J Surg 77:1205–1210

Lampel M, Kern HF (1977) Acute interstitial pancreatitis in the rat induced by excessive doses of a pancreatic secretagogue. Virchows Arch 373:97–117

Lehtola A, Kivilaasko E, Puolakkainen P, Karonen SL, Lempinen M, Schroder T (1986) Effects of dextran 70 versus crystalloids in the microcirculation of porcine haemorrhagic pancreatitis. Surg Gynecol Obstet 162:556–562

McEntee GP, Leahy A, Cottell DC, Dervan P, McGeeney KF, Fitzpatrick JM (1989) Three dimensional morphological study of the pancreatic microvasculature in caerulein induced experimental pancreatitis. Br J Surg 76:853–855

Nuutinen P, Kivisaari L, Standertskjold-Nordenstam CG, Lempinen M, Schroder T (1986) Microangiography of the pancreas in experimental oedemic and haemorrhagic pancreatitis. Scand J Gastroenterol 21:12–17

Panum PL (1862) Experimentelle Beitrage zur Lehre von der Embolie. Virchows Arch [A] 25:308–338

Papp M, Makara GB, Hajtman B, Csaki I (1966) A quantitative study of pancreatic blood flow in experimental pancreatitis. Gastroenterology 51:524–528

Papp M, Ungvari GY, Nemeth PE, Munkassi I. Zubek L (1969) The effect of bile induced pancreatitis on the intrapancreatic vascular pattern in dogs. Scand J Gastroenterol 4:681–689

Pfeffer RB, Lazzarini-Robertson A Jr, Safadi D, Mixter G Jr, Secoy CF, Hinton JW (1962) Gradations of pancreatitis, oedematous through haemorrhagic experimentally produced by controlled injection of microspheres into blood vessels in dogs. Surgery 51:764–769

Popper HB, Necheles H, Russell KC (1948) Transition of pancreatic oedema into pancreatic necrosis. Surg Gynecol Obstet 87:79–83

Rich AR, Duff GL (1936) Experimental and pathological studies on pathogenesis of acute haemorrhagic peritonitis. Bull Johns Hopkins Hosp 58:212–216

Sanfey H, Cameron JL (1984) Increased capillary permeability! An early lesson in acute pancreatitis. Surgery 96: 485–491

Sanfey H, Sarr MG, Bulkley GB, Cameron JL (1986) Oxygen-derived free radicals and acute pancreatitis: a review. Acta Physiol Scand 548:109–118

Schiller WR, Anderson MC (1975) Microcirculation of the normal and inflamed canine pancreas. Ann Surg 181:466–470

Thal A (1954) Studies on pancreatitis IV. The pathogenesis of bile pancreatitis. Surg Forum 5:391–394

Warshaw AL, O'Hara PJ (1978) Susceptibility of the pancreas to ischaemic injury in shock. Ann Surg 188:197–201

Section G

Acute Pancreatitis: Clinical Studies

Chapter 24

The Diagnosis and Assessment of Severity in Acute Pancreatitis

D. I. Heath and C. W. Imrie

Diagnosis of Acute Pancreatitis

Whilst the diagnosis of acute pancreatitis can sometimes be difficult to make, in the majority of cases it is remarkably straightforward. In spite of this, a recent study (Wilson and Imrie 1988) demonstrated that the diagnosis was missed in 42% of fatal attacks of acute pancreatitis. In almost all cases this failure could be attributed to a failure to consider the diagnosis. For this reason the first prerequisite for making the diagnosis is a high index of suspicion.

Clinical Evaluation

Clinical evaluation, whilst having a low sensitivity, may provide important indicators of the diagnosis. Almost all patients with acute pancreatitis experience severe epigastric pain passing through to the back, which may be relieved by leaning forward and is often associated with vomiting. There may in addition be a recent history of jaundice, excessive alcohol intake or drug ingestion prior to the onset of symptoms. On examination, there may be jaundice, tachypnoea, cardiovascular collapse, renal failure, a tense distended abdomen with guarding, ileus and peritoneal or pleural effusions.

Amylase

Serum and urinary amylase estimations are, at present, the most widely employed and effective diagnostic tests in acute pancreatitis. The normal range of the Phadebas test is 0–300 IU/l with a concentration greater than four times normal being considered diagnostic. Most of the enzyme is derived from the pancreas (amylase P) and salivary glands (amylase S) each of which contribute approximately 50% of the total enzyme production. The standard method of measuring serum amylase concentrations (a colorimetric assay which measures the amount of starch split by the enzyme) does not distinguish between these isoenzymes. In spite of this it is uncommon for diagnostic confusion to arise for this reason alone. This has been confirmed by a number of studies which have measured isoenzymes and have failed to demonstrate any major increase in diagnostic accuracy (O'Donnell et al. 1977; Warshaw 1977; Kolars et al. 1984). A missed or false positive diagnosis is more likely to result from the inappropriate application of the test or an alternative pathology.

Hyperlipidaemia will interfere with the amylase assay and give a false negative result. Dilution of the serum or the measurement of urinary amylase avoids this problem (Dickson et al. 1984). The most common differential diagnoses are perforated peptic ulcer and mesenteric ischaemia. Other causes of hyperamylasaemia are given in Table 1.

The sensitivity and specificity of amylase estimation depends on the aetiology of the pancreatitis (Ranson et al. 1976; MRC working party 1977), and the cut off concentration selected. In addition serum amylase concentrations will only remain elevated for 2–3 days after onset of symptoms. If there is a delay before the patient presents, the amylase concentration may be normal at the time of admission. This problem may be overcome by measurement of urinary amylase concentrations.

About 24% of the serum amylase is removed through the kidneys at a clearance rate of 2–3 ml/h, compared with a creatinine clearance of 100 ml/h (Levitt et al. 1977). From this the amylase–creatinine clearance ratio can be calculated. Although initial reports displayed a high diagnostic accuracy (Murray and McKay 1977) subsequent studies in which patients were compared against patients with other abdominal conditions rather than normal controls have failed to maintain these good results (Farrer and Calkins 1976; McMahon et al. 1982). This test is not widely used and is of doubtful clinical value (McMahon et al. 1982; Moossa 1984).

In clinical practice patients with a high amylase who do not have acute pancreatitis progress quite differently from those with acute pancreatitis. For example, mesenteric ischaemia/infarction and perforated duodenal ulcers will rapidly declare their presence by sepsis or other features. It is the combination of the clinical course of the early illness and an elevated amylase concentration which strongly indicate the diagnosis of acute pancreatitis.

Lipase

The measurement of serum lipase concentrations should be a more sensitive indicator of the presence of acute pancreatitis since production of this enzyme is almost totally confined to the pancreas. Whilst a number of studies have confirmed this (Song et al. 1970; Kolars et al. 1984), there is still the drawback that lipase concentrations are elevated in a number of other acute abdominal emergencies such as perforated peptic ulcer or mesenteric ischaemia. It has not been widely adopted into clinical practice because the assay has in the past been complex. It should, however, probably replace amylase as the diagnostic test of choice since new kits are both reliable and cheap. Lipase is not excreted in urine (Rick 1972).

Table 1. Causes of hyperamylasaemia

Pancreatic disease	Acute pancreatitis
	Trauma
	Pancreatic carcinoma
	Periampullary tumours
Hepatobiliary disorders	ERCP and ES
Gastrointestinal disorders	Perforated peptic ulcer[a]
	Acute intestinal obstruction
	Mesenteric infarction[a]
	Intestinal perforation
	Afferent loop syndrome
Gynaecological disorders	Salpingitis
	Ovarian tumour
	Ruptured ectopic pregnancy[a]
	Endometriosis
Salivary gland disorders	Mumps
	Parotitis
	Sialadenitis
	Trauma
	Tumours
	Maxillo-facial surgery
Renal disease	Acute renal failure
	Chronic renal failure
Macroamylasaemia	
Neoplasia	Lung tumours
	Ovarian cystadenocarcinoma
Miscellaneous causes	Dissecting aortic aneurysm[a]
	Post operative especially abdominal and cardiac surgery
	Diabetic ketoacidosis
	Intravenous steroids

ERCP, endoscopic retrograde cholangiopancreatography; ES, endoscopic sphincterotomy.
[a] Conditions which most commonly mimic acute pancreatitis and also show marked rise in serum amylase concentration.

Other Enzymes

Other pancreatic enzymes have been evaluated in the diagnosis of acute pancreatitis, including trypsin (Elias et al. 1977; Mero et al. 1982), phospholipase A$_2$ (Mero et al. 1982), carboxypeptidase B (Delk et al. 1985) and elastase (Umeki et al. 1985). The difficulties associated with these assays make their use in routine clinical practice impractical.

Peritoneal Aspiration and Lavage

Peritoneal aspiration and lavage have been used principally in the assessment of severity but they have also proved valuable in diagnosis (Keith et al. 1950;

Pfeffer et al. 1958). A high amylase concentration in the aspirated fluid is consistent with a diagnosis of acute pancreatitis, but the presence of blood or bile staining, a foul smell or organisms seen on Gram staining suggest an alternative diagnosis. Under these circumstances an urgent laparotomy is required (Pickford et al. 1977).

Plain Abdominal Radiographs

Plain abdominal and chest radiographs are of no value in making the diagnosis. They may, however, be important in the detection of alternative diagnoses such as a perforated viscus or ischaemic bowel.

Ultrasound

Ultrasound (US) examination may demonstrate the presence of a peritoneal effusion or a swollen pancreas. However, a clear view of the latter is frequently obscured by overlying bowel gas (McKay et al. 1982; Moossa 1982) so the diagnostic sensitivity of US is poor. In McKay et al.'s (1982) series of 114 patients the pancreas was visualised in only 85 (74.5%). There was no correlation between the severity of the attack and the findings on US, although all patients who subsequently developed pseudocysts had evidence of pancreatic oedema. More importantly, US is able to demonstrate the presence of associated gallstones with up to 96% accuracy (McKay et al. 1982), although more than one ultrasound scan may be required.

Computed Tomography (CT)

Pancreatic or peripancreatic swelling, peripancreatic collections of fluid or pus and peritoneal effusions may all be present in acute pancreatitis and can be readily detected by CT. Our personal experience suggests that almost all patients with acute pancreatitis have detectable abnormalities on CT (unpublished data) although most other series have suggested that the diagnostic sensitivity of CT is low, with 10%–29% of mild cases showing a normal gland (Silverstein et al. 1981; Nordestgaard et al. 1986; Clavien et al. 1988). The relative complexity of performing CT in all patients with a possible diagnosis of acute pancreatitis, and the greater cost of CT preclude its use as a routine diagnostic tool. It may, however, be usefully employed in cases where the diagnosis is in doubt, especially when a normal amylase could be explained by a delay in presentation.

Early Assessment of Disease Severity

The need for an accurate means of diagnosing acute pancreatitis is self-evident. The importance of an objective means of assessment of severity is not so immediately obvious. Instinctively we expect that careful clinical examination will detect those patients with severe disease, but unfortunately, this has not proved to be the case. For this reason a number of objective means of severity assessment have been developed.

The principal benefit of early assessment of severity is in the selection of patients who will require intensive monitoring and therapy. Almost all the mortality and morbidity of acute pancreatitis is concentrated in the 25% of patients classified as suffering from severe disease. Those predicted to have a mild attack have a very low mortality of only 1%–2% (Imrie et al. 1978a; Corfield et al. 1985; Leese et al. 1987). Whilst it is difficult to demonstrate in a statistically satisfactory manner that early active support measures have an appreciable effect on mortality, such support does delay what appears to be inevitable death, and in time more effective therapy should save some of these patients.

The ideal method of severity assessment should be simple and reproducible, should take account of the varying aetiologies of acute pancreatitis and the patient's pre-existing disease state, should be available as soon after admission as possible and should be capable of monitoring the disease course and any response to therapy. None of the means of assessment of severity described below fulfils all these criteria, but each has its strengths and weaknesses. Finally it should be noted that the systems of severity assessment only indicate the increased risk of a patient developing a complicated attack of acute pancreatitis, and cannot be expected to predict the type of complication.

Clinical Evaluation

Clinical assessment tends to be very subjective and is of limited value in the early detection of severe acute pancreatitis. Increasing age, cardiovascular collapse, renal impairment, tachypnoea, tetany, body wall ecchymosis, abdominal masses and prolonged paralytic ileus are all correlated with a severe outcome, but are either not present in many patients with severe disease or take a long time to assess. Body wall ecchymosis is especially specific for a complicated course, a mortality of 37% and complication rate of 96% (Dickson and Imrie 1984). The mortality of young patients with abdominal wall ecchymosis was not greater than those without it, whereas in patients over 70 years its appearance was frequently associated with an early death.

McMahon et al. (1980) and Corfield et al. (1985) reported the percentage of patients with mild disease correctly classified on admission (using clinical assessment alone) as 100% and 85% respectively. Severe attacks were correctly predicted in only 39% and 34% of cases. A delay of 24 and 48 h increased the percentage correct prediction to 73% and 83% (McMahon et al. 1980; Corfield et al. 1985), which is similar to the disease specific multifactorial scoring systems (Ranson et al. 1976; Imrie et al. 1978a).

Recently we have found that the sensitivity of clinical assessment on admission, in detecting severe attacks of acute pancreatitis was 64% (Heath and Imrie 1990) approximately twice that previously reported (McMahon et al. 1980; Corfield et al. 1985). The reasons for the increased sensitivity are unclear. By 48 h the sensitivity and specificity values were similar to the previous series.

Table 2. The original Ranson criteria for severity assessment in acute pancreatitis: a severe attack is predicted by the presence of three or more positive factors

On admission		
Age	> 55 years	
WCC	> 16 × 10⁹/l	
Blood glucose	> 10 mmol/l	
LDH	> 150 American U%	(> 350 IU/l)
AST	> 250 Sigma-Frankel U%	(> 120 IU/l)
During the first 48 h		
Fall in haematocrit of	> 10%	
Serum calcium	< 2.0 mmol/l	
Base deficit	> 4 mmol/l	
Increase in blood urea	> 5 mg/dl	(> 1.0 mmol/l)
Fluid sequestration	> 6 l	
Arterial Po_2	< 60 mmHg	(< 8.0 kPa)

AST, Aspartate aminotransferase; LDH, lactic dehydrogenase.

Multifactorial Scoring Systems

Ranson and Glasgow Scoring Systems

Ranson is credited with producing the first reliable means of predicting severe attacks of acute pancreatitis (Ranson et al. 1974a) (Table 2). The precursor of this scoring system has since been validated by further studies (Ranson et al. 1976; Ranson 1982).

A high proportion of Ranson's original study population (74%) had alcohol-related attacks. While the scoring system worked well in these patients it was less effective in those with gallstone-related disease. The system was therefore modified for those with gallstones (Ranson 1979). The measurement of arterial oxygen tension was omitted and eight of the 10 remaining parameters were modified (Table 3), thus producing a confusing "double system".

Ranson's original system was also modified and applied to patients within

Table 3. The modified Ranson criteria for severity assessment in acute pancreatitis: a severe attack is predicted by the presence of three or more positive factors

On admission		
Age	> 70 years	
WCC	> 18 × 10⁹/l	
Blood glucose	< 220 mg/ml	(> 12 mmol/l)
LDH	> 400 IU/l	
AST	> 240 Sigma-Frankel U%	(> 250 IU/l)
During the first 48 h		
Fall in haematocrit of	> 10%	
Serum calcium	< 8 mg/dl	(< 2.0 mmol/l)
Base deficit	> 5.0 meql/l	(> 5.0 mmol/l)
Increase in blood urea	> 2 mg/dl	(> 0.5 mmol/l)
Fluid sequestration	> 6 l	

AST, Aspartate aminotransferase; LDH, lactate dehydrogenase.

the UK (Imrie et al. 1978a) (Table 4). In this initial study all 14 patients who died were correctly predicted in the severe group by the presence of three or more prognostic criteria. However, the authors subsequently noted a tendency for patients with gallstone-related attacks to be inappropriately predicted as suffering from a severe attack more frequently than those with alcohol-related disease because of the association with gallstones of greater age and elevation of aspartate aminotransferase (AST). Osborne et al. (1981) modified the original Glasgow criteria (Table 5) and found improved accuracy of prediction in a relatively small number of patients.

The Glasgow system has subsequently been re-examined and further modifications suggested. Blamey et al. (1984) reviewed 405 episodes of acute pancreatitis diagnosed during a seven-year period in Glasgow. Of the nine prognostic factors only two, serum calcium less than 2 mmol/l and lactate dehydrogenase (LDH) greater than 600 IU/l had independent predictive value. AST concentration, included in the original scoring system, was not of predictive value. It was suggested that AST should be dropped from the system, leaving eight factors including age. This system has recently been used successfully in a study of early endoscopic sphincterotomy in patients with gallstone pancreatitis (Neoptolemos et al. 1986).

It should be noted that the sensitivity and specificity of these systems varies with the aetiology of the attack of acute pancreatitis. Both peritoneal lavage (see below) and clinical assessment were significantly worse at predicting severe attacks in patients with gallstones as compared with alcohol-related attacks. The modified Glasgow scoring system (Osborne et al. 1981) was equally effective in both aetiological groups of patients within a multicentre study of severe acute pancreatitis in Leeds, Bristol and Glasgow (Corfield et al. 1985).

Table 4. The Glasgow criteria for severity prediction in acute pancreatitis: a severe attack is predicted by the presence of three or more positive criteria

On admission	
Age	> 70 years
WCC	> 18 × 10⁹/l
Blood glucose	> 12 mmol/l (in the absence of diabetes mellitus)
LDH	> 400 IU/l
AST	> 240 IU/l
During the first 48 h	
Age	> 55 years
Arterial P_{O_2}	< 8.0 kPa
Serum albumin	< 32 g/l
Serum calcium	< 2.0 mmol/l
White cell count	> 15 × 10⁹/l
AST	> 100 U/l
LDH	> 600 IU/l
Blood glucose	> 10 mmol/l in the absence of pre-existing diabetes mellitus
Plasma urea	> 16 mmol/l

AST, Aspartate aminotransferase; LDH, lactate dehydrogenase. From Imrie et al. (1978a), with permission.

Table 5. The modified Glasgow criteria for severity prediction in acute pancreatitis: a severe attack is predicted by the presence of three or more positive criteria

Arterial Po_2	< 8.0 kPa
Serum albumin	< 32 g/l
Serum calcium	< 2.0 mmol/l
White cell count	$> 15 \times 10^9$/l
(AST)	> 200 U/l
(LDH)	> 600 U/l
Blood glucose	> 10 mmol/l (in the absence of diabetes mellitus)
Blood urea	> 16 mmol/l

AST, Aspartate aminotransferase; LDH, lactate dehydrogenase.
From Osborne et al. (1981), with permission.

Ranson and Pasternack (1977) improved the accuracy of prognostic assessment by multivariant analysis of 13 laboratory and clinical parameters. Using this technique it was possible to classify correctly 39% of patients using seven variables available at the time of admission or 96% of patients using nine variables recorded within 48 h. This method is somewhat complex and is not well suited to everyday clinical practice.

One of the criticisms of the disease specific multifactorial scoring systems is that they involve a delay of 48 h and on occasions even longer. Leese et al. (1991) tried to overcome these problems by measuring the Glasgow score at 6 h after admission. Unfortunately the specificity is not good enough to make such early measurements clinically useful.

The Hong Kong Criteria

Recently Fan et al. (1989) found that an "on admission" blood urea greater than 7.4 mmol/l and/or glucose greater than 11 mmol/l could detect severe attacks of acute pancreatitis with a sensitivity of 76% and specificity of 80%. We have applied these criteria to 122 patients with a diagnosis of acute pancreatitis admitted to six hospitals in the West of Scotland (Heath and Imrie 1990). With the Hong Kong criteria we were able to predict severe attacks of acute pancreatitis with a sensitivity of only 33% and specificity of 83%. By changing the cut-off concentration of urea to greater than 4.8 mmol/l and glucose to greater than 7.4 mmol/l, and utilising the peak concentrations during the first 48 h, we were able to increase the sensitivity to 65%; specificity was 77%. Even after modification these criteria were a less effective means of predicting severe attacks of acute pancreatitis than either the Glasgow scoring system (sensitivity 78% and specificity 86%) or clinical assessment at 48 h (sensitivity 82% and specificity 96%).

Non-specific Illness Scoring Systems

Drawbacks of the disease-specific multifactorial scoring systems for grading the severity of an attack of acute pancreatitis include a delay of 48 h or longer, an inability to take account of pre-existing disease states, differences in their sensitivity and specificity depending on the aetiology of the pancreatitis and their "once only" predictive ability: they cannot be used to monitor the disease course or response to therapy.

The advantages of the injury and sepsis scoring systems include their ability to take account of pre-existing illnesses and to monitor the disease course. For this reason they have recently been investigated as alternatives to the Ranson and Glasgow scoring systems (Larvin and McMahon 1989; Wilson et al. 1990). The best known of them is the APACHE II (acute physiology and chronic health evaluation) scoring system.

In 1981 Knaus and colleagues set out to develop a scoring system which could be used to predict the risk of mortality and morbidity in a group of medical and surgical patients with a diverse collection of diagnoses admitted to the intensive care unit. They used 34 physiological and laboratory parameters each of which attracted a score of 0–4 depending on its degree of deviation from normal values. The higher the score the sicker the patient. Although this system provided good stratification of disease severity, it was unwieldy to use and was subsequently modified to give the APACHE II scoring system (Knaus et al. 1985). This retains 12 of the original 34 parameters (Table 6). Its value has been confirmed on a series of 6100 patients (Knaus et al. 1984). We have applied this scoring system to 160 consecutive patients with acute pancreatitis (Wilson et al. 1990). Utilising the peak APACHE II score of ≥ 9 we were able to distinguish mild and severe attacks of acute pancreatitis with a sensitivity of 82% and specificity of 76% (figures comparable to the Ranson and Glasgow scoring systems). No deaths occurred in patients with a score < 10 and only 6% of these developed a complication (Fig. 1). Utilising a cut-off value of > 10 Larvin and McMahon (1989) produced a comparable sensitivity (72%) and specificity (92%). These authors also calculated the Medical Research Council (MRC) score and simplified acute physiology score (SAPS) in addition to the APACHE II score. The sensitivity of these scores at 48 h was too low to be of use in clinical practice.

Peritoneal Aspiration and Lavage

The first account of paracentesis in acute pancreatitis was produced by Keith et al. (1950). The authors inserted a 20 gauge needle into the abdominal cavity of 15 patients with a presumptive diagnosis of acute pancreatis and aspirated any free fluid. Although they intended to use the technique to diagnose acute pancreatitis in patients with a normal amylase they noted that "turbid yellow fluid indicates the interstitial type (mild pancreatitis), whereas reddish brown fluid denotes haemorrhagic pancreatitis". It was not until 1977 that the importance of paracentesis as a means of assessment of severity was recognised. Pickford et al. (1977) performed abdominal paracentesis and lavage with one litre of normal saline lavage in 27 patients with acute pancreatitis. The concentrations of albumin, AST, and total protein in the lavage fluid provided good discrimination between mild and severe groups and there were significant differences in the concentrations of urea, calcium, potassium, bilirubin, alkaline phosphatase, and white cell counts between groups. Severe attacks were predicted on the basis of an aspirated fluid volume of greater than 10 ml and/or darkly discoloured fluid. Using these criteria five patients who had been predicted as mild by clinical assessment were correctly classified as severe.

Table 6. The APACHE II score card for assessing illness severity

Physiological variable	High abnormal range				Low abnormal range				
	+4	+3	+2	+1	0	+1	+2	+3	+4
Temperature, rectal (°C)	≥41	39–40.9		38.5–38.9	36–38.4	34–35.9	32–33.9	30–31.9	≤29.9
Mean arterial pressure (mmHg)	≥160	130–159	110–129		70–109		50–69		≤49
Heart rate (ventricular response)	≥180	140–179	110–139		70–109		55–69	40–54	≤39
Respiratory rate (non-ventilated or ventilated)	≥50	35–49		25–34	12–24	10–11	6–9		≤5
Oxygenation: A_aDo_2 or P_aO_2 (mmHg)									
Fio_2 ≥0.5 record $AaDO_2$	≥500	350–499	200–349		<200				
Fio_2 <0.5 record only Pao_2					Po_2 >70	Po_2 61–70		Po_2 55–60	Po_2 <55
Arterial pH	≥7.7	7.6–7.69		7.5–7.59	7.33–7.49		7.25–7.32	7.15–7.24	<7.15
Serum sodium (mmol/l)	≥180	160–179	155–159	150–154	130–149		120–129	111–119	≤110
Serum potassium (mmol/l)	≥7	6–6.9		5.5–5.9	3.5–5.4	3–3.4	2.5–2.9		<2.5
Serum creatinine (mg/100ml) (Double point score for acute renal failure)	≥3.5	2–3.4	1.5–1.9		0.6–1.4		<0.6		

Haematocrit (%)	≥60		50–59.9	46–49.9	30–45.9	20–29.9	<20
White blood count (× 10^3/mm³)	≥40		20–39.9		15–19.9	3–14.9	1–2.9	<1
Glasgow coma score (GCS): Score = 15 – actual GCS					
Total acute physiology score (APS): Sum of the 12 individual variable points					
Serum HCO_3 (venous-mmol/l) (Not preferred, use if no ABGs)	≥52	41–51.9		32–40.9	22–31.9	18–21.9	15–17.9	<15

APACHE II score is given by the sum of the acute physiology score, the age points, and the chronic health points. Age points are assigned: age ≤44, zero; 45–54, 2 points; 55–64, 3 points; 65–74, 5 points; and ≥75, 6 points. Chronic health points are assigned if the patient has a history of severe organ system insufficiency or is immunocompromised as follows: for non-operative or emergency postoperative patients, 5 points; and for elective postoperative patients, 2 points. Organ insufficiency or an immunocompromised state must have been evident before hospital admission and must conform to the following criteria: *liver*, biopsy proven cirrhosis and documented portal hypertension, episodes of past upper gastrointestinal bleeding attributed to portal hypertension, or prior episodes of hepatic failure/encephalopathy/coma; *cardiovascular*, New York Heart Association Class IV (i.e. symptoms of angina or cardiac insufficiency at rest or during minimal exertion); *respiratory*, chronic restrictive, obstructive, or vascular disease resulting in severe exercise restriction, i.e. unable to climb stairs or perform household duties, or documented chronic hypoxia, hypercapnia, secondary polycythemia, severe pulmonary hypertension (> 40 mmHg), or respirator dependency; *renal*, receiving chronic dialysis; and, *immunocompromised*, the patient has received therapy that suppresses resistance to infection, e.g. immunosuppression, chemotherapy, radiation, long-term or recent high dose steroids, or has a disease that is sufficiently advanced to suppress resistance to infection, e.g. leukaemia, lymphoma, AIDS. AaDO_2, alveolar-arterial oxygen difference; P_aO_2, arterial partial pressure of oxygen; FiO_2, fraction of inspired oxygen; ABGs, arterial blood gases. Reproduced by the kind permission of the editor of Critical Care Medicine.

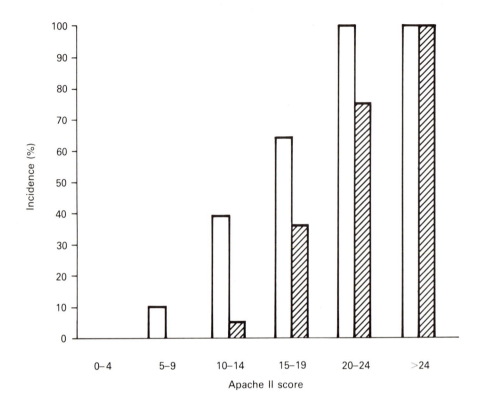

Fig. 1. The incidence of death (hatched bars) and morbidity (open bars) in 160 patients with acute pancreatitis and their relationship to the peak APACHE II score. Reproduced by the kind permission of the editor of the British Journal of Surgery.

These criteria were later refined in a larger study (McMahon et al. 1980) in which 96 patients had attempted paracentesis and lavage, and the modified criteria were used (Table 7). Fluid colour was compared with a fluid colour chart. By using these criteria 72% of severe cases were correctly predicted as severe at a mean time after admission of 7 h (standard deviation ± 6.7 h)

Table 7. The prognostic factors for peritoneal lavage which suggest a severe attack of acute pancreatitis

1. Free peritoneal fluid	Dark in colour (as per Leeds chart)
	No smell
	No organisms on Gram staining
	More than 20 ml of free fluid
2. Return lavage fluid (1 l of fluid)	Moderately dark fluid
	No smell
	No organisms on Gram staining

compared with only 39% using clinical assessment. Clinical assessment and the Ranson and Glasgow criteria produced similar levels of accuracy in prediciton only after a delay of 48 h. A multicentre study of therapeutic peritoneal lavage conducted between Leeds, Glasgow and Bristol produced similar results (Corfield et al. 1985). This study also showed that only 1 of 42 patients graded severe by this method required lavage to predict a severe attack. All others were graded by aspiration alone (greater than 20 ml of fluid or very dark fluid).

The great advantage of paracentesis and peritoneal lavage is that they are capable of predicting the severity of an attack of acute pancreatitis at the time of admission. It has also been claimed that it reduces the amount of abdominal pain experienced by the patient although this has not been demonstrated in a controlled manner. A third advantage is the identification of causes of abdominal pain other than acute pancreatitis. Macroscopic examination of the fluid obtained will identify blood, bile or intestinal contents and a Gram stain will demonstrate organisms when there is a visceral perforation (Mayer and McMahon 1985). Under these circumstances an urgent laparotomy should be performed. The disadvantages of this method include the reduced accuracy of prediction for gallstone-related attacks compared with alcohol-related attacks and the risk (about 1%) of visceral perforation. It is this latter possibility that has probably prevented this excellent technique being widely adopted into clinical practice.

Computed Tomography (CT)

There have been a number of prospective studies addressing the usefulness of CT as a means of severity assessment (Hill et al. 1982; Grabbe et al. 1982; Becker et al. 1985; Balthazar et al. 1985; Nordestgaard et al. 1986; Takada et al. 1986; Clavien et al. 1988; London et al. 1989). The signs examined were pancreatic oedema as reflected by an increase in pancreatic size, the spread of inflammation and oedema outside the pancreas into the peripancreatic fat, "phlegmon" formation, the presence of peripancreatic collections and failure of enhancement of the gland with intravenous contrast.

Whilst a number of the studies included the presence of pancreatic swelling as part of their scoring systems only three have attempted to correlate pancreatic size directly with outcome (Becker et al. 1985; Takada et al. 1986; London et al. 1989). Becker et al. compared the sagittal diameter of the pancreas to the adjacent vertebral body and London et al. determined the "pancreatic size index" by multiplying the maximum anteroposterior diameters of the pancreatic body and head. Using this index London et al. were able to distinguish mild from severe attacks with a sensitivity and specificity of 71% and 77%, respectively, which compares poorly with the values of 85% and 79% for the modified Glasgow criteria, especially as CT is considerably more expensive and time consuming than the conventional methods of prediction. Furthermore, CT may involve moving a seriously ill patient away from an intensive care setting.

The description of the extrapancreatic spread of inflammation was simplified by London et al. (1989) who simply suggested that the loss of the demarcation between the pancreas and the peripancreatic tissue indicated extrapancreatic spread. This gave a high sensitivity of 82% but an unacceptably low specificity of 45% for a prediction of a severe attack. Likewise low dose contrast enhancement (which was not intended to detect pancreatic necrosis) failed to improve assessment of severity (Grabbe et al. 1982; London et al. 1989). The presence of inflammation extending into one or more of the peripancreatic spaces has been noted by other authors to be correlated with a high morbidity and mortality. In two American studies (Hill et al. 1982; Balthazar et al. 1985) deaths only occurred where there was evidence of such extension.

Whilst the multifactorial scoring systems correlate with the degrees of abnormality on CT examination (Clavien et al. 1988) neither they nor CT used as described above is capable of selecting those patients who will develop local rather than systemic complications. It has been observed that patients with CT appearances which predict a severe outcome have had an uncomplicated recovery so it is not possible to base a decision for surgical intervention on CT appearances alone.

Single Factors

Hypocalcaemia

Edmondson and Berne (1944) were the first of several authors (Pollock 1959; Trapnell 1966; Ranson et al. 1976) to note the association between hypocalcaemia and severe pancreatitis. Much of the hypocalcaemia of acute pancreatitis is actually associated with hypoalbuminaemia and is of little physiological importance (Imrie et al. 1976). Although serum calcium concentrations less than 2.0 mmol/l are useful as part of multifactorial scoring systems (Ranson et al. 1974a; Imrie et al. 1978b) their measurement in isolation does not discriminate adequately between mild and severe attacks of pancreatitis (McMahon et al. 1980; Croton et al. 1981).

Hypoxaemia

The association between early hypoxaemia and a severe outcome is well documented (Ranson et al. 1974b; Imrie et al. 1977). The age, obesity, cigarette intake and pre-existing respiratory function of the patient will affect the level of hypoxaemia but where intubation and ventilation become necessary there is a 75% risk of death (Jacobs et al. 1977). Hypoxaemia is also an important part of the multifactorial scoring systems. Clinical detection of this feature is almost impossible and blood gas monitoring is essential.

Methaemalbuminaemia

Methaemalbumin is a complex formed by the combination of albumin and haematin (a product of the proteolytic digestion of haemoglobin). Northram et al. (1963), Winstone (1965) and Trapnell (1966) described an association between haemorrhagic pancreatitis and elevated serum levels of methaemalbumin. Experimental work in dogs has confirmed these observations. A number of clinical studies on peritoneal fluid (Geokas et al. 1974; Lankisch et al.

1978) and serum (Lankisch et al. 1978) have supported the usefulness of methaemalbumin measurements, whereas others have not found it valuable (Ranson et al. 1974a; McMahon et al. 1980; Berry et al. 1981). In McMahon et al.'s series removal of peritoneal fluid rich in methaemalbumin may have accounted for low serum concentrations. Nevertheless, adequate concentrations are not present early enough in an attack of acute pancreatitis to be of value in the prediction of severity. This test has not been adopted into routine clinical practice.

Changes in the Coagulation Cascade

Changes in the coagulation cascade, including, rarely, disseminated intravascular coagulation have been noted in association with acute pancreatitis (Goodhead 1969; Bryne et al. 1971; Kwaan et al. 1971; Murphy et al. 1977; Ranson et al. 1977) and attributed to the effects of trypsin. Platelet, fibrinogen, factors V and VIII concentrations tend to rise during severe attacks as part of the acute phase protein response (Imrie et al. 1988). These changes have been correlated with renal, respiratory and hepatic impairment (Ranson et al. 1977) but have not proved helpful in prognostication.

C-reactive Protein (CRP)

CRP is the most rapidly detectable of the acute phase proteins. It appears in the serum within 6 h of an injury, usually reaches peak levels within 48 h and, in the absence of a continuing injury, begins to fall by 60 h. The normal serum CRP level is less than 10 mg/l.

Elevation of CRP has proved a useful marker of disease activity in a variety of inflammatory, infective and ischaemic conditions (Amos et al. 1977; Kushner et al. 1981). These include pneumonia, tuberculosis, pyelonephritis, Crohn's disease, ankylosing spondylosis, rheumatoid arthritis, myocardial infarction and metastatic carcinoma of the breast. Serial measurements can warn of postoperative complications, but have proved disappointing as a means of detecting the site or severity of intra-abdominal sepsis (Mustard et al. 1977).

McMahon et al. (1984) measured CRP concentrations in 55 patients with acute pancreatitis and demonstrated a good separation between complicated and uncomplicated attacks. A more detailed analysis concluded that a persistently elevated CRP suggested continuing inflammation with the associated risk of a complication (Mayer et al. 1984). These findings have been confirmed by other workers (Buchler et al. 1986; Puolakkainen et al. 1987). In some reports (Mayer et al. 1984; Wilson et al. 1989), CRP concentrations were low on admission. However, Buchler et al. (1986) and Poulakkainen et al. (1987) found maximal concentrations in severe acute pancreatitis at the time of admission. This can be explained by the fact that many of the patients in the latter series have been referred from other centres and have therefore already undergone a delay of 24–48 h. Buchler et al. found that a CRP greater than 120 mg/l detected 95% of cases of necrotising pancreatitis confirmed at laparotomy. This resulted in an extraordinarily high incidence of pancreatic necrosis (22 of 35 or 63% of a consecutive series of patients). In these patients, Buchler et al. have demonstrated CRP concentrations greater than 120 mg/l to be a better and cheaper discriminator of acute necrotising pancreatitis than angiogram enhanced CT (95% vs 85%). These results vary markedly from recent findings from Glasgow (Wilson et al. 1989) where the incidence of pancreatic necrosis was half this figure. Wilson et al. demonstrated that CRP concentrations of greater than 210 mg/l were needed reliably to detect severe disease and that CRP was unable to discriminate between the types of complications: in particular CRP could not accurately determine the presence of pancreatic necrosis.

CRP is undoubtedly an important indicator of disease severity and is a valuable aid in monitoring the course of the disease. CRP estimation is at present under-utilised in clinical practice. Although it involves a delay similar to scoring systems in severity assessment, it is very simple to perform, cheap, objective and reproducible.

Interleukin-6 (IL-6)

Interleukin-6 is the principal mediator of the acute phase protein response (Castell et al. 1988) and therefore might be expected to provide earlier severity assessment than CRP. We have demonstrated that peak CRP concentrations of IL-6 occurred between 24 and 36 h after onset of symptoms, whereas peak CRP concentrations were seen somewhat later at between 36 and 48 h (Fig. 2) (Heath et al. 1989). IL-6 concentrations greater than 140 U/l between 24 and 36 h detected severe attacks of acute pancreatitis with a sensitivity of 90% and specificity of 83%; the corresponding values for a CRP level > 130 between 36 and 48 h are 100% and 86%. Clearly these tests have similar sensitivities and specificities although severity prediction with IL-6 was available

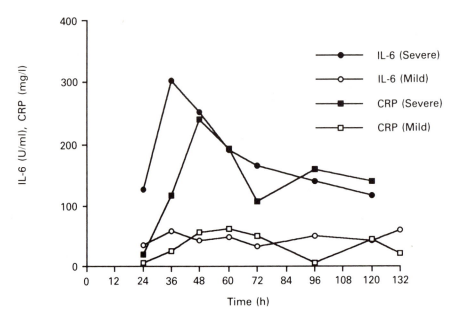

Fig. 2. Median serum concentrations of IL-6 and CRP throughout the 5 days of the study in ten patients with complicated and 14 patients with uncomplicated acute pancreatitis.

up to 24 hours earlier than with CRP. This test is expensive to perform and is not really a practical alternative to CRP at present.

Trypsinogen Activation Peptide (TAP)

Both Hermon-Taylor and Heywood (1985) and Rinderknecht (1986) have postulated that the differences between oedematous and necrotising acute pancreatitis can be explained in terms of biochemical events. They suggest that during an attack of mild or oedematous acute pancreatitis acinar cell damage leads to the release of amylase and lipase. There is, however, no activation of the zymogens and pancreatic necrosis does not develop. During an attack of severe or necrotising pancreatitis there is in addition activation of the pancreatic zymogens which is necessary for the development of pancreatic necrosis. Although this theory is plausible the importance of zymogen activation in the initiation of acute pancreatitis is difficult to assess (Katz et al. 1964) and is not universally accepted (Beck et al. 1964; Schmidt and Creutzfeldt 1969).

Attempts to relate the severity of acute pancreatitis to the degree of trypsinogen activation by the measurement of serum immunoreactive trypsin concentrations have proved unsuccessful (Elias et al. 1977; Lake-Bakaar et al. 1980; O'Connor et al. 1981). The principal problem is that the immunoassays employed are unable to distinguish between the parent zymogen and the active enzyme. Secondly, the majority of zymogen activation is thought to occur at the beginning of an attack of acute pancreatitis and measurements taken several days later will have missed this phase. Furthermore, most of the active enzyme is rapidly bound to α_2-macroglobulin and eliminated from the circulation by the reticuloendothelial system (Ohlsson and Laurell 1976). Further difficulty arises from the fact that the amount of trypsin assayed in any particular specimen will depend on the partition of trypsin between the α_1-antiprotease, α_2-macroglobulin and the "free phase".

An alternative approach has been to quantify the trypsinogen activation peptide (TAP). TAP is a small peptide with amino acid sequence tetra-aspartyl-lysine which is released in equimolar concentrations to trypsin when trypsinogen is activated. It does not have any proteolytic activity and is eliminated only slowly. TAP can be detected in the urine for several hours after intravenous injection of a bolus in a dog (Hurley et al. 1988). Hurley et al. (1988) have developed an immunoassay against the C-terminal end of TAP which will only detect TAP after it has been released from the trypsinogen molecule. The assay has the great advantage that it will not falsely detect the parent zymogen.

In a joint clinical study between St George's Hospital and Glasgow Royal Infirmary 57 consecutive patients with a diagnosis of acute pancreatitis had urinary concentrations of TAP measured every 6 h for 48 h and then every 12 h for a further 3 days (Gudgeon et al. 1990) (Fig. 3). A TAP concentration of greater than 2 nmol/l on admission predicted severe attacks of acute pancreatitis with a sensitivity of 85% and specificity of 90%. Whilst the results of this initial study require validation by other groups the measurement of urinary TAP concentrations probably represents the best means of rapid assessment of severity available at present. However a commercial kit test is not yet available.

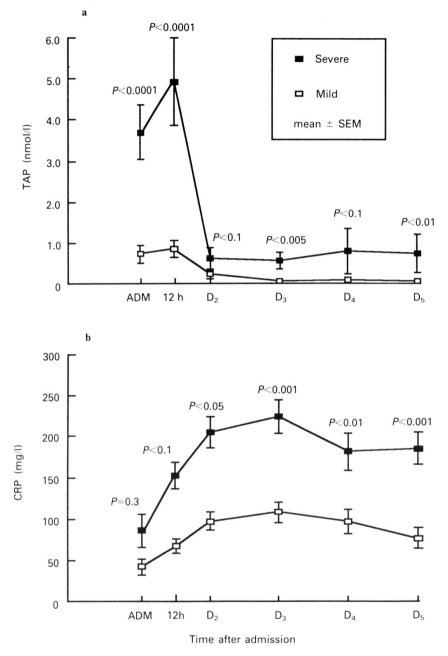

Fig. 3. Mean urinary concentration of **a** trypsinogen activation peptide (TAP) (± standard error) and **b** mean serum concentration of CRP (± standard error) over the first 5 days of admission. From Gudgeon et al. (1990), with permission.

α_2-*Macroglobulin*

Falls in the concentration of α_2-macroglobulin characterise severe acute pancreatitis, but the concentrations tend to return to normal at the end of the first weeks of illness (McMahon et al. 1984). Indeed in that study the α_2-macroglobulin concentrations of all three patients who died were in the normal range prior to death. The degree of consumption of this large molecule does reflect disease severity but not as accurately as CRP (Buchler et al. 1986; Wilson et al. 1989). It is also a more expensive test to perform than CRP measurements.

Polymorphonuclear Neutrophil (PMN) Elastase

This product of neutrophils can be measured as a marker of severity of a number of conditions including trauma, burns and acute pancreatitis (Uhl et al. 1989; Dominquez-Munoz et al. 1990). It is likely that this test will prove to be a step forward in severity assessment as the prediction is available before that provided by CRP.

Current Clinical Practice

The present practice which we undertake at Glasgow Royal Infirmary is continuously to assess all patients clinically and measure:

1. The Glasgow prognostic score
2. CRP
3. Perform contrast enhanced CT in all cases of severe acute pancreatitis (this may need to be repeated up to 3 times a week)
4. The APACHE II score
5. PMN elastase in patients being assessed in the clinical research setting

References

Amos RS, Constable TJ, Crockson RA, McKonkey B (1977) Rheumatoid arthritis: relation to serum C-reactive protein and erythrocyte sedimentation rates to radiographic changes. Br Med J 1:195–197

Balthazar EJ, Ranson JH, Naidich DP, Megibow AJ, Caccavale R, Cooper M (1985) Acute pancreatitis: Prognostic value of CT. Radiology 136:767–772

Beck JT, Khan DS, Solymar J, McKenna RD, Zylberszac B (1964) The role of pancreatic enzymes in the pathogenesis of acute pancreatitis. III Comparison of the pathologic and biochemical changes in the canine pancreas to intraductal injection with bile and trypsin. Gastroenterology 46:531–542

Becker H, Gahbauer H, Horn J, Mechler TH (1985) Korrelation klinischer und computertomographischer Befunde für die Therapie und Prognose der akuten Pancreatitis. Ghirurg 56:386–392

Berry AR, Taylor TV, Davies GC (1981) Pulmonary function and fibrinogen metabolism in acute pancreatitis. Br J Surg 68:870–873

Blamey SL, Imrie CW, O'Neill J, Gilmour WM, Carter DC (1984) Prognostic factors in acute pancreatitis. Gut 25:1340–1346

Bryne J, Migliore J, Beekley W et al. (1971) Platelet response to induction of haemorrhagic pancreatitis. Proc Soc Exp Biol Med 136:994–996

Buchler M, Malfertheiner P, Beger HG (1986) Correlation of imaging procedures, biochemical parameters and clinical stage in acute pancreatitis. In: Malfertheiner P, Ditschuneit H (eds) Diagnostic procedures in pancreatic disease. Springer-Verlag, Berlin, pp 123–129

Castell JV, Gomez-Lechon MJ, David M et al. (1988) Recombinant human interleukin-6 (IL-6/BSF-2/HSF) regulates the synthesis of acute phase proteins in human hepatocytes. FEBS Lett 232:347–350

Clavien PA, Hauser H, Mayer P, Rohner A (1988) Value of contrast enhanced computerised tomography in the early diagnosis and prognosis of acute pancreatitis. Am J Surg 155:475–466

Corfield AP, Cooper MJ, Williamson RCN et al. (1985) Prediction of severity in acute pancreatitis: a prospective comparison of three prognostic indices. Lancet ii:403–406

Croton RS, Warren RA, Scott, Roberts NB (1981) Ionised calcium in acute pancreatitis and its relationship with total calcium and serum lipase. Br J Surg 68:241–244

Delk AS, Durie PR, Fletcher TS, Largman C (1985) Radioimmunoassays of active pancreatitis enzymes in sera from patients with acute pancreatitis. 1. Active carboxypeptidase B. Clin Chem 31:1294–1300

Dickson AP, Imrie CW (1984) The incidence and prognosis of body wall ecchymosis in acute pancreatitis. Surg Gynecol Obstet 159:343–347

Dickson AP, O'Neill J, Imrie CW (1984) Hyperlipidaemia, alcohol abuse and acute pancreatitis. Br J Surg 71:685–688

Dominquez-Munoz E et al. (1990) Behaviour of the circulating levels of antiproteinases, complement factors, C-reactive protein and polymorphonuclear elastase in the early prognostication of acute pancreatitis. Revista de la Associacion Castellana de Apanato Digestiivo 6:101–108

Edmondson HA, Berne CJ (1944) Calcium changes in acute pancreatic necrosis. Surg Obstet Gynecol 79:240–244

Elias E, Redshaw M, Wood T (1977) The diagnostic importance of changes in circulating concentrations of immunoreactive trypsin. Lancet ii:66–68

Fan ST, Choi TK, Lai ECS, Wong J (1989) Prediction of severity of acute pancreatitis: an alternative approach. Gut 30:1591–1595

Farrer WH, Calkins WG (1976) A study of amylase creatinine clearance ratio in acute pancreatitis. Gastroenterology 70:883

Geokas MC, Rinderknecht H, Walberg CB, Reisman R (1974) Methaemalbumin in the diagnosis of acute haemorrhagic pancreatitis. Ann Intern Med 81:483–486

Goodhead H (1969) Vascular factors in the pathogenesis of acute haemorrhagic pancreatitis. Ann R Coll Surg 45:80–97

Grabbe VE, Dammann HG, Heller M (1982) Wert der Computertomographie für die Prognose der akuten Pankreatitis. Fortschr Röntgenstr 136:534–537

Gudgeon M, Heath DI, Hurley P et al. (1990) Trypsinogen activation peptides assay in the early severity prediction of acute pancreatitis. Lancet 335:4–8

Heath DI, Imrie CW (1990) Severity prediction in acute pancreatitis using the Hong Kong criteria. HPB Surgery 2: Suppl FP 128

Heath DI, Cruickshank AC, Shenkin A, Imrie CW (1989) Interleukin-6, a mediator of the acute phase response in acute pancreatitis? Gut 30:A1456–A1457

Hermon-Taylor J, Heywood GC (1985) A rational approach to the specific chemotherapy of acute pancreatitis. Scand J Gastroenterol 20:39–46

Hill MC, Barkin J, Isikoff MB, Silverstein W, Kalser M (1982) Acute pancreatitis: clinical vs CT findings. AJR 139:263–269

Hurley PR, Cook A, Jehanli A, Austen BM, Hermon-Taylor J (1988) Development of radioimmunoassays for free tetra-aspartyl-L-lysine trypsinogen activation peptides (TAP). J Immunol Methods 111:195–203

Imrie CW, Allam BF, Ferguson JC (1976) Hypocalcaemia in acute pancreatitis: the effect of hypoalbuminaemia. Curr Med Res Opin 4:101–116

Imrie CW, Murphy D, Ferguson JC, Blumgart LH (1977) Arterial hypoxia in acute pancreatitis. Br J Surg 64:185–188

Imrie CW, Benjamin IS, McKay AJ, Mackenzie I, O'Neill J, Blumgart LH (1978a) A single centre double blind trial of Trasylol therapy in primary acute pancreatitis. Br J Surg 65:337–341

Imrie CW, Beastall GH, Allam BF et al. (1978b) Parathyroid hormone and calcium homeostasis in acute pancreatitis. Br J Surg 65:717–720

Imrie CW, Shearer MG, Wilson C (1988) Glycoproteins as markers of pancreatic damage in acute pancreatitis. Int J Pancreatol 3:S43–S52

Jacobs ML, Daggett WM, Civetta JM et al. (1977) Acute pancreatitis: analysis of factors influencing survival. Ann Surg 185:45–63

Katz W, Silverstein M, Kobold EE, Thal AP (1964) Trypsin release, kinin production and shock: relationship in experimental and human pancreatitis. Arch Surg 89:322–331

Keith LM, Zollinger RM, McCleary RS (1950) Peritoneal fluid amylase determinations as an aid in the diagnosing of acute pancreatitis. Arch Surg 61:930–936

Knaus WA, Zimmerman JE, Wagner DP, Draper EA, Lawrence DE (1981) APACHE-acute physiology and chronic health evaluation: a physiologically based classification system. Crit Care Med 9:591–597

Knaus WA, Wagner DP, Draper EA, Zimmerman JE (1984) APACHE-II final form and national validation results of a severity of disease classification system. Crit Care Med 12:213

Knaus WA, Draper EA, Wagner DP, Zimmerman JE (1985) APACHE II: a severity of disease classification system. Crit Care Med 13:818–829

Kolars JC, Ellis CJ, Levitt MD (1984) Comparison of serum amylase, pancreatic isoamylase and lipase in patients with hyperamylasaemia. Dig Dis Sci 29:289–293

Kushner I, Gewurz H, Benson MD (1981) C-reactive protein and the acute phase response. J Lab Clin Med 97:739–749

Kwaan HC, Anderson MC, Gramatica L (1971) A study of pancreatic enzymes as a factor in the pathogenesis of disseminated intravascular coagulation during acute pancreatitis. Surgery 69:663–672

Lake-Bakaar G, McKavanagh S, Gatus B, Summerfield JA (1980) The relative values of serum immuno-reactive trypsin concentrations and total amylase activity in the diagnosis of mumps, chronic renal failure and pancreatic disease. Scand J Gastroenterol 15:97–101

Lankisch PG, Koop H, Otto J, Oberdieck U (1978) Evaluation of methaemalbumin in acute pancreatitis. Scand J Gastroenterol 13:975–978

Larvin M, McMahon MJ (1989) APACHE II score for assessment and monitoring of acute pancreatitis. Lancet ii:201–205

Leese T, Holliday M, Heath D, Hall AW, Bell PRF (1987) Multicentre trial of low volume fresh frozen plasma therapy in acute pancreatitis. Br J Surg 74:907–911

Leese T, Holliday M, Watkins M et al. (1991) A multicentre controlled clinical trial of high volume fresh frozen plasma in prognostically severe acute pancreatitis. Ann R Coll Surg 73 (in press).

Levitt MD, Johnson SG, Ellis CJ, Engel RR (1977) Influence of amylase assay technique on renal clearance of amylase/creatinine ratio. Gastroenterology 72:1260–1263

London NJM, Neoptolomos JP, Lavelle J, Bailey I, James D (1989) Contrast-enhanced abdominal computerised tomography scanning and prediction of severity of acute pancreatitis: a prospective study. Br J Surg 76:268–272

Mayer AD, McMahon MJ (1985) The diagnostic and prognostic value of peritoneal lavage in patients with acute pancreatitis. Surg Obstet Gynecol 160:507–512

Mayer AD, McMahon MJ, Bowen M, Cooper EH (1984) C-reactive protein: an aid to assessment and monitoring of acute pancreatitis. J Clin Pathol 37:207–211

McKay AJ, Imrie CW, O'Neill J, Duncan JG (1982) Is an early ultrasound scan of value in acute pancreatitis? Br J Surg 69:369–372

McMahon MJ, Playforth MJ, Pickford IR (1980) A comparative study of methods for the prediction of severity of attacks of acute pancreatitis. Br J Surg 67:22–25

McMahon MJ, Playforth MJ, Rashid SA, Cooper EH (1982) The amylase-to-creatinine clearance ratio – a non-specific response to acute illness? Br J Surg 69:29–32

McMahon MJ, Bowen M, Mayer AD, Cooper EH (1984) Relationship of α_2-macroglobulin and other antiproteases to the clinical features of acute pancreatitis. Am J Surg 147:164–170

Mero M, Schroder T, Tenhunen R, Lempinen M (1982) Serum phospholipase A_2, immunoreactive trypsin and trypsin inhibitors during human acute pancreatitis. Scand J Gastroenterol 17:413–416

Moossa AR (1982) The impact of computer tomography and ultrasound on surgical practice. Bull Am Coll Surg 67:10–14

Moossa AR (1984) Diagnostic tests and procedures in acute pancreatitis. N Engl J Med 311:639–643

MRC working party (1977) MRC working party on the treatment of acute pancreatitis: Death from acute pancreatitis. Lancet ii:632–635

Murphy D, Imrie CW, Davidson JF (1977) Haematological abnormalities in acute pancreatitis. A prospective study. Postgrad Med J 53:310–314

Murray WR, McKay C (1977) The amylase/creatinine clearance ratio in acute pancreatitis. Br J Surg 64:189–191

Mustard RA, Bohnen MA, Haseeb S, Kasina R (1977) C-reactive protein levels predict postoperative septic complications. Arch Surg 122:69–73

Neoptolomos JP, London NJ, Slater ND, Carr-Locke DL, Fossard DP (1986) A prospective study of ERCP and endoscopic sphincterotomy in the diagnosis and treatment of gallstone acute pancreatitis. Arch Surg 121:679–702

Nordestgaard AG, Wilson SE, Williams RA (1986) Early computerised tomography as a predictor of outcome in acute pancreatitis. Am J Surg 152:127–132

Northram BE, Rowe DS, Winstone NE (1963) Methaemalbumin in the differential diagnosis of acute haemorrhagic and oedematous pancreatitis. Lancet i:348–352

O'Conner CM, O'Donnell MD, McGeeney KF (1980) Problems associated with the radioimmunoassay of serum trypsin. Clin Chim Acta 114:29–35

O'Donnell MD, Fitzgerald O, McGeeney KF (1977) Differential serum amylase determination by the use of an inhibitor and design of a routine procedure. Clin Chem 23:560–566

Ohlsson K, Laurell CB (1976) The disappearance of enzyme–inhibitor complexes from the circulation of man. Clin Sci Mol Med 51:87–92

Osborne DH, Imrie CW, Carter DC (1981) Biliary surgery in the same admission for gallstone-associated acute pancreatitis. Br J Surg 68:758–761

Pfeffer RB, Mister G, Hinton JW (1958) Acute haemorrhagic pancreatitis: A safe, effective technique for diagnostic paracentesis. Surgery 43:550–554

Pickford IR, Blackett RL, McMahon MJ (1977) Early assessment of severity of acute pancreatitis using peritoneal lavage. Br Med J ii:1377–1379

Pollock AV (1959) Acute pancreatitis. Analysis of 100 patients. Br Med J i:6–14

Puolakkainen P, Valtonen V, Paananen A, Schroder T (1987) C-reactive protein (CRP) and serum phospholipase A_2 in the assessment of the severity of acute pancreatitis. Gut 28:764–771

Ranson HJC (1979) The timing of biliary surgery in acute pancreatitis. Ann Surg 189:654–662

Ranson JHC (1982) Etiology and prognostic factors in human acute pancreatitis: a review. Am J Gastroenterol 77:633–638

Ranson HJC, Pasternack BS (1977) Statistical methods for quantifying the severity of clinical acute pancreatitis. J Surg Res 22:79–91

Ranson JHC, Rifkind KM, Roses DF, Fink SD, Eng K, Spencer FC (1974a) Prognostic signs and the role of operative management in acute pancreatitis. Surg Gynecol Obstet 139:69–81

Ranson JHC, Turner JW, Roses DF, Rifkind KM, Spencer FC (1974b) Respiratory complications in acute pancreatitis. Ann Surg 179:557–566

Ranson JHC, Rifkind KM, Turner JW (1976) Prognostic signs and non-operative peritoneal lavage in acute pancreatitis. Surg Gynecol Obstet 143:209–219

Ranson JHC, Lackner H, Berman IR, Schinella R (1977) The relationship of coagulation factors to clinical complications of acute pancreatitis. Surgery 81:502–511

Rick W (1972) Chemical methods in the diagnosis of pancreatic disease. Clin Gastroenterol 1:3–25

Rinderknecht H (1986) Activation of pancreatic zymogens. Dig Dis Sci 24:180–186

Schmidt H, Creutzfeldt W (1969) The possible role of phospholipase A in the pathogenesis of acute pancreatitis. Scand J Gastroenterol 4:39–48

Silverstein W, Isikoff MB, Hill MC, Barkin J (1981) Diagnostic imaging of acute pancreatitis: a prospective study using CT and sonography. AJR 137:497–502

Song H, Tietz NW, Tan C (1970) Usefulness of serum lipase, enterase and amylase estimation in the diagnosis of acute pancreatitis. Clin Chem 16:264–268

Takada T, Yasuda H, Uchiyama K, Hasegawa H, Sitaka J, Nagai J (1986) CT findings and CT score in acute pancreatitis compared with severity. Nippon Igaku Hoshasen Gakkai Zasshi 46:1167–1173

Trapnell JP (1966) The natural history and prognosis of acute pancreatitis. Ann R Coll Surg Engl 38:265–287

Uhl W, Buchler M, Malfertheiner P, Martini M, Beger H (1989) PMN-elastase: a new serum marker for the staging of acute pancreatitis. Digestion 43:141

Umeki S, Satoh T, Ueda S (1985) Alterations in serum pancreatic elastase. 1. Content in acute and chronic pancreatitis; comparison with α-amylase activity. J Lab Clin Med 106:578–583

Warshaw AL (1977) Serum amylase isoenzyme profiles as a differential index in disease. J Lab Clin Med 90:1–3

Wilson C, Imrie CW (1988) Deaths from acute pancreatitis: why do we miss the diagnosis so frequently. Int J Pancreatol 3:273–282

Wilson C, Heads A, Shenkin A, Imrie CW (1989) C-reactive protein, antiproteases and complement factors as objective markers of severity in acute pancreatitis. Br J Surg 76:177–181

Wilson C, Heath DI, Imrie CW (1990) Prediction of outcome in acute pancreatitis: a comparative study of APACHE II, clinical assessment and multiple factor scoring systems. Br J Surg 77:1260–1264

Winstone NE (1965) Methaemalbumin in acute pancreatitis. Br J Surg 52:804–808

Chapter 25

Systemic Effects of Acute Pancreatitis

C. Wilson and C. W. Imrie

Acute pancreatitis is the most terrible of all the calamities that occur in connection with the abdominal viscera. The suddenness of its onset, the illimitable agony which accompanies it, and the mortality attendant upon it, all render it the most formidable of catastrophies.

Moynihan (1925)

Moynihan (1925) went on to describe the characteristic distribution of the pain and the collapse and shock that may occur. This classical picture of acute pancreatitis associated with pallor, sweating, cyanosis, low blood pressure and oliguria with tenderness and rigidity of the abdomen describes the characteristic systemic effects but was observed in only half the patients studied by Pollock (1959). Cyanosis is indeed very unusual, whereas tachypnoea is the normal systemic effect of hypoxaemia.

Abdominal Pain

The vast majority of patients with acute pancreatitis present with abdominal pain, the proportion ranging from 84% (Jacobs et al. 1977) to 98% (Bockus et al. 1955). There may be no pain in up to 15% of attacks (Read et al. 1976) but as such cases may not be diagnosed in life, the true prevalence is difficult to estimate.

The pain associated with acute pancreatitis is typically centred in the epigastrium (Albo et al. 1963; Romer and Carey 1966) but may be right hypochondrial in 20% of patients, or more rarely, maximal in the left hypochondrium or lower abdomen (Foster and Ziffren 1962). Radiation of pain to the back was described in 50% of patients (Romer and Carey 1966).

Pollock (1959) found the pain to be of sudden onset in 84% of patients. Durr (1979) considered that the pain was typically of sudden onset, gradually increasing in severity and reaching maximal intensity within a few hours of onset. This sudden onset of pain is clinically very similar to that found in perforated duodenal ulcer. It is unusual for severe pain to extend beyond 48 h of the commencement of intravenous fluid replacement.

Vomiting

This is a common systemic effect of acute pancreatitis occurring in between 53% (Jacobs et al. 1977) and 90% of cases (Pollock 1959). The vomiting in the early stages of the attack is probably associated with the severity of the pain. Vomiting occurring later in the course of the illness is more likely to be due to duodenal ileus. In our experience 85% of patients exhibit vomiting which may be more of an upset than the pain.

Abdominal Signs

The abdominal findings associated with acute pancreatitis are non-specific. Durr (1979) considered that tenderness and guarding were more common than rigidity and that the striking disparity between the severity of the pain and the paucity of signs was characteristic.

Features of paralytic ileus were found in between 12% and 16% of cases and 10% may have an abdominal mass (Bockus et al. 1955; Foster and Ziffren 1962; Jacobs et al. 1977).

Ascites is associated with severe attacks of pancreatitis and is typically found in the early phase of the illness. The ascites may vary from a pale straw-colour to a dark, haemorrhagic fluid; assessment of the volume and colour of the fluid has been shown to be of prognostic value, the darker the fluid the poorer the prognosis (McMahon et al. 1980; Corfield et al. 1985). Peritoneal fluid examination is much more useful in grading the severity of alcoholic pancreatitis than for attacks due to gallstones (Corfield et al. 1985).

Shock

Shock, defined as arterial blood pressure less than 100 mmHg, has previously been considered the major cause of early death in acute pancreatitis (Shader and Paxton 1966; Trapnell 1966; Storck et al. 1976). Shock is found infrequently on admission, although severe hypotension had a positive correlation with eventual death (Jacobs et al. 1977). Hypovolaemia is considered the major cause of shock, although other cardiovascular factors such as myocardial depression are thought to contribute. The major factors contributing to hypovolaemia are shown in Fig. 1.

Hypovolaemia

Plasma volume deficits in a canine pancreatitis model, calculated from the change in haematocrit, were estimated to reach a maximum deficit of 38%

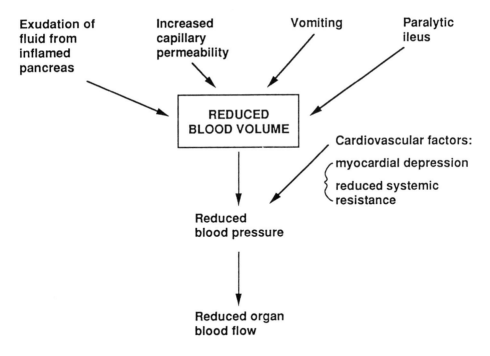

Fig. 1. Major factors contributing to hypovolaemia.

(Carey 1979). In another study intravascular volume was found to have fallen by 19% after 2 h and by 30% after 6 h; the plasma volume fell by 33% after 2 h and by 39% 6 h after the induction of pancreatitis (Anderson et al. 1967). On the basis of these findings it was calculated that in a 70 kg man with comparable pancreatitis, the intravascular volume deficit would be nearly 2 litres during the first 6 h of the illness (Anderson et al. 1967). In dogs the pancreas is an intraperitoneal organ and fluid exuded from the pancreas collects within the peritoneal cavity and accounts for over 50% of the plasma volume deficit (Carey and Rodgers 1966). Due to the anatomical position of the pancreas in man much of this fluid is sequestered in the retroperitoneal peripancreatic tissues.

There is, in addition, a more widespread capillary leak with loss of fluid into the extravascular space in tissues remote from the pancreas, including the lungs (Tahamont et al. 1982) and subcutaneous tissues. This results in a profound fall in the serum albumin concentration (Imrie et al. 1976). The proposed mechanism for this fluid leak is altered capillary permeability mediated directly or indirectly by vasoactive agents released into the circulation from the pancreas or peritoneal exudate (Takada et al. 1976; Ellison et al. 1981). It is also possible that leucocyte/pancreatic elastase (both present in high concentrations) may be important in this mechanism. The clinical situation is remarkably similar to that in a patient with extensive burns and up to 10 litres of replacement fluid may be required during the initial 24 h of therapy.

Fluid lost by vomiting and by sequestration within the bowel as a result of paralytic ileus may also contribute to the hypovolaemia.

Myocardial Depression

A myocardial depressant factor, thought to be a peptide with a molecular weight of between 800 and 1000 daltons, has been postulated to exist in the plasma of humans and experimental animals in various forms of shock and also in acute pancreatitis (Lefer et al. 1971; Lovett et al. 1971).

Haemodynamic studies in man showed myocardial depression in patients with severe acute pancreatitis (Di Carlo et al. 1981; Ito et al. 1981). Others were unable to confirm this, considering that patients with severe acute pancreatitis have a high output, low resistance picture resembling that seen in sepsis (Bradley et al. 1983; Beger et al. 1986). Cobo et al. (1984) considered that depressed myocardial function alone did not account for the hypotension in patients with acute pancreatitis, but that myocardial depression compromised cardiac compensation for the significantly diminished vascular tone.

Correction of the hypovolaemia by adequate fluid replacement remains the most important treatment for shock. Inotropes and pressor agents should be reserved for hypotension or other markers of low cardiac output that persist after ensuring adequate filling pressures have been achieved.

Renal Failure

Acute renal failure complicates acute pancreatitis in up to 15% of patients and in the majority is a consequence of hypovolaemia and shock (Balsov et al. 1962; Imrie 1974). Acute tubular necrosis is the most common form of renal failure although renal cortical necrosis may occur occasionally (Carey 1979). In the past the mortality associated with this complication has been high at 69%–100% (Beisel et al. 1959; Balsov et al. 1962; Imrie and Blumgart 1975), although all five patients in another study survived (Goldstein et al. 1976).

A better appreciation of the risk of acute renal failure and more aggressive fluid therapy, hourly monitoring of the urine output and the use of mannitol or frusemide when the urine output fell below 30 ml/h reduced the incidence of acute renal failure from 14.5% to 5.2% (Imrie and Blumgart 1975). The reported incidence subsequently fell to around 3% (Imrie et al. 1978a) and with better renal support utilising low dose dopamine and early peritoneal or haemodialysis in established cases of renal failure, the mortality from this complication is now undoubtedly lower.

Acute renal failure has usually been explained on the basis of hypovolaemia and/or hypotension although it has been reported in the absence of hypotension (Goldstein et al. 1976). In canine pancreatitis a decrease in both glomerular filtration and blood pressure was found, with a relatively greater fall in renal blood flow indicating increased renal vascular resistance (Frey and Brody 1966). A fall in glomerular filtration, renal blood flow and renal plasma flow with a simultaneous increase in renal vascular resistance was also found in a group of patients without renal failure (Werner et al. 1974). Unusually, this was associated with systemic hypertension and increased total peripheral resistance which suggests the release of a vasopressor, the nature of which was unknown, during the acute phase of the illness.

Deposits of fibrin material have also been found in the glomerular capillaries. These are thought to arise as a result of intravascular coagulation, which may contribute to the development of acute renal failure (Gupta 1971). This feature was absent in fatal attacks of pancreatitis not characterised by an association with acute renal failure.

Respiratory Complications

Respiratory complications are frequently associated with acute pancreatitis and were thought to be the most significant factor contributing to death. They may occur even where the pancreatic damage appears to be moderate in extent (Renner et al. 1985). Abnormal chest radiology was found at some time during the hospital course in 34% of patients, and nearly one quarter of these patients died (Jacobs et al. 1977). This finding, therefore, correlated strongly with death but unsuspected hypoxaemia may be even commoner. Fig. 2 shows the major factors contributing to hypoxaemia.

Ranson et al. (1974) found early evidence of hypoxaemia (Pao_2 below 76 mmHg) in 69% of his patients and in 38% the Pao_2 was below 66 mmHg. Clinical evidence of respiratory failure was usually not obvious and only nine patients (11%) had radiographic evidence of respiratory complications.

We found severe arterial hypoxaemia (Pao_2 below 60 mmHg) in 45% of patients, a further 35% having Pao_2 levels below 70 mmHg recorded at some stage during the first week of illness (Imrie et al. 1977). Only 18% of these patients had any radiological abnormality (pleural effusion in 10 and atelectasis

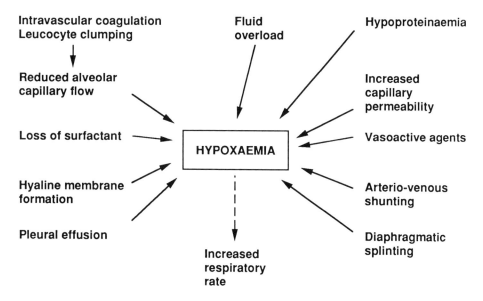

Fig. 2. Major factors contributing to hypoxaemia.

in five) and clinical features of respiratory embarrassment (except for tachypnoea) were rarely evident. In a subsequent study right to left shunting was found to be the major abnormality responsible for the hypoxia, with shunts of up to 30% of the cardiac output (Murphy et al. 1980). The recognition of this complication and the provision of humidified oxygen led to the halving of mortality in the elderly (Imrie and Blumgart 1975).

Acute pleural effusions are usually found on the left side and are most often small and self-limiting. Chronic effusions are the result of an internal pancreatic fistula which develops following pancreatic duct disruption (Cameron 1978). While acute pleural effusions rarely require treatment, chronic effusions will require surgical intervention if they fail to settle with conservative measures aimed at diminishing pancreatic secretion.

The most severe form of lung involvement in acute pancreatitis comprises pulmonary oedema, atelectasis and diffuse pulmonary infiltrates in variable degree but which may give rise to the adult respiratory distress syndrome. In one study diffuse pulmonary involvement occurred in 18% of patients of whom 56% died (Interiano et al. 1972). Among the possible causes of the lung lesion are physical factors such as aspiration, fluid overload and hypoproteinaemia, shock, local or disseminated intravascular coagulation and fat embolism (McKenna et al. 1977). Various pancreatic enzymes have also been implicated, in particular phospholipase A_2, which may have a specific action on pulmonary surfactant. Loss of surfactant with hyaline membrane formation was shown to be a feature of fatal acute pancreatitis associated with major respiratory insufficiency or failure (Lankisch et al. 1983). Finally, complement breakdown products and kinins released in acute pancreatitis may increase capillary permeability; kinins can also cause pulmonary venous hypertension and so exacerbate the increased vessel permeability (McKenna et al. 1977).

Coagulopathy

Disseminated intravascular coagulation may occur as a rare complication of acute pancreatitis, but in several reported cases other factors may have been reponsible for its occurrence (Kwaan et al. 1971; Greipp et al. 1972). A similar consumptive coagulopathy may be induced in dogs by the intravenous infusion of trypsin but not lipase or phospholipase (Kwaan et al. 1971).

Changes suggesting a hypercoagulable state were found in a study of coagulation parameters in 25 patients, of whom only one showed features of disseminated intravascular coagulation (Murphy et al. 1977). Activation of the coagulation system was manifest by raised levels of fibrin degradation products (FDPs), reduced platelet counts and increased levels of factors V, VIII and fibrinogen (Murphy et al. 1977; Imrie et al. 1988). Another group found no consistent pattern in prothrombin time, partial thromboplastin time and thrombin time, and wide individual variability in these coagulation factors (Ranson et al. 1977). Alterations in coagulation were greatest in those with severe pancreatitis. Because early coagulation measurements could be correlated with respiratory, renal and hepatic dysfunction, Ranson et al. (1977) considered that enzyme-related intravascular coagulation might be implicated in the pathogenesis of these complications.

Fulminant Acute Pancreatitis

Where gross changes in the cardiovascular and respiratory systems combine with acute renal failure or insufficiency, a fulminant picture of acute pancreatitis (not unlike the description given in the introduction to this chapter) does occur and all the resources of a modern intensive care unit are necessary to resuscitate such a patient. Quite often with such efforts, including the use of mechanical ventilation, renal support and many drugs (catecholamines, dobutamine, nitroprusside etc.) the patient is managed through this phase. When this occurs the next major concern is the development of sepsis.

Sepsis

This can occur very early in the course of the attack if the biliary tree is infected. Features of cholangitis with jaundice, high fever and rigors may necessitate urgent endoscopic sphincterotomy and duct clearance (Neoptolemos et al. 1987). Later problems of sepsis may be due to infection of intravenous lines, urinary catheters, and pleural or peritoneal aspiration sites but the main concern is infection of necrotic peripancreatic tissue. This concern is greatest in the obese patient with severe disease.

We do not routinely advocate the use of antibiotics, but where the evidence points to gallstones and infection within the biliary tree, a cephalosporin and metronidazole are given. Such antibiotic treatment is valueless in reaching infected necrotic tissue and pyrexia may persist despite their use. Sepsis should be identified at an early stage by CT-guided aspiration (Gerzof et al. 1987) and appropriate surgical intervention should be undertaken without delay. This later peripancreatic sepsis can occur from the third day of the illness onwards and typically presents between days seven and 11. It is the single most important factor in determining survival (Beger et al. 1988). CT scans outlining the typical development of sepsis are shown in Figs. 3 and 4.

Unusual Complications of Acute Pancreatitis

Other complications attributed to systemic enzyme release include subcutaneous fat necrosis (Blauvelt 1946) and osteolytic lesions in bones due to intramedullary fat necrosis (Scarpelli 1956; Keating et al. 1972).

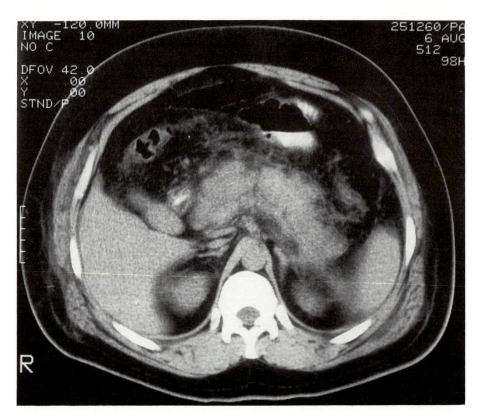

Fig. 3. CT scan of 30-year-old male patient 72 h after admission with severe acute pancreatitis. This shows marked pancreatic swelling throughout the gland.

Psychotic disturbances characterised by disorientation, confusion, delirium, delusions or hallucinations are not infrequently seen in acute pancreatitis (Durr 1979). While these may simply reflect alcohol withdrawal in alcoholic pancreatitis, there appears to exist a distinct entity of pancreatic encephalopathy. In a study of 17 patients, none of whom were alcoholics, encephalopathy was demonstrated in six (35%). This was associated with increased levels of lipase in the cerebrospinal fluid (Estrada et al. 1979).

Tetany is a consequence of hypocalcaemia and may rarely occur in acute pancreatitis. However, in one of the original descriptions it is likely that the tetany described was due to hyponatraemic convulsive movements; the sodium levels were exceedingly low whereas the calcium levels were only moderately reduced (Hernandez et al. 1961). Most of the fall in ionised calcium is rapidly corrected by parathyroid hormone (PTH) elevation of a spectacular type (Imrie et al. 1978b). The large loss of intravascular albumin that occurs results in a fall in protein-bound calcium and so reduces the measured total calcium concentration, but there is little change in ionised calcium (Imrie et al. 1976). Acid–base changes also influence ionised calcium concentrations but the initial

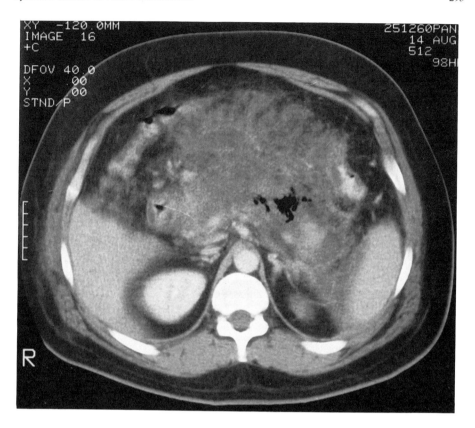

Fig. 4. The same patient 8 days later with development of focal abscess formation around the pancreas indicated by the black gas shadows on the anterior surface of the distal pancreas. A short time after this scan was taken surgical intervention was performed with a good result.

phases of severe acute pancreatitis are characterised by a metabolic acidosis with subsequent respiratory alkalosis if therapy is successful.

Conclusion

The systemic complications of acute pancreatitis are thought to be mediated indirectly, by activated pancreatic enzymes, kinins, peptides and perhaps other toxic products released from the pancreas and peritoneal exudate. These complications may occur in the absence of pancreatic necrosis and in the past have often resulted in early death from a shock-like illness associated with renal, respiratory and cardiovascular failure (Shader and Paxton 1966; Trapnell 1966). Currently, with improved understanding of the magnitude of the fluid losses and fluid shifts that may occur, fewer patients die of the consequences of hypovolaemia.

References

Albo R, Silen W, Goldman L (1963) A critical analysis of acute pancreatitis. Arch Surg 86:1032–1038

Anderson MC, Schoenfeld FB, Iams WB, Suwa M (1967) Circulatory changes in acute pancreatitis. Surg Clin North Am 47:127–140

Balsov JT, Jorgensen HE, Nielsen R (1962) Acute renal failure complicating severe acute pancreatitis. Acta Chir Scand 124:348–354

Beger HG, Bittner R, Buchler M, Hess W, Schmitz JE (1986) Hemodynamic data patterns in patients with acute pancreatitis. Gastroenterology 90:74–79

Beger HG, Buchler M, Bittner R et al. (1988) Necrosectomy and postoperative local lavage in necrotizing pancreatitis. Br J Surg 75:207–212

Beisel WR, Herndon EG, Myers JE, Stones L (1959) Acute renal failure as a complication of acute pancreatitis. Arch Intern Med 104:539–543

Blauvelt H (1946) A case of acute pancreatitis with subcutaneous fat necrosis. Br J Surg 34:207–208

Bockus HL, Kalser MH, Roth JLA, Bogoch AL, Stein G (1955) Clinical features of acute inflammation of the pancreas. Arch Intern Med 96:308–321

Bradley EL, Hall JR, Lutz J, Hamner L, Lattouf O (1983) Hemodynamic consequences of severe pancreatitis. Ann Surg 198:130–133

Cameron JL (1978) Chronic pancreatic ascites and pancreatic pleural effusions. Gastroenterology 74:134–140

Carey LC (1979) Extra-abdominal manifestations of acute pancreatitis. Surgery 86:337–342

Carey LC, Rodgers RE (1966) Pathophysiologic alterations in experimental pancreatitis. Surgery 60:171–178

Cobo JC, Abraham E, Bland RD, Shoemaker WC (1984) Sequential hemodynamic and oxygen transport abnormalities in patients with acute pancreatitis. Surgery 95:324–330

Corfield AP, Cooper MJ, Williamson RCN et al. (1985) Prediction of severity in acute pancreatitis: prospective comparison of three prognostic indices. Lancet ii:403–407

Di Carlo V, Nespoli A, Chiesa R et al. (1981) Hemodynamic and metabolic impairment in acute pancreatitis. World J Surg 5:329–339

Durr GH-K (1979) Acute pancreatitis. In: Howat HT, Sarles H (eds) The exocrine pancreas. WB Saunders, London, pp 352–401

Ellison EC, Pappas TN, Johnson JA, Fabri PJ, Carey LC (1981) Demonstration and characterization of the hemoconcentrating effect of ascitic fluid that accumulates during hemorrhagic pancreatitis. J Surg Res 30:241–248

Estrada RV, Moreno J, Martinez E et al. (1979) Pancreatic encephalopathy. Acta Neurol Scand 59:135–139

Foster PD, Ziffren SE (1962) Severe acute pancreatitis. Arch Surg 85:252–259

Frey CF, Brody GL (1966) Relationship of azotemia and survival in bile pancreatitis in the dog. Arch Surg 93:295–300

Gerzof SG, Banks PA, Robbins AH et al. (1987) Early diagnosis of pancreatic infection by computed tomography-guided aspiration. Gastroenterology 93:1315–1320

Goldstein DA, Llach F, Massry SG (1976) Acute renal failure in patients with acute pancreatitis. Arch Intern Med 136:1363–1365

Greipp PR, Brown JA, Gralnick HR (1972) Defibrination in acute pancreatitis. Ann Intern Med 76:73–76

Gupta RK (1971) Immunohistological study of glomerular lesions in acute pancreatitis. Arch Pathol 92:267–272

Hernandez IA, Powers SR, Frawley TF (1961) The role of the parathyroid glands in calcium and magnesium metabolism in acute hemorrhagic pancreatitis. Surgery 50:143–150

Imrie CW (1974) Observations on acute pancreatitis. Br J Surg 61:539–544

Imrie CW, Blumgart LH (1975) Acute pancreatitis: a prospective study on some factors in mortality. Bull Soc Int Chir 6:601–603

Imrie CW, Allam BF, Ferguson JC (1976) Hypocalcaemia of acute pancreatitis: the effect of hypoalbuminaemia. Curr Med Res Opin 4:101–116

Imrie CW, Ferguson JC, Murphy D, Blumgart LH (1977) Arterial hypoxia in acute pancreatitis. Br J Surg 64:185–188

Imrie CW, Benjamin IS, Ferguson JC et al. (1978a) A single-centre double-blind trial of Trasylol therapy in primary acute pancreatitis. Br J Surg 65:337–341

Imrie CW, Beastall GH, Allam BF et al. (1978b) Parathyroid hormone and calcium homeostasis in acute pancreatitis. Br J Surg 65:717–720

Imrie CW, Shearer MG, Wilson C (1988) Glycoproteins as markers of pancreatic damage in acute pancreatitis. Int J Pancreatol 3:S43–S52

Interiano B, Stuard ID, Hyde RW (1972) Acute respiratory distress syndrome in pancreatitis. Ann Intern Med 77:923–926

Ito K, Ramirez-Schon G, Shah PM et al. (1981) Myocardial function in acute pancreatitis. Ann Surg 194:85–88

Jacobs ML, Daggett WM, Civetta JM et al. (1977) Acute pancreatitis: analysis of factors influencing survival. Ann Surg 185:43–51

Keating JP, Shackelford GD, Shackelford PG, Ternberg JL (1972) Pancreatitis and osteolytic lesions. J Pediatr 81:350–353

Kwaan HC, Anderson MC, Gramatica L (1971) A study of pancreatic enzymes as a factor in the pathogenesis of disseminated intravascular coagulation during acute pancreatitis. Surgery 69:663–672

Lankisch PG, Rahlf G, Koop H (1983) Pulmonary complications in fatal acute hemorrhagic pancreatitis. Dig Dis Sci 28:111–116

Lefer AM, Glenn TM, O'Neill TJ, Lovett WL (1971) Inotropic influence of endogenous peptides in experimental hemorrhagic pancreatitis. Surgery 69:220–228

Lovett WL, Wangensteen SL, Glenn TM, Lefer AM (1971) Presence of a myocardial depressant factor in patients in circulatory shock. Surgery 70:223–231

McKenna JM, Craig RM, Chandrasekhar AJ, Cugell DW, Skorton D (1977) The pleuropulmonary complications of pancreatitis. Chest 71:197–204

McMahon MJ, Playforth MJ, Pickford IR (1980) A comparative study of methods for the prediction of severity of attacks of acute pancreatitis. Br J Surg 67:22–25

Moynihan B (1925) Acute pancreatitis. Ann Surg 81:132–134

Murphy D, Imrie CW, Davidson JF (1977) Haematological abnormalities in acute pancreatitis. Postgrad Med J 53:310–314

Murphy D, Pack AI, Imrie CW (1980) The mechanism of arterial hypoxia occurring in acute pancreatitis. Q J Med 49:151–163

Neoptolemos JP, Carr-Locke DL, Leese T, James D (1987) Acute cholangitis in association with acute pancreatitis: incidence, clinical features, outcome and the role of ERCP and endoscopic sphincterotomy. Br J Surg 74:1103–1106

Pollock AV (1959) Acute pancreatitis. Analysis of 100 patients. Br Med J i:6–14

Ranson JHC, Turner JW, Roses DF, Rifkind KM, Spencer FC (1974) Respiratory complication in acute pancreatitis. Ann Surg 179:557–566

Ranson JHC, Lackner H, Berman IR, Schinella R (1977) The relationship of coagulation factors to clinical complications of acute pancreatitis. Surgery 81:502–511

Read G, Braganza JM, Howat HT (1976) Pancreatitis – a retrospective study. Gut 17:945–952

Renner IG, Savage WT, Pantoja JL, Renner VJ (1985) Death due to acute pancreatitis. A retrospective analysis of 405 autopsy cases. Dig Dis Sci 30:1005–1018

Romer JF, Carey LC (1966) Pancreatitis. A clinical review. Am J Surg 111:795–798

Scarpelli DG (1956) Fat necrosis of bone marrows in acute pancreatitis. Am J Pathol 32:1077–1087

Shader AE, Paxton JR (1966) Fatal pancreatitis. Am J Surg 111:369–373

Storck G, Pettersson G, Edlund Y (1976) A study of autopsies upon 116 patients with acute pancreatitis. Surg Gynecol Obstet 143:241–245

Tahamont MV, Barie PS, Blumenstock FA, Hussain MH, Malik AB (1982) Increased lung vascular permeability after pancreatitis and trypsin infusion. Am J Pathol 109:15–26

Takada Y, Appert HE, Howard JM (1976) Vascular permeability induced by pancreatic exudate formed during acute pancreatitis in dogs. Surg Gynecol Obstet 143:779–783

Trapnell JE (1966) The natural history and prognosis of acute pancreatitis. Ann R Coll Surg Engl 38:265–287

Werner MH, Hayes DF, Lucas CE, Rosenberg IK (1974) Renal vasoconstriction in association with acute pancreatitis. Am J Surg 127:185–190

Chapter 26

The Diagnosis and Management of Pancreatic Pseudocyst

C. W. Imrie and M. G. Shearer

Pseudocyst is a relatively uncommon complication of acute pancreatitis which is not well predicted by the early determinants of severe acute pancreatitis. Neither the Ranson nor Glasgow criteria nor peritoneal aspiration have proved effective at identifying patients who will suffer from this late complication of the disease (Mayer et al. 1985; Corfield et al. 1985). This complication cannot develop in a period of less than 10–14 days because it is characterised by the presence of a dense fibrous lining without epithelial cells (which distinguishes pseudocyst from a true cyst). A working definition of a pancreatic pseudocyst is: a cystic collection of fluid (usually with a very high amylase level) enclosed by fibrous walls. Those which develop immediately after an attack of acute pancreatitis are most commonly retrogastric and a direct link to a disrupted main or major pancreatic duct can be demonstrated in almost every patient. Those which develop in association with chronic pancreatitis occasionally demonstrate this fistula-like linkage to the main duct system.

As can be seen from the above definition, it is essential to differentiate pancreatic pseudocysts which are a direct consequence of an attack of acute pancreatitis from those which occur without such a preceding episode. The French were first to recognise this important distinction. Others have emphasised this importance (Cross and Way 1981; McConnell et al. 1982; Imrie et al. 1988), but most contributions to the literature fail to do so. Analysis of the natural history and the outcome of therapy are therefore very difficult. Another difficulty is the failure of many of the papers to take into account the aetiology of the pancreatitis. It has been shown that patients with a pseudocyst after acute pancreatitis caused by alcohol abuse have a much lower mortality and morbidity than those associated with gallstones (Imrie et al. 1988).

Diagnosis of Pancreatic Pseudocyst

Clinical Features

The recent history of acute pancreatitis (AP) (or blunt abdominal trauma associated with signs and symptoms of AP) is exceedingly important. Most patients present with epigastric fullness associated with anorexia, but fullness and swelling can be in other locations when the pseudocyst is not in the retrogastric position. The overall size of the pseudocyst determines whether or not the clinical sign of a "mass" or "fullness and distension" can be detected. For the pseudocysts which arise in the retrogastric position, anorexia is often associated with both vomiting and weight loss. Large pseudocysts in this position prevent filling of the stomach with food, and readily contribute to vomiting. These two features result in weight loss, but in addition, there may be a catabolic effect of the pseudocyst which may result in weight loss of up to a kilogram every two days.

Pain is another fairly common feature of pancreatic pseudocyst, but a continual discomfort is more usual. The pain is determined by the location of the pseudocyst. Those in the common site behind the stomach present with epigastric and back pain whereas pseudocysts in the area of head of pancreas may produce many symptoms disproportionately to their overall size. In particular, vomiting and pain may be very troublesome.

Occasionally pseudocysts cause jaundice when they obstruct the common bile duct (CBD), usually with lateral distortion of the lower common hepatic duct and the CBD. Decompression of the pseudocyst relieves this complication (Imrie 1980; Warshaw and Rattner 1980).

A similar effect can occur when pseudocysts cause duodenal obstruction and this is usually effectively treated by decompression of the cystic lesion (Bradley 1982).

Finally gastrointestinal bleeding in the form of haematemesis can occur when there is bleeding down the pancreatic duct and into the duodenum from pseudocysts which decompress in this fashion. Such bleeding usually follows erosion into a major arterial branch of the celiac axis (Leger et al. 1976). Most frequently a branch of the splenic artery is involved (Wu et al. 1977). Incorporation of a vessel into the posterior wall of the pseudocyst and its subsequent rupture is the most common cause of bleeding, but we have treated one patient whose enlarging pseudocyst ruptured a moderate-sized artery stretched across the internal diameter of the pseudocyst. Rarely, arterial erosion may convert the pseudocysts into a pseudoaneurysm. Gastrointestinal bleeding may also occur from gastro-oesophageal varices when there is splenic vein thrombosis in association with a pseudocyst.

Spontaneous decompression of a pseudocyst into either the duodenum or the gastric antrum is very unusual. This results in its contents being regurgitated, followed by rapid resolution of the signs and symptoms. There may then be vomiting of blood or "cyst" contents.

Spontaneous rupture of a pseudocyst into the peritoneal cavity can cause pancreatic ascites. On two occasions we have noted subcutaneous fat necrosis associated with this entity. Each was originally thought to be erythema nodosum, but histological proof of fat necrosis was obtained. The painful skin necrosis was confined to the limbs in each patient.

Chronic pancreatitis with pseudocyst formation tends to be associated with smaller-diameter cysts and the symptoms come on less rapidly and are less commanding in nature. In addition, if the patient is still drinking alcohol then the senses are often dulled, and the patient may make little complaint.

The diagnosis of pseudocyst depends in the first instance on clinical suspicion. This should be aroused if a patient has failed to recover completely from an attack of acute pancreatitis or blunt abdominal trauma and then develops any of these clinical features, especially epigastric fullness. Persistent elevation of serum and urine amylase may also point to the diagnosis. Imaging methods, particularly ultrasound scanning, will usually identify the location and size of the pseudocyst.

Biochemical Features

It is common to find continuing elevated amylase output into the vascular compartment in patients with pseudocysts. In a series of 81 consecutive patients with a pseudocyst following acute pancreatitis gross hyperamylasaemia was present in 33% (greater than four times the upper limit of normal), while an additional 43% showed moderate hyperamylasaemia (300–1200 IU/l). Just under half of a group of 36 patients who had urinary amylase measurements had levels greater than 3000 IU/l (Imrie et al. 1988).

Imaging of Pseudocysts

Ultrasound scanning is particularly valuable as it is inexpensive and can be repeated frequently to monitor progression or regression of the pseudocyst without exposure to radiation. It is essential that the sonographer gives accurate diameters of the pseudocyst. Only in this way can consistent and accurate monitoring of its size be obtained.

Computed tomography (CT) gives particularly valuable information, but this is an expensive test and does not require to be used on a routine basis. Contrast-enhanced CT can be used to diagnose bleeding into a pseudocyst.

Endoscopic retrograde cholangiopancreatography (ERCP) can be particularly helpful immediately before a therapeutic intervention is planned (Sankaran and Watt 1975). There is an appreciable risk of introducing infection into a sterile collection, especially when the procedure is carried out in isolation from any intent at therapy. When a pseudocyst is suspected it is sensible to put an aminoglycoside antibiotic into the injection fluid. A typical pancreatogram with pseudocyst is shown in Fig. 1. A number of the abnormalities demonstrated with this investigation will be related to the pancreatic duct as it is common to find some break in the integrity of the duct system communicating with the pseudocyst. Occasionally distortion of the biliary tree will be shown.

Nordback et al. (1988) suggested a classification of pancreatogram appearances

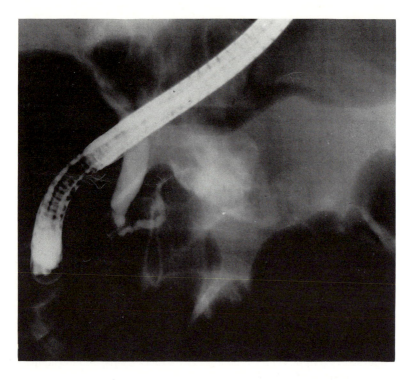

Fig. 1. ERCP showing leakage of dye from main pancreatic duct into a pseudocyst cavity.

in pseudocyst. Type I shows a normal duct with no communication with the cyst. Type II shows a normal duct opening into the cyst, and in Type III there is stenosis of the pancreatic duct. Type I cysts may be managed by external drainage with good results, but Type III cysts usually require internal drainage. Two cases of Type II cysts resolved spontaneously.

It is noteworthy that, in the rare instance when ultrasound is unavailable, a lateral erect barium meal examination will usually show anterior displacement of the stomach by a retrogastric pseudocyst or distortion of the duodenum by a cyst in the head of the gland. This was formerly the standard approach to investigation but gave no information as to the exact nature of the structure causing the displacement (Anderson 1972; Frey 1978).

Imaging investigations should be able to give information not only on the size of a pseudocyst, but also the thickness of the wall. However, a decision on therapy is not necessarily guided by the overall size of the pseudocyst, but rather by the combination with symptoms and whether the pseudocyst is enlarging or decreasing in overall size. It is very important not to confuse the diagnosis of pancreatic pseudocyst with that of a peripancreatic collection arising within the first two weeks of an episode of acute pancreatitis. At this stage there has been insufficient time for development of a fibrous wall (Bradley et al. 1979).

Therapy

Conservative

A "wait and see policy" is perfectly justifiable in all pancreatic pseudocysts, but particularly those arising in the period after an episode of acute pancreatitis. It is difficult to interpret the current literature because of the mixing of patients whose pseudocyst follows acute pancreatitis and those with chronic pancreatitis. However, both in a study in the 1970s (Duncan et al. 1976) and more recently (Shearer and Imrie 1990), we have documented spontaneous regression occurring in pseudocysts in approximately 50% of patients. A particular guideline which recommends intervention after six weeks' documentation of a pseudocyst derived from an important study in Atlanta (Bradley et al. 1979). In that study patients were randomised to interventional surgery at six weeks after diagnosis, or to continued conservative management. Pseudocyst rupture, abscess formation or obstruction of the CBD occurred in 41% of 54 patients allocated to the conservative management group. This occurred at an average time of 13.5 weeks after diagnosis. Bradley et al. concluded that "unfortunately, even in retrospect, no specific clinical warning of impending complications could be identified in the group of patients treated expectantly". They identified a 20% rate of spontaneous resolution of pseudocyst before six weeks and only a 3% rate after this time (Bradley et al. 1979). Thus this important piece of work has become the lynchpin for the policy that active measures be taken at six weeks from diagnosis of pseudocyst.

Other authors have supported Bradley's view that six weeks be used as a guide (Aranha et al. 1983; Agha 1984; Beebe et al. 1984; Wade 1985). Most of those groups have also inferred that pseudocysts of diameter 6 cm or greater are unlikely to resolve spontaneously. We have recently re-examined this question (Shearer and Imrie 1990) and found grounds for considerable caution in using the guidelines of a 6 cm diameter pseudocyst and six weeks' duration to indicate the requirement for therapeutic intervention. It was certainly true that the larger pseudocysts more frequently warranted intervention. The median size of those requiring drainage was 10×7 cm, whereas the median size of those resolving spontaneously was 8×5 cm. However, pseudocysts of greater than 6 cm maximum diameter did resolve spontaneously. In an initial series of 85 patients, 25 (29%) resolved spontaneously and 12 of these measured greater than 6 cm. Furthermore, we found that only 33% of pseudocysts resolved within six weeks of development and, in contrast to Bradley's experience, no patient experienced complications during the time to resolution. We believe, therefore, that, providing the clinical condition of a patient with a pancreatic pseudocyst is not deteriorating, repeated clinical and ultrasound monitoring should be continued up to 12 weeks from the time of diagnosis before embarking on some form of drainage.

Interventional Therapy

This can broadly be divided into non-surgical and surgical drainage of pancreatic pseudocyst. There are a number of options in both main categories. These range from percutaneous aspiration of the pseudocyst, through various forms of endoscopic drainage to major surgical procedures under general anaesthetic.

Percutaneous Aspiration

This technique is usually performed under local anaesthesia using ultrasound to determine the most direct route to the collection in order to minimise the risk of damage to the colon, liver and spleen (Bernardine and Amerson 1984; Peng et al. 1984). As much fluid as possible is withdrawn and then the needle is removed. Ultrasound scanning determines the completeness of aspiration. This technique is particularly valuable for older patients, and to reduce the need for surgery in a particularly ill patient. In our own experience of over 20 patients complete success was only found in 29%, with refilling of the pseudocyst occurring quite rapidly in the remainder. Repeat aspiration can be performed but this is rarely successful. However, a combination of percutaneous aspiration with subcutaneous or intravenous somatostatin therapy may prove useful in the future.

Percutaneous Catheter Drainage

This is depicted in Fig. 2 which shows the typical dark fluid which can be found in a pseudocyst being aspirated. There is obviously an increased risk with indwelling catheters which may cause infection within the pseudocyst

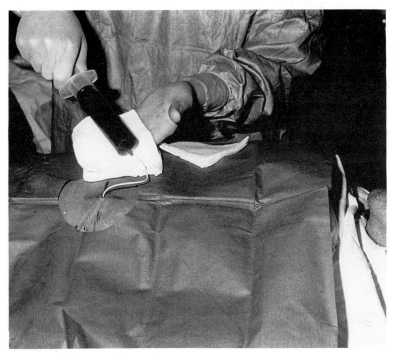

Fig. 2. An elderly patient with percutaneous catheter drainage of pseudocyst being established.

cavity and our own experience is limited. Others have found this a very successful form of treatment. In particular, Hancke and Henriksen (1985) have reported an 85% success rate in over 30 patients drained with a double pigtail catheter technique. This uses a combined percutaneous and endoscopic placement of the catheter into retrogastric pseudocysts, using the endoscope to grip the central part of the catheter with biopsy forceps in the stomach in order to leave one end of the catheter located in the pseudocyst and the other in the stomach. These drains are left in place for approximately 9 months and have been used almost exclusively in patients with pseudocyst associated with chronic pancreatitis.

Percutaneous catheter drainage has also been employed quite successfully by the Seattle group both in sterile and infected peripancreatic collections (Freeny et al. 1988). In 16 patients with loculated single collections the median drainage time was 29 days, whereas more complicated collections had a median drainage time of 96 days by catheter technique. Of a total of 23 patients, 15 (65%) were successfully managed without surgery. It is fair to say that this does not reflect general experience but rather that of a highly specialised group containing an individual (Dr Freeny) with a vast experience of percutaneous catheter and tube drainage. This does indicate what is possible and points the general direction for others.

Endoscopic Drainage Techniques

In addition to upper gastrointestinal endoscopes being used to steady the catheter as described above, they have been employed to direct needle knife diathermy equipment to burn a hole in the most prominent aspect of the bulge of a pseudocyst (Kozarek et al. 1985). Laser techniques have also been employed and these approches have met with variable success. At the present time it is quite difficult to assess the overall place of such techniques as the numbers of patients in any individual report are still quite small. There is obviously great difficulty in controlling the sudden rush of a large volume of fluid from a tense pseudocyst and a major calamity could ensue if the pseudocyst was filled with blood and no provision had been made for angiographic, therapeutic or direct surgical help. There is also the major problem of the presence of peripancreatic necrotic tissue in the pseudocyst content in patients who develop this complication after an attack of acute pancreatitis. Such necrotic material is an ideal medium for the growth of bacteria. In the authors' opinion, when ultrasound or CT demonstrate necrotic material within the cyst it should be removed surgically.

Surgical Techniques

The most popular and safer operations are those of internal surgical drainage either to the posterior wall of the stomach (cystogastrostomy) or drainage into a Roux loop of jejunum (cystojejunostomy).

Cystogastrostomy

This is the most popular operation and the simplest as most pseudocysts lie behind the stomach. In carrying out this technique it is important to observe that in the largest pseudocysts it may be quite difficult initially to identify the stomach which may appear as only a ribbon of tissue stretched over the anterior surface of the pseudocyst. Direct aspiration of the content of the pseudocyst into a syringe at an early stage of the operation identifies the nature of the contents which may range from clear pancreatic juice to very dark fluid or even blood. It is wise to use an aspiration identification technique at all operations for pseudocyst so that untimely surprises are avoided. When blood is encountered dissection around the pseudocyst should identify and control the major feeding vessels. Where this is difficult cross-clamping of the aorta may be required to control bleeding. A preoperative angiogram can forewarn of such potential problems and a therapeutic angiographic blocking of local vessels may be possible. It is, therefore, good clinical practice to obtain such angiographic information before operation.

In the standard operation of cystogastrostomy a longitudinal incision is made in the anterior surface of the stomach and then a similar incision is made in the posterior wall, cutting through the anterior wall of the pancreatic pseudocyst which will usually be in direct continuity and firmly adherent to that part of the stomach. Aspiration of the pseudocyst content and removal of any necrotic material using gentle finger dissection is advised. The size of the posterior gastric wall anastomosis with the front of the pseudocyst should be between 5 and 8 cm, but a larger anastomosis may be indicated in the biggest pseudocysts. Recurrence of the original pseudocyst is associated with smaller anastomoses. It is our technique to use interrupted sutures of polyglycolic acid (Ovicryl or Dexon) for this anastomosis to minimise the risk of postoperative haemorrhage.

Postoperatively, there is usually a very rapid fall in the hyperamylasaemia and complete resolution of major symptoms occurs very soon. Inspection of the cystogastrostomy anastomosis can be carried out endoscopically if there are any postoperative complications. It is usual to find that there is difficulty entering the previous pseudocyst cavity more than two weeks from the operation. This rate of resolution can be confirmed by imaging procedures.

Cystojejunostomy

Although cystojejunostomy can be carried out using a loop of jejunum to the pseudocysts which are away from the retrogastric position, it is accepted practice to use a Roux loop drainage technique. Similar mortality and recurrence rates are reported after cystogastrostomy and cystojejunostomy (Table 1). The majority of the papers involved in the collection of these data have been from American series in which alcohol-induced chronic pancreatitis predominates.

Cystoduodenostomy

This operation is the most logical for smaller pseudocysts occurring close to the curve of the duodenum in the area of the head of pancreas. A technique similar to that for cystogastrostomy is employed, only the cyst and consequently

Table 1. Results of surgical management of pancreatic pseudocysts (collected series)

Operation	No. of patients	Mortality (%)	Recurrence (%)
Cystogastrostomy	342	15 (4.4)	19 (5.5)
Cystojejunostomy	263	16 (6.1)	16 (6.1)
Cystoduodenostomy	57	4 (7.0)	3 (5.3)
Excision	187	18 (9.6)	8 (4.3)
External drainage	516	38 (7.4)	118 (22.9)[a]

[a] Highly significant difference.

the anastomosis tends to be much smaller. Again the results are similar to those for other forms of internal drainage and superior to the external drainage techniques (Table 1).

Pseudocyst Excision

This is particularly recommended in pseudocysts arising towards the tail of the pancreas in which there is a great deal of distortion of the local anatomy. It is most commonly practised in patients with chronic pancreatitis. The overall results are generally satisfactory, although a higher mortality is to be expected with more extensive operation (Table 1).

External Drainage

This is only necessary when the pseudocyst wall is immature and unable to "take" suture material. This was more common in the past and with the increase in percutaneous interventional techniques the numbers of patients being treated by external drainage will probably drop appreciably. Our own experience has been that external drainage has been a much more dangerous approach for the patient with both a higher mortality and morbidity (Imrie et al. 1988), although the collected data shown in Table 1 indicate a mortality of under 10%, but with a very high recurrence rate of over 20%. It is certainly the least desirable approach and is frequently complicated by the development of a pancreatic fistula.

Haemorrhage Associated with Pseudocyst

The causes of this have been mentioned earlier in the chapter. Where spontaneous haemorrhage develops a grave emergency exists. Pain and discomfort may disappear very rapidly to be replaced by cardiovascular collapse. Treatment options include

1. Therapeutic angiographic embolisation
2. Surgical control including the use of aortic cross-clamping and total excision of the diseased tissue (Leger et al. 1976)
3. Opening of the pseudocyst and oversewing of the bleeding point (Bradley 1982)

The blood loss may be abrupt and very dramatic. Unless a temporary tamponade occurs within the cyst then death may take place before any effective therapy can be arranged. The most attractive proposition from a therapeutic standpoint is effective control by interventional radiology with arterial embolisation (Huizinga et al. 1984).

Importance of Aetiology

From the data of patients treated in our own hospital, we found a mortality of under 4% for patients with alcohol-related pseudocyst developing after acute pancreatitis whereas the mortality in patients with gallstone-associated pseudocysts was over 20% (Imrie et al. 1988). We believe that the increased mortality in the patients with gallstone pancreatitis was related to the greater age of these patients and also the tendency for surgeons not to perform definitive biliary surgery at the time of pseudocyst drainage. Failure to carry out such definitive biliary surgery, we believe, increased the risk of postoperative sepsis. Our recommendation is always to carry out biliary surgery under antibiotic cover at the same time as the pseudocyst surgery.

Conclusion

At present there is a changing situation in the diagnosis and management of these complications of acute pancreatitis. Percutaneous and catheter drainage techniques will increasingly be employed, but are not without danger. The results from highly specialised centres, and particularly of small series of patients, must be interpreted with caution. There will be continued interest in and expansion of non-surgical interventional techniques. It is very important to remember that spontaneous resolution of a pseudocyst may occur up to 12 weeks and that both surgical and non-surgical interventional methods can safely be withheld for a longer time than was previously appreciated. This can only be considered safe in association with regular monitoring by sonography and clinical assessment.

At the present time the best type of therapeutic intervention will depend on local expertise. When the pathology follows an episode of acute pancreatitis, it should be remembered that peripancreatic necrotic material will not be removed by any other technique than surgical drainage, that infection may complicate percutaneous approaches and that excellent results have followed careful internal surgical drainage procedures. In an individual patient the age and general health of the patient will greatly influence the therapeutic approach.

Finally, great care must be taken not to employ percutaneous methods when there is any suspicion of an alternative diagnosis such as cystadenoma or cystadenocarcinoma because dissemination of the disease and delay in effective therapy may well prove very costly to the patient (Warshaw and Rutledge 1987).

References

Agha FP (1984) Spontaneous resolution of acute pancreatitic pseudocysts. Surg Gynecol Obstet 158:22–26

Anderson MC (1972) Management of pancreatic pseudocysts. Am J Surg 123:209–221

Aranha GV, Prinz RA, Esguerra AC, Greenlee HB (1983) The nature and course of cystic pancreatic lesions diagnosed by ultrasound. Arch Surg 118:486–488

Beebe DS, Bubrick MP, Onstad GR, Hitchcock CR (1984) Management of pancreatic pseudocysts. Surg Gynecol Obstetrics 159:562–564

Bernardine ME, Amerson JR (1984) Percutaneous gastrocystostomy: a new approach to pancreatic pseudocyst drainage. AJR 143:1096–1097

Bradley EL (1982) Complications of pancreatitis. Medical and surgical management. WB Saunders, Philadelphia, pp 124–153

Bradley EL, Clements JL, Gonzales AC (1979) The natural history of pancreatic pseudocysts: a unified concept of management. Am J Surg 137:135–141

Corfield AP, Cooper MJ, Williamson RCN et al. (1985) Prediction of severity in acute pancreatitis: prospective comparison of three prognostic indices. Lancet ii:403–407

Cross RA, Way LW (1981) Acute and chronic pancreatic pseudocysts are different. Am J Surg 142:660–663

Duncan JG, Imrie CW, Blumgart LH (1976) Ultrasound in the management of acute pancreatitis. Br J Radiol 49:858–862

Freeny PC, Lewis GP, Traverso LW, Ryan JA (1988) Infected pancreatic fluid collections: percutaneous catheter drainage. Radiology 167:435–441

Frey CF (1978) Pancreatic pseudocyst – operative strategy. Ann Surg 188:652–662

Hancke S, Henriksen FW (1985) Percutaneous pancreatic cystogastrostomy guided by ultrasound scanning and gastroscopy. Br J Surg 72:916–917

Huizinga WKJ, Kalideen JM, Bryer JV, Bell PSH, Baker LW (1984) Control of major haemorrhage associated with pancreatic pseudocysts by transcatheter arterial embolization. Br J Surg 71:133–136

Imrie CW (1980) In: Sircus W, Smith A (eds) Scientific foundation of gastroenterology. Heinemann, London, pp 622–629

Imrie CW, Buist LJ, Shearer MG (1988) The importance of etiology in the outcome of pancreatic pseudocyst. Am J Surg 156:159–162

Kozarek RA, Brayko CM, Harlan J, Sanowski RA, Cintora I, Kovac A (1985) Endoscopic drainage of pancreatic pseudocysts. Gastrointest Endosc 31:322–328

Leger L, Lenriot JP, Hovasse P (1976) Les hemorrhagies intra-kystiques des pseudokysts pancreatiques. J Chir (Paris) 111:137–162

Mayer AD, McMahon MH, Corfield AP et al. (1985) Controlled clinical trial of peritoneal lavage for the treatment of severe acute pancreatitis. N Engl J Med 312:399–404

McConnell DB, Gregory JR, Sasaki TM, Vetto RM (1982) Pancreatic pseudocyst. Am J Surg 143:599–601

Nordback I, Auvinen O, Airo I, Islauri J, Teerenhovi O (1988) ERCP in evaluating the mode of therapy in pancreatic pseudocyst. HPB Surg 1:35–44

Peng SY, Chi YG, Yu MK, Peng SG (1984) Sequential external and internal drainage of pancreatic pseudocyst. Br J Surg 71:317

Sankaran S, Watt AJ (1975) The natural and unnatural history of pancreatic pseudocysts. Br J Surg 62:37–44

Shearer MG, Imrie CW (1990) Spontaneous resolution of pancreatic pseudocysts. Digestion 46:177–178 (abstract)

Wade JW (1985) Twenty five year experience with pancreatic pseudocysts. Are we making progress? Am J Surg 149:705–708

Warshaw AL, Rattner DW (1980) Facts and fallacies of common bile duct obstruction by pancreatic pseudocyst. Ann Surg 192:33–37

Warshaw AL, Rutledge PL (1987) Cystic tumours mistaken for pancreatic pseudocysts. Ann Surg 205:393–398

Wu TK, Zaman SN, Gullick HD, Powers SR (1977) Spontaneous haemorrhage due to pseudocysts of the pancreas. Am J Surg 124:408–410

Chapter 27

"Idiopathic" Pancreatitis: Do We Need to Know the Cause?

C. D. Johnson

In the United Kingdom about half the attacks of acute pancreatitis are related to gallstones and about one-quarter to alcohol consumption (Table 1). Other aetiological agents have been reviewed elsewhere (Tables 2 and 3). This chapter is concerned with the search for an aetiology in patients in whom initial assessment has shown no evidence of gallstones and no excessive alcohol consumption (non-gallstone non-alcohol related (NGNA) pancreatitis). Patients

Table 1. Aetiological factors in acute pancreatitis identified in two reports from the United Kingdom (Bristol/Leeds/Glasgow: Corfield et al. 1985a; North East Scotland: Thomson et al. 1987)

	Bristol/Leeds Glasgow			North East Scotland[a]		
	M	F	Total	M	F	Total
Gallstones (%)	42	62	54	30	53	41
Alcohol (%)	33	4	20	26.5	3	15
Idiopathic (%)	21	30	27	19	22	20
Other (%)			4	24.5	22	23
Pancreas cancer	3	2	5			6
Trauma	1		1	9	3	12
Postoperative	1	2	3	24	21	45
ERCP	1	4	5			4
Hyperparathyroid		1	1			
Drugs	2		2			7
Hypothermia						3
Viral infection						4
Sepsis						2
Total in sample	237	217	454	189	170	359

[a] Includes all patients with hyperamylasaemia.

Table 2. Possible causes of acute pancreatitis other than gallstones and alcohol

Metabolic	Hyperlipoproteinaemia
	Hypercalcaemia
	Drugs
	Scorpion venom
	Genetic
Mechanical	Postoperative (gastric, biliary)
	Post-traumatic
	Retrograde pancreatography
	Pancreatic duct obstruction
	Pancreatic tumour
	Ascaris infestation
	Duodenal obstruction
Vascular	Postoperative (cardiopulmonary bypass)
	Periarteritis nodosa
	Atheroembolism
Infections	Mumps
	Coxsackie virus
Drugs (see Table 3)	

Adapted from Ranson (1984).

Table 3. Drugs which may cause acute pancreatitis

Definite association	Probable association	Possible association
Ethanol	Chlorothiazide	Amphetamines
Azathioprine	Hydrochlorothiazide	Cholestyramine
Oestrogen	Tetracycline	Cyproheptadine
	Frusemide	Propoxyphene
	Sulphonamides	Diazoxide
	L-Asparaginase	Histamine
	Chlorthalidone	Indomethacin
	Corticosteroids	Isoniazid
	Ethacrynic acid	Mercaptopurine
	Phenformin	Opiates
	Procainamide	Rifampicin
		Salicylates
		Cimetidine
		Acetominophen

From Clemens and Cameron (1989).

with recurrent NGNA pancreatitis deserve particularly thorough investigation, to forestall further attacks, although these patients have a similar distribution of aetiology to primary cases (Table 4).

The starting point for this discussion is the patient in whom a careful history has excluded alcohol (or a pharmaceutical) as a factor in the illness, and in

Table 4. Causes of recurrent attacks of pancreatitis in the Bristol area.

	Primary attack	Recurrent attacks
Gallstones	319 (50)	41 (51)
Alcohol	51 (8)	13 (16)
Idiopathic	148 (23)	21 (26)
Steroids	14 (2.2)	1 (1)
Hyperlipidaemia	6 (0.9)	1 (1)
Pancreas divisum	1 (0.2)	1 (1)
Postoperative	20 (3.1)	
Neoplasia	11 (1.7)	
Total	638	80

From Corfield at al. (1985b).
Figures in parentheses are percentages.

whom initial and follow-up ultrasound examinations have failed to reveal gallstones. This position is usually achieved five to seven days after admission to hospital, when the attack is resolving. Investigation from this point is concerned with the search for gallstones and the need to identify other rare causes of acute pancreatitis. It is safe to assume a biliary aetiology until another cause is demonstrated.

The Search for Gallstones

Despite initial negative investigations, undetected gallstones remain the most likely cause of acute pancreatitis. Faecal sieving during the acute phase consistently diagnoses more cases of gallstones than any other method (Acosta and Ledesma 1974; Kelly 1976). Goodman et al. (1985) found gallstones in seven patients out of 33 who underwent endoscopic retrograde cholangiopancreatography (ERCP) after initial negative ultrasonography and oral cholecystography. They also demonstrated that biochemical analysis on admission could give a good indication of the presence of gallstones (Goodman et al. 1985). Computed tomography (CT) may give useful information if gallstones are demonstrated, although the sensitivity is poor (about 34%) and CT cannot be recommended specifically for the diagnosis of gallstones (London et al. 1989).

Ultrasonography will detect gallbladder stones reliably, but bile duct stones are more difficult to diagnose with this imaging technique. Several authors have demonstrated the value of ERCP for the diagnosis of gallstones and other lesions in patients with normal ultrasonography after pancreatitis (Table 5). After recovery from the acute attack of pancreatitis, ERCP is likely to give images of both bile duct and pancreatic duct, with useful diagnostic information of previously unsuspected and potentially remediable disease in one-third to one-half of patients (Cooperman et al. 1981; Feller 1984). Neoptolemos et al. (1988a) demonstrated the safety of ERCP during the initial hospital admission, either within the first 72 h (urgent ERCP) or after resolution of the attack but

Table 5. Diagnosis at ERCP in patients with NGNA pancreatitis

	Reference	
	Cooperman et al. (1981)	Feller (1984)
Pancreas divisum	8 (23)	5 (7)
Papillary stenosis	3 (8)	5 (7)
Pancreatic duct obstruction	3 (8)	4 (5)
Gallstones	2 (6)	9 (12)
Normal	19 (55)	44 (60)
Total	35	73

Figures in parentheses are percentages.

before discharge from hospital (early ERCP). They stress, however, that pains should be taken to avoid injection of contrast into the pancreatic duct during urgent or early ERCP. The important point is to obtain a cholangiogram and deal with any common bile duct stones by endoscopic sphincterotomy. Pancreatography was usually successful and safe more than 30 days after the acute attack (delayed ERCP).

Bile Crystals and "Microcalculi"

One possible explanation for failure of ultrasonography to detect gallstones is that the stones are smaller than the limit of resolution of the technique. Farinon et al. (1987) defined "microlithiasis" as stones of homogeneous size with a diameter of 3 mm or less. They excluded biliary sand and microscopic crystals from this report. They studied 44 patients prospectively and found 31 of these to have microlithiasis by this definition. Haemorrhagic pancreatitis and necrosis were more frequent in the patients with microlithiasis (8/31) compared with those with large stones (1/13). Thus it seems that small stones can cause big trouble in the pancreas, which is why investigations to detect gallstones must be repeated several times.

Gallstones are thought to arise when nucleating factors lead to the precipitation of crystals of cholesterol or bile pigment. These crystals then increase in size by crystal propagation, with the final result being a gallstone. Can the presence of crystals in bile predict gallstones? Feller (1984) performed ERCP in 73 patients with negative initial investigations. Seven of these had common bile duct stones and two had gallbladder stones. Duodenal aspiration of bile for microscopic examination revealed no evidence of cholesterol or pigment crystals in these patients.

In contrast Neoptolemos et al. (1988b) examined duodenal bile in patients undergoing ERCP. The bile was collected after intravenous injection of cholecystokinin (CCK). In 11 patients with gallstone pancreatitis, crystals were found in seven. None of 15 patients with alcohol-related pancreatitis had crystals in the bile. The bile of five of 14 patients with NGNA pancreatitis contained calcium bilirubinate crystals. One patient without crystals subsequently developed gallstones. Three of the five patients with positive crystal analysis underwent cholecystectomy and gallstones were confirmed in all three, so it does appear that there is a strong correlation between crystals and stones. These authors recommend duodenal bile crystal analysis as a specific and easily performed test for the further elucidation of patients with NGNA pancreatitis.

It is most likely that bile will crystallise within the gallbladder where it is concentrated and may be static. Duodenal bile aspiration depends on ejection of bile from the gallbladder following CCK stimulation. An alternative approach to obtain gallbladder bile uses direct percutaneous needle aspiration from the gallbladder. We are now convinced of the safety and feasibility of ultrasound-guided percutaneous aspiration of bile (S. W. Hosking, personal communication). A total of 44 patients have undergone gallbladder aspiration under local anaesthesia immediately prior to elective cholecystectomy for gallstones. The procedure was successful in 40 of these. The four failures were associated with a contracted thick-walled gallbladder containing little bile. There were four complications (10%). Three patients were found to have bile in the abdominal cavity following transperitoneal gallbladder puncture. One patient had persistent bleeding from the liver after transhepatic gallbladder puncture. Paired analysis showed that in patients with crystals the aspirated bile had been obtained from the gallbladder in every case. We now perform percutaneous transhepatic gallbladder aspiration under local anaesthesia as part of the diagnostic examination of patients with NGNA pancreatitis but experience is so far too limited to allow an evaluation of its usefulness.

Non-gallstone Causes of Pancreatitis

Duct Abnormalities or Obstruction

ERCP is useful for the diagnosis of remediable causes of pancreatitis other than gallstones (Table 5). Pancreas divisum (isolated dorsal pancreas) can only be diagnosed with this technique. Ampullary stenosis (Feller 1984) or sphincter spasm (Toouli et al. 1985) can be diagnosed and treated.

A rare cause of pancreatitis, but one which is important to diagnose is pancreatic duct obstruction secondary to ampullary carcinoma. Robertson and Imrie (1987) found ampullary carcinoma to be more frequently associated with pancreatitis than hyperparathyroidism. The importance of making this diagnosis lies in the possibility of resection with reasonable hope of 5-year survival or, if the patient is unfit for resection, endoscopic "sphincterotomy" may be performed to relieve pancreatic and bile duct obstruction.

There are case reports of pancreatitis secondary to a duodenal duplication cyst (Waldron et al. 1985), and to obstruction of the bile duct by calculous material impacted in a periampullary duodenal diverticulum (Heath et al. 1987). Modern ultrasonography should be capable of diagnosing choledochal and duodenal replication cysts in the periampullary region. At the least, ultrasonography will demonstrate dilated bile ducts with low obstruction, which should alert the clinician to the need for cholangiography.

Drugs

A considerable list of therapeutic agents has been associated with acute pancreatitis (Table 3). It is not sufficient to note that the patient is taking such an agent to be able to ascribe the pancreatitis to this cause. If treatment has been prolonged before the onset of pancreatitis it is unlikely that there is a causal relationship. Such a causal relationship seems more likely if there is a short latent period, and the pancreatitis recurs with reintroduction of the supposed aetiological agent.

Lipids

Hyperlipidaemia is associated with acute pancreatitis. It has been suggested (Dickson et al. 1984) that many cases of hyperlipidaemia are secondary to alcohol consumption, and that the pancreatitis is caused by the alcohol rather than the hyperlipidaemia. Nevertheless, hyperlipidaemia unrelated to alcohol intake is present in 1%–2% of cases in most large series of pancreatitis although precise details of the lipid abnormality and its relationship to acute pancreatitis are often lacking. I have seen four patients with recurrent attacks of acute pancreatitis with hypertriglyceridaemia; three of these patients were of Indian origin. The attacks abated in all cases with control of the hypertriglyceridaemia, and recurred in two cases when lipid-lowering treatment was discontinued.

Admission to hospital, the acute illness of acute pancreatitis, and the hospital diet in the early recovery phase may all affect serum lipid levels. For this reason measurement of fasting triglyceride and cholesterol levels should be delayed until the patient has fully recovered and is re-established on his normal diet. It is convenient to perform this test after the first post-admission outpatient visit.

Guzman et al. (1985) suggested that there might be impaired lipid clearance in patients following acute pancreatitis. They studied 40 patients with normal fasting serum triglycerides who had had an attack of acute pancreatitis. The incidence of gallstones and alcoholism were similar to most other series, but nine patients had diabetes mellitus. Following ingestion of 100 g of vegetable oil these patients had elevated serum triglycerides for 24 h, when compared with healthy controls. The mechanism for this impaired lipid clearance is unclear. The authors postulate a pre-existing defect in lipid metabolism. Such a predisposition might interact with other causes of pancreatitis such as alcohol ingestion or administration of steroids, or even with a high fat diet. However, the practical usefulness of this test has not been established.

Infections

Several virus and other infections have been associated with acute pancreatitis. The patient may have loose stools at the time of presentation (Imrie et al. 1977). Viral infections may be detected by comparison of acute and convalescent antibody titres, but there is limited positive value to making this diagnosis. The infections are generally self-limiting and the diagnostic information comes too late to affect management of the acute attack. It is useful, however, to exclude alcohol as a cause, and to prevent a series of unnecessary tests in the search for an aetiology. It is also useful in studies of acute pancreatitis to have information on viral infections, to allow completeness in diagnosis and to minimise the size of the "idiopathic" group.

Calcium

Hypercalcaemia has been proposed by many authors as a cause of acute pancreatitis. The incidence of hypercalcaemia in patients with pancreatitis varies greatly in different series, but many authors find 1%–2% of patients with this condition. Similarly the incidence of pancreatitis in patients with hyperparathyroidism presenting with hypercalcaemia is of the order of 1%–2%. These figures are not greatly different from the corresponding incidence in the normal population. Sitges-Serra et al. (1988) claimed to demonstrate an association between hypercalcaemic hyperparathyroidism and different types of pancreatitis. They reported seven cases of acute pancreatitis and three of chronic pancreatitis in 86 patients with primary hyperparathyroidism. However, three of these patients were receiving steroids and azathioprine following renal transplantation (out of a total of 236 transplant patients). One patient had had a recent gastrectomy. There were thus only three cases of idiopathic acute pancreatitis in the hyperparathyroid patients and one of these had been treated and was hypocalcaemic at the time of presentation with pancreatitis. There is in fact little evidence to support the contention that hypercalcaemia is associated with acute pancreatitis.

A Plan for Investigation

The initial management of patients with pancreatitis will include a full history to exclude alcohol and drugs as causes, and an early ultrasound examination to exclude gallstones. Ultrasonography is repeated after five to seven days, to exclude gallstones and to detect any fluid collection which might be developing. If these investigations have been normal, how should the patient be investigated?

CT is indicated at this stage if the patient's condition is not improving (London et al. 1989), but there is little value in CT for diagnosis of the aetiology.

Our management plan is shown in Fig. 1. Blood is taken before discharge from hospital for acute phase viral titres. After recovery of the acute attack the patient is allowed to go home from hospital, and is re-admitted after two to three weeks for further investigation. Blood is sent for viral titres and a fasting sample is analysed for lipids. Abnormalities on these blood tests may diagnose the aetiology, but do not preclude further imaging investigation, as viral infections may coexist with other pathologies, and lipid abnormalities may predispose to gallstones. Chronic pancreatitis may also be a consequence of hypertriglyceridaemia, so pancreatography is required in these patients.

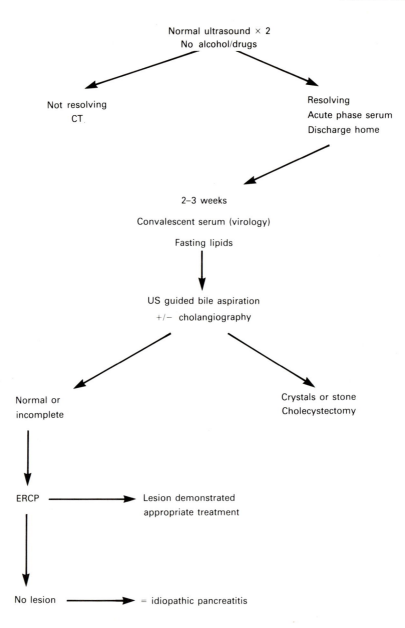

Fig. 1. Plan for investigation of NGNA pancreatitis.

During this second admission percutaneous ultrasound-guided gallbladder aspiration is performed for bile crystal analysis. If possible, a cholangiogram is also obtained by this route. The presence of bile crystals, or stones on cholangiography is an indication for cholecystectomy. Negative bile aspiration with inadequate cholangiography is followed by endoscopic cholangiography.

Pancreatography is attempted only with great caution less than four weeks after the acute attack. Any lesion demonstrated is treated on its merits. If ERCP is normal the pancreatitis may be truly idiopathic.

References

Acosta JM, Ledesma CL (1974) Gallstone migration as a cause of acute pancreatitis. N Engl J Med 290:484–487
Clemens JA, Cameron JL (1989) The pathogenesis of acute pancreatitis. In: Carter DC, Warshaw AL (eds) Pancreatitis. Churchill Livingstone, Edinburgh, pp 1–30
Cooperman M, Ferrara JJ, Carey LC, Thomas FB, Martin EW, Fromkes JJ (1981) Idiopathic acute pancreatitis: the value of endoscopic retrograde cholangiopancreatography. Surgery 90:666–670
Corfield AP, Cooper MJ, Williamson RCN et al. (1985a) Prediction of severity in acute pancreatitis: prospective comparison of three prognostic indices. Lancet ii:403–407
Corfield AP, Cooper MJ, Williams RCN (1985b) Acute pancreatitis: a lethal disease of increasing incidence. Gut 26:724–729
Dickson AP, O'Neill J, Imrie CW (1984) Hyperlipidaemia, alcohol abuse and acute pancreatitis. Br J Surg 71:685–688
Farinon AM, Ricci CL, Sianesi M, Percudani M, Zanella E (1987) Physiopathologic role of microlithiasis in gallstone pancreatitis. Surg Gynecol Obstet 164:252–256
Feller ER (1984) Endoscopic retrograde cholangiopancreatography in the diagnosis of unexplained pancreatitis. Arch Intern Med 144:1797–1799
Goodman AJ, Neoptolemos JP, Carr-Locke DL, Finaly DBL, Fossard DP (1985) Detection of gallstones after acute pancreatitis. Gut 26:125–132
Guzman S, Nervi F, Llanos O, Leon P, Valdivieso V (1985) Impaired lipid clearance in patients with previous acute pancreatitis. Gut 26:888–891
Heath D, Leese T, Carr-Locke DL, Thornton Holmes J (1987) Obstructing calculous material in a periampullary duodenal diverticulum associated with primary common bile duct calculi and acute pancreatitis. Br J Surg 74:648
Imrie CW, Ferguson JC, Sommerville RG (1977) Coxsackie and mumps virus infection in a prospective study of acute pancreatitis. Gut 18:53–56
Kelly TJ (1976) Gallstone pancreatitis: pathophysiology. Surgery 80:488–492
London NJM, Neoptolemos JP, Lavelle J, Bailey I, James D (1989) Serial computed tomography scanning in acute pancreatitis: a prospective study. Gut 30:397–403
Neoptolemos JP, Carr-Locke DL, London N, Bailey I, Fossard DP (1988a) ERCP findings and the role of endoscopic sphincterotomy in acute gallstone pancreatitis. Br J Surg 75:954–960
Neoptolemos JP, Davidson BR, Winder AF, Vallance D (1988b) Role of duodenal bile crystal analysis in the investigation of "idiopathic" pancreatitis. Br J Surg 75:450–453
Ranson HC (1984) Acute pancreatitis: pathogenesis, outcome and treatment. Clin Gastroenterol 13:843–863
Robertson JFR, Imrie CW (1987) Acute pancreatitis associated with carcinoma of the ampulla. Br J Surg 74:395–397
Sitges-Serra A, Alonso M, de Lecea C, Gores PF, Sutherland DER (1988) Pancreatitis and hyperparathyroidism. Br J Surg 75:158–160
Thomson SR, Hendry WS, McFarlane GA, Davidson AI (1987) Epidemiology and outcome of acute pancreatitis. Br J Surg 74:398–401
Toouli J, Roberts-Thomson IC, Deut J, Lee J (1985) Sphincter of Oddi motility disorders in patients with idiopathic recurrent pancreatitis. Br J Surg 72:859–863
Waldron R, Drumm J, McCarthy CF, Murray JP, Murphy B (1985) Surgically correctable recurring pancreatitis. Br J Surg 72:203

Chapter 28

Cystic Fibrosis

R. Dinwiddie

Cystic fibrosis (CF) is the commonest recessively inherited condition in the population of the UK. It affects in 1 in 2500 live-born infants in this country (Dodge et al. 1988), approximately 85% of patients have pancreatic deficiency leading to significant malabsorption of protein, fat, carbohydrates and vitamins. The primary defect appears to be due to an abnormality of chloride secretion across secretory cell surfaces (Quinton 1983). These abnormalities cause unusually viscid intestinal secretions which result in pancreatic obstruction and distended pancreatic ducts (Grand et al. 1966). The pathophysiology of this process involves other abnormalities of pancreatic secretion, including decreased protease activity and reduced flow of pancreatic secretions which again predispose to intestinal obstruction (Durie and Forstner 1989). The cardinal features of pancreatic deficiency in cystic fibrosis consist of reduced enzyme secretion and a very low bicarbonate level (Gaskin et al. 1982; Coupleman et al. 1988).

Genetic Aspects

The gene for CF has been specifically cloned to chromosome 7 and the most common mutation ($\triangle$F508 – a phenylalanine deletion) has been identified (Kerem et al. 1989). Since then a large number of other mutations have also been described (Dean et al. 1990). CF patients may, therefore, be homozygous or heterozygous for the $\triangle$F508 gene. In the UK population the incidence of homozygosity of the $\triangle$F508 gene in CF patients is 57% (McMahon et al. 1990) and heterozygosity for $\triangle$F508 was found in 30% of patients. There is some evidence to suggest that the presence of $\triangle$F508 is associated with more severe pancreatic disease than other genotypes (Kerem et al. 1990; Stuhrmann et al. 1990). Meconium ileus is also more common among $\triangle$F508 homozygotes (European Working Group 1990). Adequate pancreatic function is thought to be more common among $\triangle$F508 heterozygotes (Kerem et al. 1990). A recent study from Denmark has shown that homozygous ▲F508 patients had a higher enzyme requirement than heterozygotes (Johansen et al. 1991).

Meconium Ileus

Approximately 10% of children with cystic fibrosis present with this complication at birth (Donnison et al. 1966). This condition is thought to result from intrauterine pancreatic insufficiency and has been detected by ultrasound examination as early as 17–18 weeks' gestation (Muller et al. 1985). During fetal life there may be intrauterine bowel perforation, or meconium within the bowel may cause obstruction secondarily to volvulus or gut atresia (Mabogunje et al. 1982). These complications arise from inspissated meconium within the bowel. The obstruction may also lead to microcolon. After birth the infant presents with abdominal distension and failure to pass stools (Dinwiddie 1983). Nowadays this is initially treated by gastrograffin enema which resolves the problem in 10%–15% of cases. Those who do not respond require laparotomy with resection of gangrenous or atretic bowel, followed by an end-to-end anastomosis. This usually results in restoration of bowel function. The continuity of the gut avoids the large fluid, electrolyte and nutritional losses associated with an ileostomy (Dinwiddie 1991).

Pancreatic Disease

The pathological changes within the pancreas have been delineated by Imrie et al. (1975). These workers showed that there is poor development of the pancreatic acini with increasing connective tissue deposition with age and enlargement of the intraluminal ductal volume due to the accumulation of viscid secretions within the pancreatic ducts.

Clinical Features of Pancreatic Insufficiency

Pancreatic insufficiency in CF presents in a number of ways (Table 1). In most studies, 85% of CF patients require pancreatic enzymes in order to control

Table 1. Pancreatic insufficiency in CF

Meconium ileus
Elevated immunoreactive trypsin
Steatorrhoea
Rectal prolapse
Distal intestinal obstruction syndrome
Pancreatitis
Diabetes mellitus

their symptoms of insufficiency (Park and Grand 1981). Between 10% and 15% of babies with cystic fibrosis will present with meconium ileus, as a result of intrauterine pancreatic insufficiency. Most babies present with abdominal distension and bile-stained vomit at birth, if they have not already developed complications. Infants with meconium ileus used to have a worse prognosis than others with CF, but this mortality has now been abolished and the long-term outcome for these children is as good as for those who present later in other ways.

The clinical features of exocrine or endocrine pancreatic insufficiency are well known, but in children there is the added consideration that inadequate nutrition may lead to growth retardation. A few babies with CF present in the early months with hypoproteinaemia and oedema (Chase et al. 1979) which usually responds to initial replacement with albumin and red blood cells followed by resolution as the diet and pancreatic enzyme replacement improve nutrient absorption.

Immunoreactive Trypsin (IRT)

In the neonatal period CF may not necessarily be manifest by obvious symptoms but there is elevation of the circulating trypsin levels in the blood during the first 2–3 months of life. This has been utilised as a screening test. One disadvantage of the use of immunoreactive trypsin is a significant false positive rate in the first two weeks of life; Kuzemko (1986) found an elevated IRT in 0.5% of 93 000 infants sampled. Wilcken and Chalmers (1985) suggested that infants diagnosed by screening had better growth in the early years, initially had fewer symptoms and spent less time in hospital than unscreened patients. This probably reflects better care generally and earlier diagnosis of milder cases.

The outcome of longer-term follow-up of screened and unscreened populations is awaited although there is as yet no conclusive evidence that it significantly affects outcome in adult life. The ability to start treatment regimes designed to prevent or slow down long-term damage is, however, facilitated following diagnosis at a presymptomatic stage of the disease. Genetic advice and prenatal diagnosis for future pregnancies can also be offered at the most appropriate time for each family.

Energy Requirements

Patients with CF are known to have an increased energy requirement (Buchdahl et al. 1988). This is partly due to the basic biochemical defect which involves ATP binding domains that affect ion transport across the cell membrane (Riordan et al. 1989). In addition there are large energy losses in the stools due to malabsorption if pancreatic function is poor and enzyme replacement is not optimised. Patients who have active chest infection also have increased energy requirements both to deal with the infection itself and also to support the extra work of breathing against increasing stiffness of the lungs (Pencharz et al. 1984). These patients may have energy requirements 25%–80% above those of healthy controls. A further problem may be anorexia: although the young infant with relatively good lungs and significant malabsorption may have a large appetite, those with chronic infection commonly have a poor appetite and decreased energy intake (Bell et al. 1984).

It is important, therefore, that an adequate intake of calories is provided for CF patients especially those with chronic lung disease. A high protein, high carbohydrate, unrestricted fat diet should be given to achieve an energy intake of 120% to 150% of normal recommended daily requirements (Littlewood and MacDonald 1987). The importance of a relatively high fat intake as a source of extra calories should be emphasised. In the past most CF patients were unable to tolerate the high fat intake because of poor enzyme availability. The new enteric coated preparations such as Creon® have helped greatly to overcome this problem.

Some CF patients continue to have major abdominal problems despite modern pancreatic enzyme preparations. These include excessive bile salt loss which can be partially overcome by enzyme replacement (Watkins et al. 1977). The mucus lining of the gut itself is also abnormal and this may impair the ability to absorb nutrients properly. Those who have frequent chest infections often take broad-spectrum antibiotics which can affect the microflora of the gut, another factor which can influence bile acid loss (Roy et al. 1979).

Vomiting as a result of coughing is another frequent complication in CF. Meals should be timed after physiotherapy sessions in order to avoid this complication. Oesophagitis and heartburn are often underrecognised associated features. These may be exacerbated if the patient it taking oral steroids as part of the treatment of chest complications.

The effects of gastric acid are also important, since pancreatic lipase works less efficiently at low pH. Bile acids may also be precipitated at low pH (Zentler-Munro et al. 1985). Gastric acidity can be reduced with the use of H_2-receptor antagonists such as cimetidine or ranitidine. This is a useful approach to adopt empirically in patients who have extremely high enzyme replacement requirements.

Reduction of the total bile salt pool is another important contributory factor in the maldigestion of CF. Bile salts can bind to protein or neutral lipids within the gut. Oral taurine supplementation, which alters the glycocholate to taurocholate ratio, can be helpful in patients with this problem (Belli et al. 1987).

Essential fatty acid deficiency is another feature of pancreatic deficiency in CF patients, although this appears to be most relevant only in patients with the most severe defects where pancreatic function is less than 6% of normal (Durie and Pencharz 1989). The effects of this essential fatty acid deficiency are not clear but could contribute to increasing susceptibility to infection, poor wound healing and possibly impaired growth potential.

The many factors contributing to energy imbalance in CF are outlined in Fig. 1.

Nutritional Management

Pancreatic replacement therapy plays a central role in the maintenance of adequate nutrition in CF patients. It must, however, form only a part of an

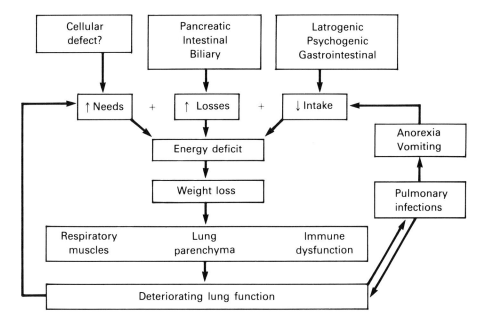

Fig. 1. Interdependent factors which may give rise to progressive energy deficit as lung function deteriorates in CF.

overall strategy for care and management. In addition, requirements of growth must always be carefully accounted for in nutritional assessment of infants and children with CF.

An adequate nutritional intake is vital and should be sustained at all times. Anorexia may be a direct effect of pulmonary infection and also may be secondary to swallowed sputum. Depression and anxiety about the long-term outcome also contribute to poor intake. A high energy intake is required, consisting of 35% calories derived from fat, 15% from protein and 50% from carbohydrates. The exact regime to be followed varies with the child's age, nutritional preferences and the severity of the pulmonary and pancreatic disease. The best approach is to individualise the nutrition to the patient's needs. This requires the expertise of a specialist CF clinic dietitian who is central to the team approach for these patients. Children and young adults often benefit from the opportunity to "calorie count", which enables them to choose high calorie foods of their own liking to achieve the desired level of energy intake (Dinwiddie and Madge 1988).

Infants have different nutritional requirements depending on type of presentation and age at diagnosis. Those who present with meconium ileus may require initial support with intravenous feeding until full oral feeds are established. Thereafter they can be successfully breast fed (Dinwiddie 1991) with the addition of pancreatic supplements, either as pancreatin powder or one of the newer enteric-coated microsphere preparations. Bottle-fed babies are now fed on a standard infant formula with enzyme supplementation. Some patients develop disaccharide intolerance after surgery and may require more elemental feeds such as Pregestimil. Weaning is encouraged in the normal way and is introduced at an early stage, from 3 months of age, if tolerated, in order to allow a higher energy intake.

Pancreatic Enzymes

As many as 90% of CF patients of all ages require enzyme supplements. The amount required varies from one individual to another and depends on the degree of residual pancreatic function as well as the overall nutritional intake. The aim of replacement is to achieve adequate weight gain and growth, a normal stool pattern and to decrease the fat malabsorption to a level below 15% of ingested fat. Apart from very young infants, all patients can now take enteric-coated microspheres – Creon, Pancrease or Nutrizyme GR, which are superior to the preparations previously available (Beverley et al. 1987; Stead et al. 1987; Vyas et al. 1990). These preparations are resistant to gastric acid and are released in the duodenum at pH levels of 5.0–5.5 or above. The way in which they are taken is also important. If they are to be effective they should be taken at the same time as the meal, most commonly half at the start and half in the middle. It is best to take the capsule directly so as not to chew it; if it is opened the granules are taken with only a small portion of food so that enzyme activity is not lost through the microspheres being destroyed in the mouth. The dosage should be individualised and will vary from an average of 6–8 capsules per meal up to 12–16 per large meal. Patients who need more than this number are seen from time to time; they may well have hyperacidity and could benefit from the addition of an H_2-receptor antagonist.

If too much enzyme is given this can lead to constipation. If excessive enzyme comes through the bowel a typical circumscribed perianal rash and soreness occurs. Should too much powdered enzyme be used or the enteric coated microspheres be chewed, irritation and redness in the mouth may also occur due to "digestion" of the mucosal lining of the buccal cavity. Some patients or young infants also become allergic to the powdered preparations and may develop a contact skin rash or nasal irritation when handling the preparation. This can be overcome by the wearing of gloves or a face mask, but it is easier to transfer the infant to one of the enteric-coated preparations as soon as this can be tolerated.

The modern enteric coated preparations are usually very well tolerated by most patients and have proved to be a major advance in the management of pancreatic disease in CF patients.

Distal Intestinal Obstruction Syndrome (DIOS)

Despite optimal pancreatic enzyme replacement and careful attention to diet, a small number of patients still have persisting problems due to inadequate digestion, particularly of protein in the gut. This is usually associated with abnormally viscid intestinal mucus and leads to the accumulation of sticky, putty-like intestinal secretions in the terminal ileum and ascending colon (Weller and Williams 1986). The term "meconium ileus equivalent" has often been used to describe this condition but DIOS is more accurate. The incidence previously reported was 10%–20%; however with the new enteric-coated enzyme preparations this has almost disappeared as a major complication of CF gut disease.

Acute episodes are best managed initially by a combination of lactulose and Fabrol (acetylcysteine) given orally. If this does not relieve the obstruction then oral diatrigoate and subsequently an enema will be effective in most patients with symptoms short of complete obstruction. Where there are more persistent features, short of total bowel obstruction, then intestinal lavage with propylene glycol balanced intestinal solution (Golytely®) is effective. Other causes of intestinal obstruction or a right iliac fossa mass should not be forgotten. These include an appendix mass, intussusception, adhesion obstruction and stricture. If there is any doubt about aetiology, abdominal X-ray, ultrasound and contrast enema can be helpful.

Diabetes Mellitus

Diabetes mellitus is an increasingly recognised complication of CF as the patients get older. In the paediatric age group this amounts to 2%–3% with an increasing prevalence in adolescence. As many as 57% of all CF patients have abnormal glucose tolerance (Rodman and Matthews 1981), although this only causes clinical problems in a relative minority of cases. The incidence in adult CF patients is approximately 8% (Finkelstein et al. 1988). The use of steroids in the treatment of the underlying lung disease frequently precipitates glycosuria and this is one of the major disadvantages to this approach to the control of lung disease in CF.

The onset of diabetes may be subtle, especially in adolescence, as the pancreatic islet cells are slowly destroyed by fibrosis. It is useful to test the urine for glucose when any adolescent or adult CF patient attends the clinic with weight loss, since polyuria and polydipsia are not always obvious. Insulin therapy is usually necessary to ensure optimal control. Finkelstein et al. (1988) reported significantly reduced survival for CF patients with diabetes, fewer than 25% surviving beyond 30 years, whereas nearly 60% of non-diabetic CF adults reached this age. There is clearly room for improvement in the management of CF patients with diabetes mellitus.

Conclusion

Pancreatic involvement remains one of the major complications in infants, children and adults with CF. There is, however, a much greater understanding of the underlying pathophysiology than previously and the recent genetic and biochemical advances have considerably improved our knowledge in this area. The introduction of the enteric-coated microsphere pancreatic enzyme preparations has proved a major advance in treatment. These preparations allow much better control of the steatorrhoea and a return to a normal or indeed high fat, high calorie diet for these patients.

The improved nutritional state enables better growth and development in children, increased ability to cope with the associated pulmonary infections and a greater sense of physical and emotional well-being at all ages because of the more normal lifestyle that is possible.

References

Bell L, Durie P, Forstner GG (1984) What do children with cystic fibrosis eat? J Pediatr Gastroenterol Nutr 3 (suppl 1):137–146

Belli DC, Levy E, Darling P et al. (1987) Taurine improves the absorption of a fat meal in patients with cystic fibrosis. Pediatrics 80:417–523

Beverley DW, Kelleher J, MacDonald A, Littlewood JM, Robinson T, Walters MP (1987) Comparison of four pancreatic extracts in cystic fibrosis. Arch Dis Child 62:564–568

Buchdahl RM, Cox M, Fulleylove C et al. (1988) Increased energy requirement in cystic fibrosis. J Appl Physiol 64 (5):1810–1816

Chase PM, Long MA, Lavin MH (1979) Cystic fibrosis and malnutrition. J Pediatr 95:337–347

Coupleman HR, Corey M, Gaskin KJ, Durie P, Forstner GG (1988) Impaired chloride secretion as well as bicarbonate secretion underlies the fluid secretory defect in cystic fibrosis pancreas. Gastroenterology 95:349–355

Dean M, White M, Gerrard B et al. (1990) Identification of cystic fibrosis mutations. Pediatr Pulmonol. Suppl 5:203

Department of Health and Social Security (1985) Recommended daily amounts of food energy and nutrients for groups of people in the UK (revision). Report No 15. HMSO, London

Dinwiddie R (1983) The management of the first years of life. In: Hodson ME, Norman AP, Battern JC (eds) Cystic fibrosis. Ballière Tindall, London, pp 197–208

Dinwiddie R (1991) Cystic fibrosis. Yesterday, today and tomorrow. J R Soc Med 84 (suppl 18):36–40

Dinwiddie R, Madge S (1988) Intensive calorie counting in CF: an effective way of achieving weight gain? Excerpta Medica, Asia Pacific Congress Series 74:165

Dodge JA, Goodall J, Geddes D et al. (1988) Cystic fibrosis in the United Kingdom 1977–85. An improving picture. British Paediatric Association Working Party on Cystic Fibrosis. B Med J 297:1599–1602

Donnison AB, Schwachman H, Gross RE (1966) A review of 164 children with meconium ileus seen at the Children's Hospital Medical Centre, Boston. Pediatrics 37:833–837

Durie PR, Forstner GG (1989) Pathophysiology of the exocrine pancreas in cystic fibrosis. J R Soc Med 82:2–10

Durie PR, Pencharz PB (1989) A rational approach to the nutritional care of patients with cystic fibrosis. J R Soc Med 82 (suppl 16):11–20

European Working Group on CF Genetics (EWGCFG) (1990) Obedient of distribution in Europe of the major CF mutation and of its associated haplotype. Hum Genet 85:436–445

Finkelstein SM, Wielinski CL, Elliott GR et al. (1988) Diabetes mellitus associated with cystic fibrosis. J Pediatr 112:373–377

Gaskin KJ, Durie P, Corey M, Wei P, Forstner GG (1982) Evidence of a primary defect of bicarbonate secretion in cystic fibrosis. Paediatr Res 16:554–557

Grand RJ, Schwartz RH, Di Sant'Agnese PA, Gelderman AH (1966) Macroscopic cyst of the pancreas in a case of cystic fibrosis. J Pediatr 69:393–398

Imrie J, Fagan D, Sturgess J (1975) Quantitative evaluation of the development of the exocrine pancreas in cystic fibrosis and controlled subjects. Am J Pathol 95:697–708

Johansen HK, Nir M, Hoiby N, Koch C, Schwartz M (1991) Severity of cystic fibrosis in patients homozygous and heterozygous for ▲F508 mutation. Lancet 337:631–634

Kerem BS, Rommens JM, Buchanan JA et al. (1989) Identification of the cystic fibrosis gene: genetic and analysis. Science 245:1073–1080

Kerem E, Corey M, Kerem BS et al. (1990) The relationship between genotype and phenotype in cystic fibrosis. Analysis of the most common mutation (▲F508). N Engl J Med 323:1517–1522

Kuzemko JA (1986) Screening early neonatal diagnosis and prenatal diagnosis. J R Soc Med 79 (12):225–227

Littlewood JM, MacDonald A (1987) Rationale of modern dietary recommendations in cystic fibrosis. J R Soc Med 80 (suppl 15):16–24

Mabogunje OA, Wang Chun I, Mahour GH (1982) Improved survival of neonates with meconium ileus. Arch Surg 117:37–40

McMahon CJ, Genet SA, Middleton-Price HR et al. (1990) The major cystic fibrosis mutation in the British population. Hum Genet 86:236–237

Muller F, Aubrei MC, Gasser B, Duchatel F, Boue J, Boue A (1985) Prenatal diagnosis of cystic fibrosis II: meconium ileus in affected fetuses. Prenat Diagn 5:104–117

Park RW, Grand RJ (1981) Gastrointestinal manifestations of cystic fibrosis. A review. Gastroenterology 81:1143–1161

Pencharz P, Hill R, Archibald E, Levy L, Newth C (1984) Energy needs and nutritional rehabilitation in undernourished adolescents and adults with cystic fibrosis. J Pediatr Gastroenterol Nutr 3 (suppl 1):S147–153

Quinton PM (1983) Chloride impermeability in cystic fibrosis. Nature 301:431–432

Riordan JR, Rommens JM, Kerem B et al. (1989) Identification of the cystic fibrosis gene: cloning and characterisation of complementary DNA. Science 1066–1073

Rodman HM, Matthews LW (1981) Hyperglycaemia in cystic fibrosis: a review of the literature and our own experience. In: Warwick WJ (ed) 1000 years of cystic fibrosis. University of Minnesota, p 69

Stead RJ et al. (1987) Enteric coated microspheres of pancreatin in the treatment of cystic fibrosis: comparison with a standard enteric coated preparation. Thorax 42:533–537

Stuhrmann M, Macek MJ, Reis A et al. (1990) Genotype analysis of cystic fibrosis patients in relation to pancreatic sufficiency. Lancet i:783–789

Vyas H, Matthew DJ et al. (1990) A comparison of enteric coated microspheres with enteric coated tablet pancreatic enzyme preparations in cystic fibrosis. Eur J Pediatr 149:241–243

Watkins JB, Tercyak AM, Szczepanik P, Klein P (1977) Bile salt kinetics in cystic fibrosis: influence of pancreatic enzyme replacement. Gastroenterology 73:1023–1028

Weller PH, Williams J (1986) Clinical features, pathogenesis and management of meconium ileus equivalent. J R Soc Med 79 (suppl 12):36–37

Wilcken B, Chalmers G (1985) Reduced mortality in patients with cystic fibrosis detected by neonatal screening. Lancet ii:1319–1321

Zentler-Munro PL, Fine DR, Batten JC, Northfield TC (1985) Effect of cimetidine on enzyme inactivation, bile acid precipitation and lipid solubilisation in pancreatic steatorrhoea due to cystic fibrosis. Gut 16:892–901

Chapter 29

Surgical Treatment of Pancreatic Disease in Childhood

M. Davenport and E. R. Howard

Introduction

A wide range of congenital, inflammatory and neoplastic aetiologies may be implicated in a group of "surgical" disorders of the pancreas in childhood (Table 1). All of them are unusual and because of their rarity diagnosis is often delayed. Consequently the morbidity associated with many of these conditions can be severe.

This chapter starts with a consideration of disorders of embryology which explains an interesting group of anatomical pancreatic anomalies which may be present at any age, including early infancy.

Development

The normal pancreas develops as a dorsal and ventral outgrowth at the junction of fore- and midgut. These two structures are diametrically opposed at first but eventually the ventral portion rotates around its duodenal axis in a clockwise direction (as viewed from above) to converge and coalesce on the left side with the dorsal outgrowth. The superior mesenteric vessels are in the centre of this rotational process and become surrounded by glandular tissue. The main pancreatic duct (of Wirsung) is finally composed of a long segment of the dorsal duct in the distal gland and the original ventral duct in the proximal gland (head of pancreas). The accessory pancreatic duct (of Santorini) is a portion of the original dorsal duct. This coalescence of the two duct systems occurs at around six weeks' gestation (Fig. 1).

The common bile duct joins the original ventral pancreatic duct outside the duodenal wall and sphincter-choledochus before eight weeks of gestation (Wong

Table 1. An outline of surgical pancreatic disease in childhood

Congenital	Annular pancreas
	Pancreas divisum
	Pancreatic heterotopia
Inflammatory	
Acute pancreatitis	Common pancreaticobiliary channel and choledochal cyst
	Gallstones
	Mumps
	Ascariasis
	Trauma (accident, abuse, surgical)
	Multisystem disease (e.g. Reye's syndrome)
	Idiopathic
Chronic pancreatitis	Acute pancreatitis as above
	Hereditary type
	Hypercalcaemia
	Hyperlipidaemia
Hyperplasia and neoplasia	
Benign	Nesidioblastosis
	Islet cell adenomas
	Cysts (congenital and traumatic)
Malignant	Adenocarcinoma
	Pancreatoblastoma
	Papillary-cystic tumour
Trauma	

and Lister 1981). The junction migrates toward the duodenal wall as development proceeds and comes to lie within the sphincter muscle complex. Some movement of the junction into the wall of the duodenum has been noted after birth. Failure of migration into the muscle sphincter has been termed anomalous pancreaticobiliary ductal union (APBD) and is estimated to occur in up to 3.2% of the population (Kimura et al. 1985; Misra and Dwivedi 1990). This anomaly is found in association with approximately 70% of choledochal cysts and has been implicated in the aetiology of carcinoma of the gallbladder in adults (Kimura et al. 1985).

Abnormalities in pancreatic embryology give rise to three conditions which may present in childhood; annular pancreas, pancreas divisum and pancreatic heterotopia.

Annular Pancreas

Two theories have been suggested for the formation of this anomaly. Tieken (1901) described right and left elements to the ventral analage and believed that as rotation occurs the left half is drawn around the duodenum separately as a tongue of glandular tissue. Lecco (1917), on the other hand, suggested that the tip of the rotating ventral gland remains fixed to the ventral duodenum and therefore persists along the right side of the duodenum as rotation occurs.

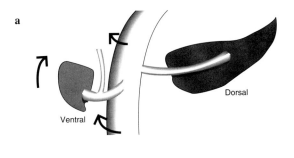

Common bile duct

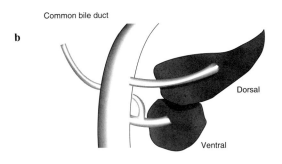

Common bile duct

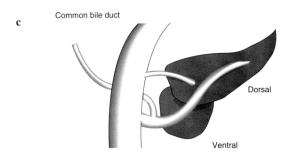

Fig. 1. Diagrammatic representation of stages in the embryological development of the pancreas. **a** Ventral and dorsal pancreatic outgrowths from the foregut. **b** Clockwise rotation of the ventral portion around the duodenal axis. **c** Coalescence of the duct systems to form the main duct of Wirsung and the accessory duct of Santorini.

The importance of annular pancreas is its association with abnormal duodenal development (Irving and Rickham 1978). An annular pancreas is present in approximately one-third of the infants treated for duodenal stenosis or atresia (Fig. 2). Chromosomal abnormalities, particularly Down's syndrome, are not infrequently associated with duodenal atresia and annular pancreas although the explanation for this is not clear. Although the association of annular pancreas and pancreatitis has not been described in children, Drey (1957) noted that in a collective review of 62 cases of symptomatic annular pancreas in adults 15 (24%) had had pancreatitis at some time.

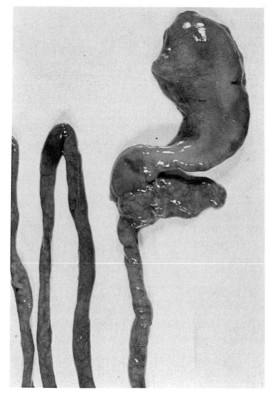

Fig. 2. Post-mortem specimen of upper gastrointestinal tract showing an annular pancreas surrounding the second part of the duodenum, from a 10-day-old infant who died of congenital heart disease and bilateral aspiration pneumonia.

Surgical treatment is directed towards the underlying duodenal pathology and a duodenoduodenostomy is the operation of choice without division of pancreatic tissue.

Pancreas Divisum

A failure of coalescence of the two embryological duct systems results in two independently draining pancreatic segments; the larger segment of pancreatic body and tail drains through the accessory duct whilst the main duct drains only the uncinate process. Other anomalies include an incomplete communication between the ductal systems and occasionally a complete absence of the ventral duct. The term "dominant dorsal duct syndrome" has been suggested for all these anomalies to indicate that most pancreatic secretion occurs via the accessory or dorsal duct (Warshaw et al. 1990). These are not uncommon anomalies and they occur in 6%–10% of the population (Cotton 1980; Warshaw et al. 1990). Although ductal anomalies are described in patients with both acute and chronic pancreatitis there is no proof that the anomaly is the causative factor. However, stenosis of the accessory pancreatic

duct as it enters the duodenal wall has been described in patients with
pancreatitis and chronic pancreatic pain (Cotton (1980) (Fig. 3 a,b). Although
ductal anomalies are malformations they are not usually diagnosed until adult
life and two recent large series of pancreatitis in children did not mention the
association in any patient (Synn et al. 1987; Vane et al. 1989). However, in
children who present with "idiopathic" pancreatitis particularly if recurrent,
we suggest endoscopic pancreatography (ERCP) to exclude this anomaly when
the disease is quiescent (Wagner and Golladay 1988; Adzick et al. 1989).
ERCP in children is now possible at all ages including infancy.

Experience in a series of 100 adult patients with pancreas divisum included
a diagnostic technique which utilised ultrasonography and secretin stimulation
of the pancreas to show functional accessory duct obstruction. With this
technique it may be possible to select patients who would benefit from a duct
drainage procedure (Warshaw et al. 1990). Experience of this type has not
been reported in children and reports of surgical intervention remain anecdotal
although usually favourable (Wagner and Golladay 1988; Adzick et al. 1989).
Although endoscopic sphincterotomy has been tried it has generally been

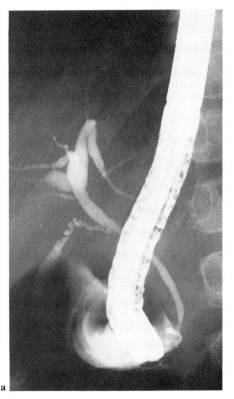 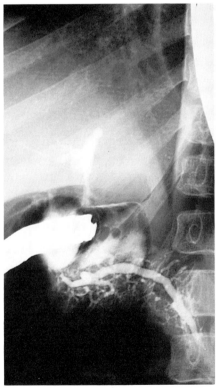

a   b

Fig. 3. ERCP in a 9-year-old boy who had a history of recurrent pancreatitis. **a** Normal bile duct
and gall bladder with minute ventral pancreatic duct suggestive of pancreas divisum. **b** Cannulation
of the accessory duct showing dilatation. (There was no communication between the accessory
duct and a small pseudocyst in the tail of the pancreas.)

unsuccessful and therefore, if indicated, a transduodenal sphincterotomy or sphincteroplasty is the correct procedure (Russell et al. 1984).

Pancreatic Heterotopia

Pancreatic tissue may be found in ectopic sites particularly within the stomach, duodenum and jejunum. Rarer sites include Meckel's diverticulum, gallbladder (Qizblash 1976), umbilicus (Carbewell et al. 1977), and Fallopian tube (Mason and Quagliarello 1976). Histologically the tissue is predominantly of acinar and ductal origin. Although it is an incidental finding in a majority of cases, overlying mucosal ulceration may cause gastrointestinal bleeding, intussusception, epigastric pain and gastric outlet obstruction (Synn et al. 1988; Lai and Tompkins 1986). Of 37 patients with heterotopic pancreatic tissue six were children (Lai and Tompkins 1986). Surgical excision is the treatment of symptomatic lesions.

Pancreatitis in Childhood

Acute Pancreatitis

Acute pancreatitis is an uncommon cause of abdominal pain in children but the clinical features, natural history and complications are similar to those seen in adult patients. However, some of the aetiological factors in childhood are rare in adults. Drug therapy (e.g. steroid, L-asparaginase, azathioprine), blunt abdominal trauma (e.g. seat-belts, child abuse) and congenital abnormalities of the pancreatic duct (e.g. pancreas divisum, common pancreaticobiliary channel (Tan and Howard 1988) and anomalous drainage of the common bile duct into the fourth part of duodenum (Doty et al. 1985) (Figs. 4 and 5) are well-recognised associations. Acute pancreatitis may also complicate multisystem diseases such as Reye's syndrome (hepatic failure, encephalopathy and renal failure), haemolytic uraemic syndrome, cystic fibrosis and Wilson's disease (Weizman and Durie 1988; Weizman et al. 1988), hyperlipidaemia (Types I, IIa and IV) and hypercalcaemia. Pancreatitis occurs in up to two-thirds of the cases of Reye's syndrome but may be masked by the associated neurological symptoms. Mumps pancreatitis is rare in childhood as is gallstone-induced pancreatitis but may be seen occasionally in haemolytic disorders such as sickle cell anaemia and spherocytosis.

Blockage of the pancreatic duct can cause pancreatitis and Dabadie et al. (1989) reported a case of acute pancreatitis caused by impaction of a paper-clip in the ampulla in a 14-month-old child. The commonest cause of pancreatic duct obstruction in children is helminthic infestation of the common bile duct with ascariasis (Sultan Khuroo et al. 1990). The worms infect the upper gastrointestinal tract and may migrate through the duodenal ampulla into the biliary or pancreatic ducts to cause biliary colic, cholangitis and acute pancreatitis. For example 31 of 500 patients (adults and children) from Kashmir

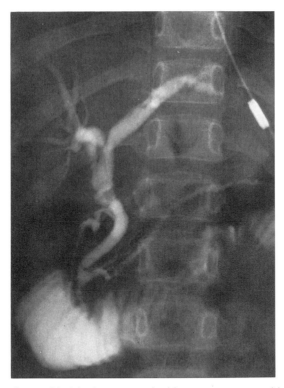

Fig. 4. ERCP in a 7-year-old girl who presented with recurrent pancreatitis. A long common pancreaticobiliary channel is demonstrated. Treatment by division of the bile duct and hepaticojejunostomy gave complete relief from symptoms. (The pancreas was swollen and hard at laparotomy.)

province, India, with documented hepatobiliary or pancreatic ascariasis presented with acute pancreatitis (Sultan Khuroo et al. 1990). ERCP and sphincterotomy as well as antihelminthic therapy (e.g. mebendazole) have a therapeutic role in the management of these patients. The worms are removed from the ampulla and ducts with biopsy forceps and endoscopic baskets in episodes of acute pancreatitis.

Intrapancreatic enteric duplication cysts are rare anatomical anomalies which may present as recurrent pancreatitis possibly due to aberrant ductal communication (Akers et al. 1972; Welch 1986).

Pancreatitis may follow surgical or endoscopic trauma to the pancreatobiliary duct system, for example after dissection of a choledochal cyst or after ERCP examination. Leijala and Louhimo (1988) have recorded an extraordinary prevalence of hyperamylasaemia and clinical acute pancreatitis in 54 children who had undergone open-heart surgery. The aetiology of this is not clear.

An association between mental retardation, cerebral palsy and "idiopathic" pancreatitis has been noted and seen as a complication of gastric surgery (fundoplication) for oesophageal reflux for these patients (Vane et al. 1989).

Trapnell (1990) has described a group of adolescent patients with pancreatitis labelled as "teenage pancreatitis". He noted an unusually high risk of chronic

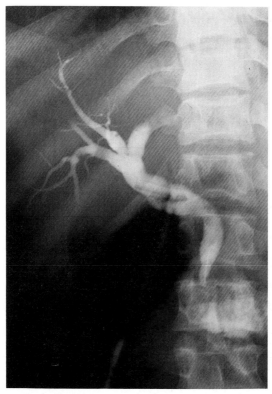

Fig. 5. Operative cholangiogram in a 15-year-old male with sickle cell disease who complained of recurrent biliary colic. The common bile duct is dilated and there is poor flow of contrast material through the ampulla which is at the junction of the third and fourth parts of the duodenum. The gall bladder contained pigment stones. Treatment consisted of cholecystectomy and sphincteroplasty.

relapsing pancreatitis when a first attack occurs during adolescence, but again the aetiology is not known. Perhaps these are cases of hereditary chronic pancreatitis.

The principles of management of acute pancreatitis in children do not differ from those in adult patients; complications are similar and most series still report significant mortality rates of 15%–20% (Synn et al. 1988; Weizman and Durie 1988).

Pseudocyst formation following pancreatitis is well described in children (Fig. 6). In a series of 25 children who developed pseudocysts, a third were managed conservatively with satisfactory resolution, half had a cystogastrostomy and the remainder a cystojejunostomy-en-Roux (Millar et al. 1988).

Chronic Pancreatitis

Chronic pancreatitis is probably under-recognised as a cause of chronic abdominal pain in childhood. Food avoidance, weight loss, growth retardation and even developmental delay may occur before pancreatic exocrine and

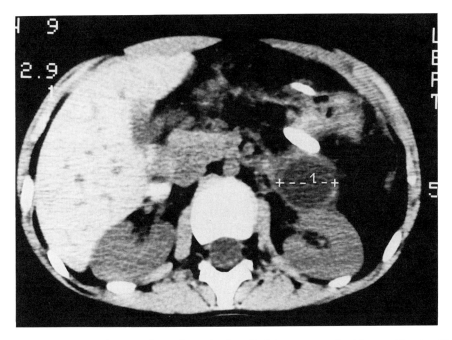

Fig. 6. CT demonstrating a small pseudocyst in the tail of the pancreas of a 16-year-old male with a history of pancreatitis.

endocrine failure becomes apparent (Ghishan et al. 1983). All the causes discussed in relation to acute pancreatitis may be implicated. Hereditary pancreatitis transmitted as an autosomal dominant disease with variable penetrance usually presents in childhood. Approximately 80% of cases have developed symptoms by 20 years of age with 10 years as the usual age of onset. It is important to exclude other hereditary metabolic disorders such as alpha-1-antitrypsin deficiency, hyperparathyroidism with hypercalcaemia and hyperlipidaemia. Pancreatic calcification on plain abdominal radiographs may be seen in some of these patients (Vane et al. 1989) (Fig. 7a) and abnormally dilated pancreatic ducts and occasionally strictures may be recognised on ERCP (Fig. 7b). It is not clear whether duct strictures are primary and causative or whether they are secondary to the inflammatory process. Although reports of surgical intervention in childhood are few and necessarily limited by the rarity of the disease, both Scott et al. (1984) and Crombleholme et al. (1990) have reported good results using the Puestow procedure (longitudinal pancreaticojejunostomy) to achieve retrograde duct drainage and relief of symptoms. This does suggest that mechanical obstruction of the ducts is perhaps an aetiological factor in some cases.

Choledochal Cyst

Cystic dilatation of the biliary tree is considered in this chapter because of its relationship with biliary-pancreatic duct anomalies and pancreatitis.

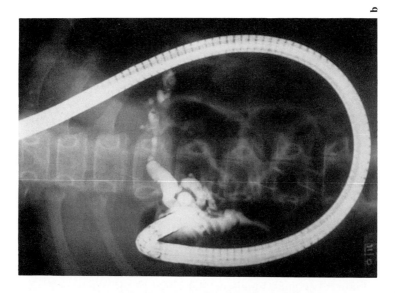

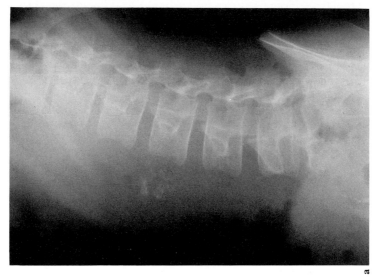

Fig. 7. An 11-year-old girl presented with a history of recurrent pancreatitis of unknown aetiology. **a** Plain abdominal radiograph showing calcification typical of chronic pancreatitis. **b** Retrograde pancreatogram demonstrating dilatation and stricturing of the main pancreatic duct. Treatment consisted of distal pancreatectomy and pancreaticojejunostomy.

There is a female preponderance with a female:male ratio of about 4:1 and an unexplained increased prevalence in oriental races. The commonest type is a cystic dilatation of the common bile duct which frequently extends behind the duodenum to the junction of the common bile duct and pancreatic duct. Other variations such as fusiform dilatation and involvement of the intrahepatic duct system occur with much less frequency.

The classical clinical triad of jaundice, pain and an abdominal mass occurs infrequently and was recorded in only seven out of 29 (24%) in the King's College Hospital series (Tan and Howard 1988). Cholangitis, cyst rupture and secondary biliary cirrhosis as well as acute pancreatitis may complicate the condition.

True pancreatitis should be differentiated from so-called fictitious pancreatitis. Free reflux of pancreatic juice will occur through any common pancreaticobiliary channel – an anomaly present in about 70% of cases. Amylase is absorbed through the cyst wall which has an incomplete epithelial lining and hyperamyl-asaemia may therefore be detected without inflammation of the gland. Malignant transformation of the cyst epithelium is a well-recognised complication in adult life. Komi et al. (1986) were able to show age-related progression from destruction of the epithelium, through metaplasia to adenocarcinoma in a histological analysis of cysts excised from different age groups.

It has been suggested that choledochal cysts are caused by a weakness of the bile duct wall which leads to bile stasis, infection, distal duct stenosis and further dilatation. On the other hand Babitt (1969) and Altman et al. (1978) postulated that the dilatation is an acquired condition caused by a common distal channel with free pancreatic reflux into the extrahepatic bile duct and they suggested that unopposed enzyme action might cause bile duct damage and dilatation. The incidence of a common channel is certainly much higher in choledochal cysts than would be expected by chance (Wiedmeyer et al. 1989).

The diagnosis of a choledochal cyst is usually obvious on ultrasonography and delineation of the distal common bile duct and its junction is achieved with ERCP examination.

Radical excision of the choledochal cyst is now the treatment of choice. Cystenterostomy no longer has a place in management except in the rare situation of non-resectability (e.g. in the presence of severe portal hypertension) for although drainage is established, the remaining cyst wall has a potential for malignant change. We have also seen recurrent pancreatitis in three of four cases treated with cystenterostomy, all of whom had a common pancreaticobiliary channel. No further attacks of pancreatitis occurred after a second laparotomy and cyst excision. The most difficult point of choledochal cyst dissection during radical excision is at the retropancreatic union of the bile and pancreatic ducts.

A high intraoperative bile amylase measurement indicates the presence of a common channel and the need for caution during the completion of the dissection. Cholecystectomy should also be carried out to complete the procedure. There were no complications during a mean follow-up period of 3.5 years in the senior author's series of 22 cases of complete cyst excision carried out as a primary procedure (Tan and Howard 1988).

Hyperplastic, Neoplastic and Allied Disorders of the Pancreas

Nesidioblastosis (Greek: nesidion – islet)

This condition is characterised clinically by persistent hyperinsulinaemic hypoglycaemia which usually presents during the neonatal period. Although it is usually an isolated, sporadic condition it may occur as part of the multiple endocrine neoplasia syndrome (Vance et al. 1972; Thompson et al. 1989) and may be familial (Vance et al. 1972; Moreno et al. 1989). Pathologically it is divisible into two types, focal and diffuse; both occurring with about equal frequency (Goossens et al. 1989). Nesidioblastosis, islet cell hyperplasia and other allied adenomatoses, including islet cell adenoma, can be thought of as a spectrum of disease and the term islet cell dysmaturation syndrome has been applied to the conditions (Bjerke et al. 1990).

The diagnosis must be rapid as poorly treated neonatal hypoglycaemia may result in cerebral damage and mental retardation. Placement of a central venous line is mandatory if the diagnosis is suspected, to ensure rapid correction of hypoglycaemia.

Radiological investigations are of limited benefit in most cases although an occasional focal nesidioblastosis may be demonstrated.

Medical therapy includes diazoxide, glucagon and the somatostatin analogue octreotide (Battershill and Clissold 1989). Surgery is recommended for patients who fail medical treatment. It is unusual to find a macroscopic abnormality at laparotomy and the surgeon must be prepared to perform a near-total pancreatectomy. The amount of pancreatic tissue that should be resected is controversial. Subtotal pancreatectomy (about 75%) is associated with a significant failure rate of at least 50% and therefore a near-total pancreatectomy, as advocated by Harken et al. (1971), should be performed. About 95% of the pancreas is removed but a small portion is left to protect the common bile duct and duodenal vascular arcade (Warden et al. 1988). The spleen is preserved if at all possible because of its immunological benefit in childhood. Although exocrine and endocrine failure may follow this operation it is surprisingly uncommon. Dunger et al. (1988) noted clinical exocrine failure in only one of seven children following near-total pancreatectomy although the secretion of enzyme and bicarbonate was low in about half of the remainder.

Islet Cell Adenomas

Functioning insulin-secreting islet cell adenomas occur in an older age group who present with hypoglycaemic episodes. The features of Whipple's triad may be seen, that is, symptoms occurring during fasting with demonstrable hypoglycaemia, and relieved by the administration of glucose. It is worthwhile attempting a precise preoperative localisation of the tumour using selective arteriography and venous insulin sampling, if available, as limited pancreatic resections may be adequate for treatment. Adenomas are found in the body and tail in about 75% of cases and multicentric tumours are seen in about

14% of all cases. At operation the islet cell tumour is usually pink and well-encapsulated. Enucleation or distal pancreatectomy are satisfactory procedures for single tumours but tumour in the pancreatic head or multiple lesions may need more major gland excision. Rebound hyperglycaemia is noted after successful surgery and completeness of excision can be confirmed with a rapid insulin assay.

Although islet cell tumours are usually an isolated finding they may be associated with multiple endocrine neoplasia (Type I; parathyroid hyperplasia or adenomas and pituitary tumours) and have also been described in a family with Von Hippel–Lindau disease (retinal haemangiomas, cerebellar cysts or tumours and pheochromocytomas, Hull et al. 1979).

Islet cell tumours producing other hormones have been recorded in childhood. Vasoactive intestinal polypeptide (VIP)-producing tumours, for example, may occur although in contrast to the adult experience the majority have been found in ectopic sites in association with neurogenic tumours such as ganglioneuromas and neuroblastomas (Grosfeld et al. 1990). There are, however, records of two cases arising from the pancreas: one in a non-beta-cell islet adenoma in the tail (Brenner et al. 1986) and one associated with generalised islet cell hyperplasia (Ghishan et al. 1979). We have not found reports of somatostatinoma or glucagonoma in children.

The Zollinger–Ellison (ZE) syndrome may occur in childhood and of the 44 cases in the Childhood Disease Registry of the United States, 38 were in boys with a mean age at presentation of 11.7 years (Grosfeld et al. 1990). Of these 44 cases 41 were due to a pancreatic gastrinoma of which 65% were malignant. The treatment of the ZE syndrome is discussed elsewhere and accords with adult practice.

Cystic Lesions

Cystic lesions of the pancreas are rare in childhood. The commonest is pseudocyst formation following blunt abdominal trauma. Table 2 is a classification based on the nature of the epithelial lining and the congenital or acquired origin (Howard, 1989). Developmental or true congenital cysts are lined by epithelium with a deeper layer of acinar tissue. Although usually confined to the body or tail and therefore usually asymptomatic they can cause obstructive jaundice if situated in the head of the pancreas (Pilot et al. 1964). Multiple pancreatic cysts may occur as part of a multisystem disorder or syndrome such as von Hippel–Lindau disease (Seitz et al. 1987), polycystic kidney disease and cystic fibrosis. These are usually clinically silent. A few cases of dermoid cyst of pancreas have been recognised, typically containing thick sebaceous material, teeth and cartilage (Assawamatiyanont and King 1977).

Protein-calorie malnutrition in developing countries may produce fibrocalcareous changes in the pancreas leading to cyst formation. Olurin (1971) has described two such cases in severely malnourished Nigerian children.

Proliferative and neoplastic cysts rarely present in childhood but a few cases, particularly of mucinous cystadenoma have been reported (Gundersen and Jarvis 1969). Grosfeld et al. (1990) consider these to be premalignant as the

Table 2. Classification of cysts of the pancreas

Congenital
Single
Multiple
      (a) Pancreas alone
      (b) as part of systemic disorder,
      e.g. Von Hippel–Lindau, polycystic kidney, cystic
      fibrosis
Dermoid

Neoplastic
Serous cystadenoma
Mucinous cystadenoma – cystadenocarcinoma
Papillary–cystic neoplasm

Acquired
Parasitic, e.g. hydatid disease
Retention cysts
Tropical fibrocalcareous disease

Pseudocysts
Trauma
Acute pancreatitis

development of both cystadenocarcinoma and sarcoma have been reported in adult life (Tsukimoto et al. 1973; Hodgkinson et al. 1978).

Malignant Lesions of the Pancreas

Malignant tumours of the pancreas are rare in childhood. Histologically the majority are adenocarcinoma derived from acinar tissue or islet cell carcinoma. A few cases of rhabdomyosarcoma have been reported. Adenocarcinoma tends to present late with advanced local disease and all 12 cases reviewed by Welch (1986) were dead within ten months of presentation despite a variety of treatments. Tsukimoto et al. (1973) described the Japanese experience with this tumour and just under half of their patients had metastases or were unresectable at presentation. Neither chemotherapy nor radiotherapy had any effect on survival in the non- or incomplete resection group.

The term pancreatoblastoma has been used to describe a particular type of tumour which occurs in infants and young children. It is characterised by a more differentiated histological pattern with organoid and rosette pattern formation and a surrounding capsule. Complete resection has been followed by long-term survival (Horie et al. 1977). An association with the Beckwith–Wiedemann syndrome (exomphalos, macroglossia, gigantism) has been reported (Drut and Jones 1988) although the syndrome is more commonly associated with nephroblastoma and hepatoblastoma. A papillary–cystic neoplasm of the pancreas (Frantz's tumour) occurs predominantly in young women and girls. It is an unusual low-grade neoplasm which occasionally metastasises and of 116 cases reviewed by Todani et al. (1988) half were under 19 years at presentation and only two occurred in males. A majority of the tumours presented with a slowly growing abdominal mass and calcification may be seen on an abdominal radiograph. The typical operative findings are of a well-demarcated pancreatic mass with a thick capsule, calcification and a mixed solid and cystic appearance with a varying degree of haemorrhage and necrosis (Matsunou and Konishi 1990). The cell of origin is thought to be a totipotent primordial pancreatic cell capable of differentiating along exocrine or endocrine lines. Todani et al. (1988) have reported excellent results and long-term survival after complete resection.

Pancreatic Trauma in Childhood

Accidents and trauma from child abuse are well-recognised causes of pancreatic trauma in children; in a series of 22 cases for example, cycle handlebar injuries accounted for ten (45%) and child abuse for four (18%) (Smith et al. 1988). Ultrasonography, CT and retrograde pancreatography may be necessary to delineate major duct damage, but this may be more difficult to achieve in children than in adults (Smith et al. 1988). Serial amylase levels can be useful in differentiating major from minor trauma.

As in adult practice, a formal distal pancreatectomy with spleen preservation is recommended for distal duct disruption, but damage to the head of the pancreas and duodenum may demand formal pancreatectomy (Whipple's procedure).

Unrecognised trauma may present late as a palpable pseudocyst mass. Presentation may be delayed; this is a particular problem in victims of child abuse. In about half the reported cases there has been spontaneous resolution of these cysts (Gorenstein et al. 1987). Bass et al. (1988) reported spontaneous resolution in five of their ten cases and they also recorded success with percutaneous drainage in three other cases. Percutaneous drainage is not universally successful, however, and Rescorla et al. (1990) failed in three of four children. In the same paper they describe ERCP as the most satisfactory investigation for the assessment of major duct damage in childhood pseudocysts although many authors still regard CT as a sufficient guide to management (Bass et al. 1988).

Cystogastrostomy remains a useful procedure for pseudocyst drainage and Ford et al. (1990) suggested that these cysts mature at an earlier stage in children and that drainage may be contemplated at about 3–4 weeks after injury. In their series eight of 16 children underwent cystogastrostomy without complication.

References

Adzick NS, Shamberger RC, Winter HS, Hendren WH (1989) Surgical treatment of pancreas divisum causing pancreatitis in children. J Pediatr Surg 24:54–58
Akers DR, Favara BE, Franciosi RA, Nelson JM (1972) Duplication of the alimentary tract.

Report of three unusual cases associated with the bile and pancreatic ducts. Surgery 71:817–823

Altman MS, Halls JM, Douglas AP, Penner IC (1978) Choledochal cyst presenting as acute pancreatitis: evaluation with ERCP. Am J Gastrol 70:514–519

Assawamatiyanont S, King AD Jr (1977) Dermoid cysts of the pancreas. Am Surg 43:503–504

Babitt DP (1969) Congenital choledochal cyst: new etiological concept based on anomalous relationship of the common bile duct and pancreatic bulb. Ann Radiol 12:231–240

Bass J, Di-Lorenzo M, Desjardins JG, Grignon A, Ouimet A (1988) Blunt pancreatic injuries in children: the role of percutaneous external drainage in the treatment of pancreatic pseudocysts. J Pediatr Surg 23:721–724

Battershill PE, Clissold SP (1989) Octreotide. A review of pharmacodynamic and pharmacokinetic properties and therapeutic potential in conditions associated with excessive peptide secretion. Drugs 38:658–702

Bjerke HS, Kelly RE, Geffner ME, Fonkalsrud EW (1990) Surgical management of islet cell dysmaturation syndrome of young children. Surg Gynecol Obstet 191:321–325

Brenner RW, Sank LI, Kerner MB et al. (1986) Resection of a vipoma of the pancreas in a 15 year old girl. J Pediatr Surg 21:983–985

Carbewell D, Kogan SJ, Levitt SB (1977) Ectopic pancreas presenting as an umbilical mass. J Pediatr Surg 12:593–599

Cotton PB (1980) Congenital anomaly of pancreas divisum as cause of obstructive pain and pancreatitis. Gut 21:105–114

Crombleholme TM, deLorimier AA, Way LW, Adzick NS, Longaker MT, Harrison MR (1990) The modified Puestow procedure for chronic relapsing pancreatitis in children. J Pediatr Surg 25:749–754

Dabadie A, Roussey M, Betremieux P, Gambert C, Lefrancois C, Darnault P (1989) Acute pancreatitis from a duodenal foreign body in a child. J Pediatr Gastroenterol Nutr 8:533–535

Doty J, Hassall E, Fonkalsrud EW (1985) Anomalous drainage of the common bile duct into the 4th part of the duodenum. Arch Surg 120:1077–1079

Drey NW (1957) Symptomatic annular pancreas in the adult. Ann Intern Med 46:750–772

Drut R, Jones MC (1988) Congenital pancreatoblastoma in Beckwith–Wiedemann syndrome: an emerging association. Pediatr Pathol 8:331–339

Dunger DB, Burns C, Ghale GK, Muller DPR, Spitz L, Grant DB (1988) Pancreatic exocrine and endocrine function after subtotal pancreatectomy for nesidioblastosis. J Pediatr Surg 23:112–115

Ford EG, Hardin WD Jr, Mahour GH, Wooley MM (1990) Pseudocysts of the pancreas in children. Ann Surg 56:384–387

Ghishan FK, Soper RT, Nassif EG et al. (1979) Chronic diarrhea of infancy: non beta-cell hyperplasia. Pediatrics 64:46–49

Ghishan FK, Greene HL, Avant G, O'Neil JA, Neblett W (1983) Chronic relapsing pancreatitis in childhood. J Pediatr 102:514–518

Goossens A, Gepts W, Saudubray JM et al. (1989) Diffuse and focal nesidioblastosis. A clinicopathological study of 24 patients with persistent hyperinsulinaemic hypoglycemia. Am J Surg Pathol 13:766–775

Gorenstein A, O'Halpin D, Wesson DE, Daneman A, Filler RM (1987) Blunt injury to the pancreas in children: selective management based on ultrasound. J Pediatr Surg 22:1110–1116

Grosfeld JL, Vane DW, Rescorla FJ, McGuire W, West KW (1990) Pancreatic tumours in childhood: analysis of 13 cases. J Pediatr Surg 25:1057–1062

Gundersen AE, Jarvis JF (1969) Pancreatic cystadenoma in childhood. J Pediatr Surg 4:478–481

Harken AH, Filler RM, AvRuskin TW, Crigler JF (1971) The role of "total" pancreatectomy in treatment of unremitting hypoglycemia of infancy. J Pediatr Surg 6:284–289

Hodgkinson DJ, ReMine WH, Weiland LH (1978) A clinicopathologic study of 21 cases of pancreatic cystadenocarcinoma. Ann Surg 188:679–684

Horie A, Yano Y, Kotoo Y, Miwa A (1977) Morphogenesis of pancreatoblastoma, infantile carcinoma of the pancreas. Report of two cases. Cancer 39:247–254

Howard JM (1989) Cystic neoplasms and true cysts of the pancreas. Surg Clin North Am 69:651–665

Hull MT, Warfel KA, Muller J, Higgins JT (1979) Familial islet cell tumours in Von Hippel–Lindau disease. Cancer 44:1523–1526

Irving IM, Rickham PP (1978) Duodenal atresia and stenosis; annular pancreas. In: Rickham PP, Lister J, Irving IM (eds) Neonatal surgery, 2nd edn. Butterworths, London, pp 355–370

Kimura K, Ohta M, Saisho A et al. (1985) Association of gallbladder carcinoma and anomalous pancreaticobiliary duct union. Gastroenterology 89:1258–1265

Komi N, Tamura T, Tsuge S, Miyoshi Y, Udaka H, Takhara H (1986) Relation of patient age to premalignant alterations in choledochal cyst epithelium: histochemical and immunohistochemical studies. J Pediatr Surg 21:430–433

Lai EC, Tompkins RK (1986) Heterotopic pancreas. Review of a 26 year experience. Am J Surg 151:697–700

Lecco TM (1917) Zur morphologie des pankreas annulare. Sher Akad Wiss Wien 119:391

Leijala M, Louhimo I (1988) Pancreatitis after open heart surgery in children. Eur J Cardiothorac Surg 2:324–328

Mason TE, Quagliarello JR (1976) Ectopic pancreas in the Fallopian tube: report of a first case. Obstet Gynecol 48:705–755

Matsunou H, Konishi F (1990) Papillary-cystic neoplasm of the pancreas. A clinicopathological study concerning the tumor aging and malignancy of nine cases. Cancer 65:283–291

Millar AJW, Rode H, Stunden RJ, Cywes S (1988) Management of pancreatic pseudocysts in children. J Pediatr Surg 23:122–127

Misra SP, Dwivedi M (1990) Pancreaticobiliary ductal union. Gut 31:1144–1149

Moreno LA, Turck D, Gottrand F, Fabre M, Manouvier HS, Farriaux JP (1989) Familial hyperinsulinism with nesidioblastosis of the pancreas: further evidence for autosomal recessive inheritance. Am J Med Genet 34:584–586

Olurin EO (1971) Pancreatic cysts: a ten year review. Br J Surg 58:502–508

Pilot LM, Gooselaw JG, Issacson PG (1964) Obstruction of the common bile duct by a pancreatic cyst. Lancet 84:204

Qizblash AH (1976) Acute pancreatitis occurring in heterotopic pancreatic tissue in the gallbladder. Can J Surg 19:413–414

Rescorla FJ, Cory D, Vane DW, West KW, Grosfeld JL (1990) Failure of percutaneous drainage in children with traumatic pancreatic pseudocysts. J Pediatr Surg 25:1038–1042

Russell RC, Wong NW, Cotton PB (1984) Accessory sphincterotomy (endoscopic and surgical) in patients with pancreas divisum. Br J Surg 71:954–957

Scott HW Jr, Neblett WW, O'Neil JA Jr, Sawyers JL, Avant GS, Starnes VA (1984) Longitudinal pancreaticojejunostomy in chronic pancreatitis with onset in childhood. Ann Surg 199:610–622

Seitz ML, Shenker IR, Leonidas JC, Nussbaum MP, Wind ES (1987) Von Hippel–Lindau in an adolescent. Pediatrics 79:632–637

Smith S, Nakayama DK, Gantt N, Lloyd D, Rowe MI (1988) Pancreatic injuries in childhood due to blunt trauma. J Pediatr Surg 23:610–614

Sultan Khuroo M, Ali Zargar S, Mahajan R (1990) Hepatobiliary and pancreatic ascariasis in India. Lancet 335:1503–1506

Synn AY, Mulvihill SJ, Fonkalsrud EW (1987) Surgical management of pancreatitis in childhood. J Pediatr Surg 22:628–632

Synn AY, Mulvihill SJ, Fonkalsrud EW (1988) Surgical disorders of the pancreas in infancy and childhood. Am J Surg 156:201–205

Tan KC, Howard ER (1988) Choledochal cyst: a 14-year surgical experience with 36 patients. Br J Surg 75:892–895

Thompson NW, Bondeson AG, Bondeson L, Vinik A (1989) The surgical treatment of gastrinoma in MEN I syndrome patients. Surgery 106:1081–1086

Tieken T (1901) Annular pancreas. Am J Med 2:826

Todani T, Shimada K, Watanabe Y, Toki A, Fujii T, Urushihara N (1988) Frantz's tumor: a papillary and cystic tumor of the pancreas in girls. J Pediatr Surg 23:116–121

Trapnell JE (1990) Chronic relapsing pancreatitis in adolescents. World J Surg 14:48–52

Tsukimoto I, Watanabe K, Lin JB, Nakajima T (1973) Pancreatic carcinoma in children in Japan. Cancer 31:1203–1207

Vance JE, Stoll RW, Kitabachi AE, Buchanan KD, Hollander D, Williams RH (1972) Familial nesidioblastosis as the predominant manifestation of multiple endocrine adenomatosis. Am J Med 52:211–227

Vane DW, Grosfeld JL, West KW, Rescorla FJ (1989) Pancreatic disorders in infancy and childhood: experience with 92 cases. J Pediatr Surg 24:771–776

Wagner CW, Golladay ES (1988) Pancreas divisum and pancreatitis in children. Am Surg 54:22–26

Warden MJ, German JC, Buckingham BA (1988) The surgical management of hyperinsulinism in infancy due to nesidioblastosis. J Pediatr Surg 23:462–465

Warshaw AL, Simeone JF, Schapiro RH, Flavin-Warshaw B (1990) Evaluation and treatment of the dominant dorsal duct syndrome (pancreas divisum redefined). Am J Surg 159:59–66

Weizman Z, Durie PR (1988) Acute pancreatitis in childhood. J Pediatr 113:24–29

Weizman Z, Picard E, Barki Y, Moses S (1988) Wilson's disease associated with pancreatitis. J Pediatr Gastroenterol Nutr 7:931–933

Welch KJ (1986) The pancreas. In: Welch KC, Randolph JG, Ravitch MM, O'Neil JA, Rowe MI (eds) Pediatric surgery, 4th edn. Year Book Medical Publishers, Chicago, London, pp 1086–1106

Wiedmeyer DA, Stewart ET, Dodds WJ, Geenen JE, Vennes JA, Taylor AJ (1989) Choledochal cyst: findings on cholangiopancreatography with emphasis on ectasia of the common channel. AJR 153:969–972

Wong KC, Lister J (1981) Human fetal development of the hepato-pancreatic duct junction – a possible explanation of congenital dilatation of the biliary tract. J Pediatr Surg 16:139–145

Transplantation

Chapter 30

Pancreatic Transplantation

L. Fernández-Cruz, E. Astudillo, H. Sanfey,
M. López-Boado and A. Sáenz

Introduction

Over the last few years pancreas transplantation, in comparison with other
solid organs, has experienced a most spectacular improvement in terms of graft
and patient survival. This remarkable achievement is due to a number of
factors including better surgical technique, more appropriate patient selection,
use of stronger immunosuppressive therapy and the application of new methods
for the diagnosis of rejection.

Figs 1 and 2 show survival curves for patients and grafts from the time of

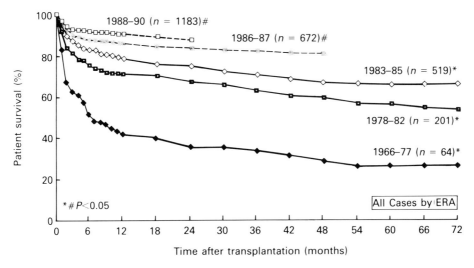

Fig. 1. Patient survival after pancreas transplantation from 16 December 1966 to 15 June 1990.
Data from the international pancreas transplant registry (University of Minnesota).

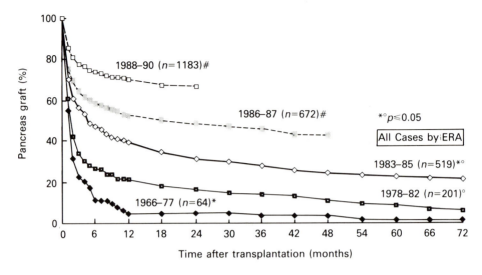

Fig. 2. Pancreas graft function after transplantation from 1 December 1966 to 15 June 1990. Data from the international pancreas transplant registry (University of Minnesota).

pancreatic transplantation (World Transplant Register, University of Minnesota). These data demonstrate the progressive improvement in success to equal that obtained in transplantation of other solid organs.

Indications for Pancreas Transplantation

Pancreas transplantation has been performed in two groups of patients; those that are uraemic type I diabetic recipients (in combination with a renal graft) and more recently, non-uraemic diabetics suffering from preproliferative or proliferative retinopathy with a high risk of blindness and neuropathy, and occasional other indications.

Combined Pancreas and Kidney Transplantation

Transplantation should be carried out in patients with end-stage renal failure. As this complication develops after 20–30 years of insulin dependency the mean age of the patients varies between 25 and 45 years. These patients also have generalised large and small vessel disease and about 20% are blind (Sutherland 1988). Pancreatic transplantation can be carried out at the same time as kidney transplantation (synchronous) or after kidney transplantation (asynchronous) once a period of time has been allowed for renal function to stabilise. The advantage of simultaneous renal and pancreatic transplantation is that both grafts are taken from the same donor so that the changes in renal function may be used as markers of a rejection process which frequently affects both organs. One therapeutic suppressor could control both immunological insults. The disadvantage of simultaneous pancreas and kidney transplantation is that these uraemic, debilitated patients have a long complicated postoperative course. On the other hand, the disadvantage of asynchronous transplantation is the need to carry out two distinct surgical procedures both of which will require aggressive immunosuppressive therapy.

In recipients of simultaneous pancreas and kidney transplants during the period 1984–89 recorded in the World Pancreas Transplant Registry (Sutherland, personal communication), the overall 1-year kidney graft survival rate was 74%, similar to that reported by the UCLA Kidney Transplant Registry of Terasaki for uraemic diabetic recipients of kidney transplants alone treated with cyclosporin (Terashita and Cook 1987).

With the addition of a pancreas graft to a kidney graft it is possible to resolve many of the problems of renal transplantation in diabetic patients, such as recurrence of nephropathy in the transplanted kidney, the difficulty of diagnosis of pancreatic rejection and reversal or arrest of the degenerative complications of diabetes mellitus (Ulbig et al. 1987).

Pancreas Transplantation Alone

There is abundant evidence to support the concept that the complications of diabetes are secondary to disordered metabolism. Whether the lesions can be influenced once they have arisen is another question, but pancreas transplantation does establish a euglycaemic state, which is impossible to achieve by exogenous insulin. Thus, pancreas transplantation should be performed before the patient develops severe secondary complications such as advanced retinopathy, disabling neuropathy, end-stage nephropathy or extensive macrovascular or microvascular disease. However, the potential benefits of a pancreas transplant should outweigh the side effects and complications of immunosuppressive therapy. The selection process must be more rigorous for non-uraemic patients who do not require a kidney transplant. There is no absolutely reliable marker to indicate which cases are prone to develop secondary complications before the earliest lesions appear. Once nephropathy, neuropathy and retinopathy are present, however, these lesions can be used as markers to predict progression.

Nephropathy

Different studies have demonstrated that the mortality for insulin-dependent diabetes mellitus (IDDM) during the first two years of renal failure is equal to or greater than 25%. The overall mortality after the diagnosis of renal failure is 17%–37% in the first year and 39%–58% at two years. One has to bear in mind that established renal failure is often accompanied by blindness, amputations and cerebrovascular insufficiency; 27% and 34% of kidney transplant recipients and patients on dialysis respectively will suffer myocardial infarction each year. Likewise the progression of retinopathy is accelerated after the onset of renal failure. Given this sequence of events and with the aim of avoiding them, the patients who will benefit from pancreas transplantation will be those patients with nephropathy in whom proteinuria ranges between 150 mg/24 h and 3 g/24 h. Above this level, pathological lesions are so advanced as to be irreversible by transplantation (Editorial 1988; Sutherland 1988). Patients should have adequate creatinine clearance of at least 60 ml/min.

Neuropathy

This occurs in 17%–40% of patients with diabetes. Recent clinical studies have revealed that 44% of diabetics with symptomatic neuropathies die within 2–5 years (Zola et al. 1986).

The reasons for advising pancreatic transplantation in this type of patient arise from data obtained at the University of Minnesota. These investigators have demonstrated an improvement in the spread of conduction of motor and sensory nerves in patients with functioning pancreatic transplants, and a deterioration in 50% of those whose grafts have failed and who once more require treatment with insulin (Van Der Vliet et al. 1988).

Symptomatic gastroparesis is also an indication for transplantation, because its appearance is considered to be the result of an extension of the neural lesion and is associated with a gloomy short-term prognosis. The mortality at 3 years in diabetics with gastroparesis is 35% (Editorial 1988). Diabetics with symptomatic orthostatic hypotension are also candidates for transplantation since this change indicates advanced neuropathy (Van der Vliet et al. 1988).

Retinopathy

At the present time controversy persists regarding the prevention and/or the reversibility of retinopathy with transplantation. In a recent study, the group at the University of Minnesota compared the results between one group of patients who had functioning grafts for more than one year with another group in whom transplantation only maintained patients insulin-free for less than three months (Ramsay et al. 1988). In the first 2–3 years after transplantation retinopathy stabilised in 70% and progressed in 30% of patients; there was no difference between the groups with or without functioning grafts. However, after three years, retinopathy remained stable in the insulin-free group and continued to progress in the group whose grafts failed to function.

Poorly Controlled Diabetics

This is a group of patients with such rapid variation in blood glucose that frequent hospitalisations are required for hypo- or hyperglycaemia. Candidates for transplantation will be those diabetics who in the preceding year required hospitalisation for more than 90 days for difficulties in glucose control, who have presented with six or more episodes of hypoglycaemia and have had four or more unexplained attacks of ketoacidosis (Fishbein 1984; Editoral 1988).

Contraindications

Pancreatic transplantation is contraindicated in those patients who are older than 55 years, patients with progressive gangrene of the extremities, and in diabetics with severe coronary artery disease which is not amenable to surgical correction. The same general contraindications as for other types of organ transplantation, such as silicosis or untreatable malignancy, apply here also.

HLA Typing

Recently, there has been a lot of interest in analysing graft survival results in relation to the similarity or disparity of the HLA–AB locus. According to the World Register, HLA–DR matching appears to influence the results, and the highest pancreas graft survival rates were with no DR mismatches. The group from the University of Minneapolis (Moudry-Munns and Minford 1990), have demonstrated in a study of 243 patients that graft survival at 2 years is 74% when there are two similar DR antigens and only 46% when there is no similarity. Also it has been shown that when the donor differs by two DR antigens, patient survival is 43% and when there is no difference, survival increases to 80%. According to these data one can conclude that one or two identical DR antigens or a difference in none or one DR antigen improves graft survival in cadaveric pancreatic transplantation (Sutherland et al. 1990).

Graft Procurement and Preservation

Most donors who are suitable for kidney donation are also acceptable for pancreas donation. The upper age limit for donors is 45 years, however, because problems can arise with advanced atherosclerosis which extends beyond the origin of the celiac and superior mesenteric (SMA) arteries. Contraindications to pancreas donation are diabetes mellitus (types I and II), chronic pancreatitis, and previous pancreatic surgery or trauma. Several groups have demonstrated the feasibility of carrying out combined pancreaticoduodenal and liver procurement from the same donor. The liver and pancreas have a common blood supply from the celiac axis. The pancreas is supplied by the splenic and gastroduodenal arteries from the celiac axis, and by the inferior pancreaticoduodenal arteries from the SMA. Two techniques are available to maintain the blood supply to the pancreatic graft. (a) The pancreas graft is removed with the origins of both the celiac axis and the SMA together with a patch of aorta, leaving the common hepatic artery to supply the liver graft. (b) In the second technique, which is most commonly used, the celiac axis and the aortic patch remain with the liver graft. The duodenal cuff and the head of the pancreas have a dual blood supply from the superior pancreaticoduodenal branch of the gastroduodenal artery and the inferior pancreaticoduodenal branch of the SMA, which divides into anterior and posterior branches thereby forming a rich vascular arcade. This allows safe ligation of the gastroduodenal branch if the inferior pancreaticoduodenal branch is preserved. The whole pancreas graft includes the splenic artery from the celiac axis and the SMA, together with the aortic cuff and portal vein. The vessels may be reconstructed using one of the following techniques (Fig. 3).

1. The splenic artery may be anastomosed end-to-side into the SMA with its Carrel patch.

2. The donor common iliac artery and bifurcation may be used for reconstruction. Usually the internal iliac artery is anastomosed end-to-end to the splenic artery, the external iliac artery is anastomosed end-to-end to the SMA and the common iliac from the graft is anastomosed end-to-side to the iliac of the recipient.

3. Where it is not possible to use the donor iliac vessels, end-to-end anastomosis is performed between the distal end of the SMA (after ligation of the two proximal jejunal arteries) and the proximal end of the splenic artery. The proximal SMA with aortic patch is then anastomosed end-to-side to the iliac artery of the recipient (Fig. 4).

One aspect of pancreas transplantation in which considerable progress has been made is in the area of graft preservation. With the use of Collin's solution preservation time was limited to 6 h, and was associated with increased thrombosis probably due to ischaemia of the pancreatic graft. With the development of silica gel-filtered plasma and the University of Wisconsin (UW) solution, pancreas allografts are now routinely stored for 18–24 h. Some groups have reported a zero thrombosis rate with these solutions which appear to decrease the incidence of oedema in the pancreatic graft.

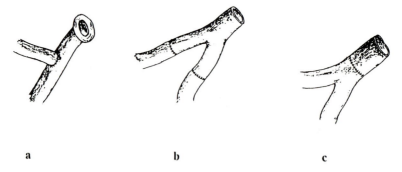

a   b   c

Fig. 3. Pancreatic vessels may be reconstructed using one of the following techniques: **a**, end-to-side anastomosis of the splenic artery into the superior mesenteric artery with its Carrel patch; **b**, the donor common iliac artery and bifurcation may be used for reconstruction; **c**, elongation of the portal vein using the donor common iliac vein.

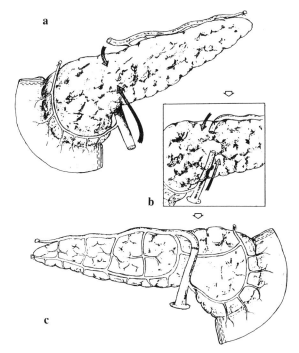

Fig. 4. Our original technique in cases where it is not possible to use the donor iliac vessels: end-to-end anastomosis is performed between the distal end of the SMA and the proximal end of the splenic artery.

Surgical Technique

There is still no standard surgical procedure for pancreatic transplantation. Some surgeons still use part of the gland in the form of a segmental graft. However, the whole pancreas–duodenum transplant offers several advantages. A larger mass of pancreatic tissue with an increased vascular bed can be transplanted, thus reducing the risk of graft thrombosis. The papilla of Vater can be preserved which should reduce the risk of later ductal obstruction. Also with the whole organ graft the duodenum is available for use as a conduit for exocrine secretions.

The optimal technique for exocrine drainage of the pancreatic duct is still a matter of controversy. According to the International Pancreas Transplant Registry the functional survival rates were significantly higher for urinary drainage than for enteric drained or duct-injected grafts, and the functional survival rate with polymer injection was significantly higher than that of enteric drainage. All three methods have inherent advantages and disadvantages.

Duct Injection

Various polymers have been used for duct injection such as neoprene, prolamine and silicon. This procedure produces early necrosis and degeneration of the ductal epithelium and later necrosis and atrophy of the acinar cells. This fibrosis is a long-lasting event (3–6 months) which finally leaves vascularised islets embedded in a matrix of fibrous tissue. This simple method has several drawbacks. Shortly after transplantation a significant number of patients (20%–50%) have been reported to develop a pancreatic fistula and wound complications. The major concern with the ductal occlusion technique is whether or not this method will eventually lead to cessation of endocrine function in the graft.

Enteric Drainage

The Stockholm group currently use enteric drainage as the most physiological approach but this is associated with a high incidence of postoperative complications requiring re-exploration (Groth et al. 1988).

Urinary Drainage

Pancreaticoduodenal transplantation with drainage into the bladder is also widely used (Sollinger et al. 1984). With this technique a 10 cm segment of duodenum is removed with the graft and both ends are closed with staples. The ends are then buried using inverting Lembert sutures. Pancreaticocystostomy is carried out by performing a one layer anastomosis between the antimesenteric border of the duodenum and the dome of the bladder (Fig. 5). Minor

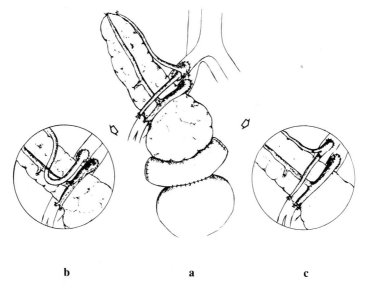

b   a   c

Fig. 5. Pancreaticoduodenal transplantation with pancreaticoduodenocystostomy. The venous anastomosis is performed end-to-side between the portal vein and the iliac vein. The arterial anastomosis can be performed using one of the following techniques: **a**, the celiac axis and the SMA together with a patch of aorta is anastomosed end-to-side to the iliac artery; **b**, the proximal SMA with aortic patch is anastomosed end-to-side to the iliac artery; **c**, the common iliac from the graft is anastomosed end-to-side to the iliac artery of the recipient.

complications such as dysuria and urinary tract infections are common after this procedure. Many of the patients develop a metabolic acidosis secondary to fixed losses of bicarbonate through the urine. In all cases this problem can be corrected by the administration of sodium bicarbonate and in most cases this supplement can be discontinued after several weeks. We, in common with other groups, have also noted an increased incidence of metabolic acidosis particularly during episodes of renal graft dysfunction due to acute tubular necrosis, acute renal allograft rejection or cyclosporin nephrotoxicity (Fernández-Cruz et al. 1987).

Immunosuppression and Diagnosis of Rejection

Another of the recent advances in pancreas transplantation has been an improved understanding of the use of immunosuppressive drugs. The use of the classical treatment of azathioprine and prednisolone is associated with an actuarial graft survival of 43%, contrasting with 54% when these drugs are combined with cyclosporin (CsA). The group of the University of Madison have introduced quadruple therapy adding antilymphocyte globulin (ALG) to CsA, azathioprine and prednisolone. Immediately postoperatively 1–2 mg/kg of CsA is administered intravenously for two to three days. Thereafter, CsA is given by mouth in a dose of between 4 and 8 mg/kg adjusted to renal function. Prednisolone is initially given at a dose of 120 mg/day for 3 days and is then tapered by 30 mg increments to 30 mg/day. After three months the dose is reduced to 10 mg/day. Azathioprine is administered at a dose of approximately 1 mg/kg per day and ALG is started on day 2 after transplant at a dose of 20 mg/kg per day and is usually given until the 14th postoperative day. Sollinger (1990) has reported a 2-year survival of 83% and 84% for pancreas and kidney transplantation respectively with this new regime. The optimal treatment of rejection is still unknown. The mainstay of antirejection therapy is increased immunosuppression. Most centres employ pulsed corticosteroids and/or ALG or OKT_3 (a monoclonal anti T_3 antibody). The best treatment of rejection is prevention. The single reason for the higher rate of pancreatic graft survival when combined pancreas and kidney transplantation is used lies in the ability to use serum creatinine and renal biopsy as indicators of rejection of the pancreas as well as the kidney. Although a sustained elevation of blood sugar is a reliable indicator of rejection, when it occurs most of the gland may already be destroyed and reversibility of the process may be more difficult.

One of the major theoretical advantages of urinary tract diversion is the ability to monitor exocrine function directly by urinary determinations (Fig. 6). Our experimental and clinical studies have shown that reductions in urinary amylase levels are an early marker of rejection (Prieto et al. 1987a, b; Fernández-Cruz et al. 1987). Along with urinary amylase content, urinary lipase, protein, bicarbonate and pH monitoring have been utilised to evaluate graft viability and predict rejection. Imaging modalities including nuclear scans, ultrasound, computed tomography and magnetic resonance imaging have not

Table 1. Stability of metabolic status with time. Mean serum glucose, insulin and C-peptide after oral glucose tolerance test (75 g glucose) in one patient with a functioning graft

Time after transplantation	0 min			60 min			90 min			120 min		
	Glucose (mg%)	Insulin (µU/ml)	C-peptide (ng/ml)	Glucose (mg%)	Insulin (µU/ml)	C-peptide (ng/ml)	Glucose (mg%)	Insulin (µU/ml)	C-peptide (ng/ml)	Glucose (mg%)	Insulin (µU/ml)	C-peptide (ng/ml)
1 year	76	16	2.5	135	—	4.4	136	—	5.7	97	—	5
3 years	58	19	2.3	95	155	6.7	98	113	7.3	107	104	7.3
5 years	58	10	1.9	164	47	8.3	144	63	11.4	128	51	11.1
7 years	86	9.8	2.5	138	74	8.0	84	44	8.8	87	34	7.4
7.5 years	76	13	2.1	126	68	8.2	110	47	8.0	95	38	8.1

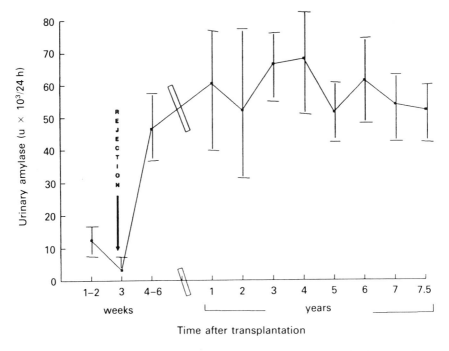

Fig. 6. Mean urinary amylase level plotted against time after transplantation in one patient with the graft functioning for more than 7.5 years. A drop was observed at the time of rejection. The preservation of the normal physiological relationship between acinar and islet cell function is clearly demonstrated.

demonstrated a great sensitivity in the diagnosis of rejection. However, combined ultrasonography and Doppler examination increase the accuracy of diagnosis when considered together with determination of amylasuria (Gilabert et al. 1988; Batink et al. 1990). Other methods which may prove to be promising are urinary/pancreatic juice cytology and fine needle biopsy (Allen et al. 1990).

Quality of Life

This has been investigated after combined kidney–pancreas transplantation by Nakache et al. (1989). These patients require less sickness pension than patients with a kidney transplant alone, more patients have full-time employment, and there is a 44% reduction in days lost from work. In addition, patients who receive a combined kidney–pancreas transplant experience an average of 13 fewer days in hospital per year than patients who receive a kidney transplant alone.

Survival Rates in the University of Barcelona

Pancreas transplantation has been performed in 40 type I diabetic recipients up to December 1990 (35 simultaneous pancreas and kidney transplantation and five pancreas alone). In January 1989 we introduced major modifications in selection and technique: restrictive recipient selection; whole organ and duodenocystostomy, and a quadruple immunosuppressive regimen.

The graft survival rates in the whole group are shown in Fig. 7. The actuarial survival rate has improved in the period 1989–1990. Of 40 transplants, current survival of the pancreatic graft is as follows: less than 6 months = 5; 6–12 months = 3; 1–2 years = 3; 2–3 years = 1; 4 years = 1; more than 7.5 years = 2.

Because our definition of successful pancreatic transplantation is no further requirement of exogenous insulin with good glucose control, all our patients with functioning grafts are by definition free of insulin therapy. Successful grafts show stable glucose homeostasis over many years (Table 1).

Conclusions

Pancreatic transplantation is the only therapeutic method which allows normal maintenance of glucose homeostasis. It frees the diabetic patient from the dietary and physical restrictions of insulin therapy. There is, however, a price

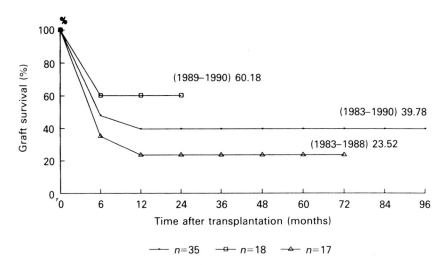

Fig. 7. Actuarial graft survival in the 35 patients who underwent pancreas and kidney transplantation up to December 1990. The actuarial 1-year and 2-year survival for all 35 patients was 39% but improved to 60% in the period 1989–1990. The numbers under the graph refer to the numbers of patients in each time period.

to be paid for these achievements in that immunosuppression is not entirely
free of side effects. In uraemic patients the benefit of simultaneous kidney and
pancreas transplantation lies in the remarkable improvement in the quality of
life and in halting the progression of diabetic pathological lesions. In non-
uraemic diabetics, the aim is to benefit the patient by the prevention of vascular
and systemic complications. For the future, pancreatic transplantation should
concentrate on those diabetic recipients who suffer aggressive disease at an
early age. Restoration of normal glucose homeostasis in these patients
slows down the development of terminal renal insufficiency, blindness and
arteriosclerosis.

References

Allen R, Wilson T, Grieson J et al. (1990) Percutaneous biopsy of the pancreas transplant. XIII
    International Congress of the Transplantation Society. Book of Abstracts, San Francisco, p 153
Batink T, Carpenter H, Morton M et al. (1990) Correlation of pancreas allograft biopsy with
    radionuclide and ultrasoundimaging of pancreas allografts. XIII International Congress of the
    Transplantation Society. Book of Abstracts, San Francisco, p 740
Editorial (1988) Pancreatic transplantation in treatment for IDDM. Proposed candidate criteria
    before end stage nephropathy. Diabetes Care 11:669–675
Fernández-Cruz L, Esmatges E, Andreu J et al. (1987) Advantages and disadvantages of urinary
    tract diversion in clinical pancreas transplantation. Transplant Proc. 19:3895–3898
Fishbein HA (1984) Diabetic ketoacidosis, hyperosmolar nonketotic coma, lactic acidosis and
    hypoglycemia. In: Diabetes in America. US Dept of Health and Human Services, Washington
    DC. NIH publ. no. 85–1468.
Gilabert R, Fernández-Cruz L, Bru C et al. (1988) Duplex–Doppler ultrasonography in monitoring
    clinical pancreas transplantation. Transplant Int 1:172–177
Groth CG, Tyden G, Brattstroin C (1988) Pancreatic transplantation for diabetes mellitus: the
    Stockholm experience. Transplant Proc 20 (Suppl 1):862–865
Moudry-Munns K, Minford S So (1990) Effect of matching or mismatching at the HLA–DR loci
    in cadaver pancreas. XIII International Congress of the Transplantation Society. Book of
    Abstracts, San Francisco, p 301
Nakache R, Tydén G, Groth CG (1989) Quality of life in diabetic patients after combined
    pancreas-kidney or kidney transplantation. Diabetes 38 (suppl 1):40–42
Prieto M, Sutherland DER, Fernández-Cruz L et al. (1987a) Experimental and clinical experience
    with urinary amylase monitoring for early diagnosis of rejection in pancreas transplantation.
    Transplantation 43:71–79
Prieto M, Sutherland DER, Fernández-Cruz L, Heil J, Najarian J (1987b) Rejection in pancreas
    transplantation. Transplant Proc 19:2348–2350
Ramsay RC, Goetz FC, Sutherland DER et al. (1988) Progression of diabetic retinopathy after
    pancreas transplantation for insulin-dependent diabetes mellitus. N Engl J Med 318:208–214
Sollinger H (1990) Lessons learned from 100 consecutive simultaneous kidney–pancreas transplants
    with bladder drainage. XIII International Congress of the Transplantation Society. Book of
    Abstracts, San Francisco, p 128
Sollinger HW, Cook K, Kamps D et al. (1984) Clinical and experimental experience with
    pancreatic-cystostomy for exocrine pancreatic drainage in pancreas transplantation. Transplant
    Proc 16:749–751
Sutherland DER (1988) Who should get a pancreas transplant. Diabetes Care 11:681–685
Sutherland DER, Moudry-Munns K, Gillingham K (1990) Solitary pancreas transplantation: alone
    in non-uremic and after a kidney in uremic. XIII International Congress of the Transplantation
    Society. Book of Abstracts, San Francisco, p 302
Terashita GY, Cook JD (1987) Original disease of the recipient. In: Terasaki PI (ed.) Clinical
    transplants, UCLA Tissue Typing Laboratory, Los Angeles, pp 373–379
Ulbig M, Kampik A, Landgraf R, Land W (1987) The influence of combined pancreatic and renal

transplantation on advanced diabetic retinopathy. Transplant Proc 19:3554–3556

Van der Vliet JA, Navarro X, Kennedy WR et al. (1988) The effect of pancreas transplantation on diabetic polyneuropathy. Transplantation 45:368–370

Zola B, Kahn JK, Juni JE, Vinik AL (1986) Abnormal cardiac function in diabetic patients with autosomic neuropathy in the absence of ischemic heart disease. J Clin Endocrinol Metab 63:208–214

Conclusion

Chapter 31

Progress and Prospects

C. D. Johnson

The various contributions to this book record the remarkable progress that has been made in the understanding and management of pancreatic diseases over the last decade. The improvement in understanding has led in some cases to better management with improved outcome for the patient, whereas in other areas the way is now clear towards a better prospect for the future.

One area above all has made a significant contribution to several disorders of the pancreas. The tools of molecular biology are allowing us to begin to unravel the complexities of pancreatic carcinogenesis. Experimental studies which demonstrate regulatory mechanisms for pancreatic cell lines perhaps point the way to future progress, but at present there has been little clinical benefit.

In contrast, the determination of the specific genetic defect responsible for cystic fibrosis opens up enormous possibilities for management. We can expect to see over the next few years a tremendous research effort directed towards achieving control of the regulation of this gene, with attempts to insert genetic material into the cells of patients suffering from the condition. This approach will strike at the root cause of the problem and could offer a permanent cure.

Other advances in the care of patients with cystic fibrosis are essentially based in improved clinical care. Patients with this condition now live much longer, so that the paediatrician with an interest in this disease finds that his clinics accumulate adolescents and adults who may feel out of place in a child-orientated environment. The point at which such patients should be transferred to the care of a medical gastroenterologist or chest physician is poorly defined. There is room for greater co-operation between adult and paediatric physicians in the management of these patients.

Pancreatic Cancer

Traditional therapy for pancreatic cancer has achieved much over the last decade, but there is still a long way to go. It is now clear that all units practising pancreatic surgery should aim to achieve a morbidity for pancreatic resection below 5%. The remarkable reduction in operative mortality is as clear cut and widespread as it is difficult to explain fully. Many factors probably contribute, including better nutrition of the patients, better general health, better preoperative care, improved surgical techniques (possibly); probably most important of all is improved intensive care and postoperative management, and the concentration of cases into the hands of specialists.

While the figures for operative survival have improved, the long-term outlook for pancreatic cancer after resection remains depressingly poor. We are now entering an era of adjuvant therapy as an obligatory consequence of resection of the pancreatic cancer and it is hoped that the proposed European Multicentre Trial of adjuvant therapy will be the first of a series of well planned and well supported investigations designed to determine the optimum treatment combination. Surgery can remove the primary tumour, but it must be supported by additional treatment aimed at micrometastases in the surrounding tissues, liver and elsewhere.

The palliation of pancreatic cancer is numerically more important. There has to date been little interest in chemotherapy as a palliative treatment. This is clearly because the costs to the patient far outweigh the benefits. Care must be given to investigate combinations of radiotherapy and chemotherapy which may favourably influence the rate of growth and perhaps depth of invasion of pancreatic primary tumours. If a partial response can be obtained, it may be possible to convert some tumours from inoperable to resectable, in the same way that can be achieved for fixed rectal cancers.

The majority of patients with pancreatic cancer require only palliative treatment. Most of these present with obstructive jaundice, but we must not forget that duodenal obstruction and pancreatic duct obstruction may also cause significant symptoms and can be corrected.

Endoscopic stenting has proved a remarkable advance in the management of obstructive jaundice. New instruments and techniques are constantly being developed, with the most promising appearing to be the Wallstent which can be placed either percutaneously, transhepatically, or by an endoscopist, with minimum morbidity and good long-term function.

Internal biliary drainage by endoscopic stenting offers several advantages over percutaneous biliary drainage in the preoperative management of patients for resection of pancreatic tumours. There is no firm evidence yet available to support the practice of preoperative internal drainage, although several experienced surgeons use this technique when possible.

Chronic Pancreatitis

Chronic pancreatitis has been extensively studied over the last 20 years, and is now clearly recognised as a separate disease entity from acute pancreatitis. The classification of chronic pancreatitis has been refined, with the identification of small groups such as those with obstructive pancreatitis who may be helped by pancreatic duct drainage or resection.

Improvements in the presentation of enzyme extracts, and better medical management all round have given these patients a better quality of life, and perhaps reduced the need for operation. The criteria for selection for surgery, and the choice of surgical procedure in chronic pancreatitis are now well defined. There remains controversy over the best surgical procedure. When resection of the pancreatic head is required, pylorus-preserving pancreaticoduodenectomy is now the choice of most surgeons, but one of the various forms of duodenum-preserving resection might offer some advantages. The Beger procedure, for example, appears to have good results in the hands of its originator, that compare well with the experience of others for pancreatic head resection. However, before this procedure can be recommended it must be evaluated by other surgeons.

Acute Pancreatitis

The outcome for the patient with severe acute pancreatitis has improved. To some extent this may reflect much better clinical care and in particular intensive monitoring and therapy in the intensive therapy unit. Despite advances in imaging and the detection of pancreatic and peripancreatic necrosis, and the ability to sample these areas for bacteriological examination, the decision to operate in severe acute pancreatitis remains a clinical one. The multiple scoring systems which allow monitoring of the patient's condition, such as APACHE-II, can probably help in this clinical decision.

Application of biochemical understanding to the assessment of severity has led to the studies of trypsinogen activation peptide (TAP) in acute pancreatitis. This molecule appears to provide a reliable indicator of a severe attack in a very early stage in the disease. We await with interest the general availability of a dipstick test that can be used on the urine of patients with suspected acute pancreatitis.

Early endoscopic sphincterotomy has been shown to reduce mortality in severe gallstone pancreatitis. Confirmation of this observation is now beginning to appear.

Diabetes

The chapter on pancreatic transplantation for diabetes records the progress that has been made. This technique is currently most suitable for patients receiving a renal transplant for diabetic neuropathy, but if the problems of immunosuppression and graft survival can be overcome then there is a potentially enormous application in the management of diabetes in general.

This review has demonstrated that our understanding of pancreatic disease is advancing on several fronts, and that the prospects are good for improvement in patient care in a large number of pancreatic diseases.

Index